Sports Nutrition: Training, Recovery and Performance

Sports Nutrition: Training, Recovery and Performance

Editor: Israel Barnardiston

AMERICAN
MEDICAL PUBLISHERS
www.americanmedicalpublishers.com

AMERICAN
MEDICAL PUBLISHERS
www.americanmedicalpublishers.com

Cataloging-in-Publication Data

Sports nutrition : training, recovery and performance / edited by Israel Barnardiston.
p. cm.
Includes bibliographical references and index.
ISBN 979-8-88740-468-4
1. Athletes--Nutrition. 2. Physical fitness--Nutritional aspects. 3. Sports--Physiological aspects.
4. Physical education and training. 5. Sports injuries--Treatment. 6. Performance. I. Barnardiston, Israel.
TX361.A8 S66 2023
613.202 479 6--dc23

American Medical Publishers,
41 Flatbush Avenue,
1st Floor, New York,
NY 11217, USA

ISBN 979-8-88740-468-4 (Hardback)

Contents

Preface

Sports nutrition refers to the study and application of diet and nutrition to enhance athletic performance. Nutrition plays a significant role in many sports training regimens, particularly in endurance sports and strength sports. The study of sports nutrition focuses on the type and amount of food and fluids consumed by athletes. It also addresses the consumption of nutrients like supplements, vitamins, minerals and organic substances like fats, carbohydrates and proteins. The supplements such as protein and amino acid are frequently used by athletes to recover from exercise. The consumption of fresh vegetables and fruits is the most efficient way to receive the natural nutrients required by the body for physiological performance and maximum health. The factors that can influence an athlete's nutritional requirements include gender, height, type of activity, body mass index, time of day, weight and stage of the activity or workout. This book provides comprehensive insights on sports nutrition. It covers the role of sports nutrition in training, recovery and performance. This book will prove to be immensely beneficial to students and researchers in this field.

This book has been the outcome of endless efforts put in by authors and researchers on various issues and topics within the field. The book is a comprehensive collection of significant researches that are addressed in a variety of chapters. It will surely enhance the knowledge of the field among readers across the globe.

It gives us an immense pleasure to thank our researchers and authors for their efforts to submit their piece of writing before the deadlines. Finally in the end, I would like to thank my family and colleagues who have been a great source of inspiration and support.

Editor

1

Dietary Intakes of Professional and Semi-Professional Team Sport Athletes do not Meet Sport Nutrition Recommendations

Sarah L. Jenner [1,2,*], Georgina L. Buckley [3], Regina Belski [3], Brooke L. Devlin [1] and Adrienne K. Forsyth [1]

1 Department of Rehabilitation, Nutrition and Sport, La Trobe University, Bundoora, VIC 3068, Australia; B.Devlin@latrobe.edu.au (B.L.D.); A.Forsyth@latrobe.edu.au (A.K.F.)
2 Carlton Football Club, Ikon Park, Carlton, VIC 3053, Australia
3 School of Health Sciences, Swinburne University of Technology, Hawthorn, VIC 3122, Australia; gbuckley@swin.edu.au (G.L.B.); rbelski@swin.edu.au (R.B.)
* Correspondence: s.jenner@latrobe.edu.au

Abstract: Background: to develop sport-specific and effective dietary advice, it is important to understand the dietary intakes of team sport athletes. This systematic literature review aims to (1) assess the dietary intakes of professional and semi-professional team sport athletes and (2) to identify priority areas for dietetic intervention. Methods: an extensive search of MEDLINE, Sports DISCUS, CINAHL, Web of Science, and Scopus databases in April–May 2018 was conducted and identified 646 studies. Included studies recruited team sport, competitive (i.e., professional or semi-professional) athletes over the age of 18 years. An assessment of dietary intake in studies was required and due to the variability of data (i.e., nutrient and food group data) a meta-analysis was not undertaken. Two independent authors extracted data using a standardised process. Results: 21 (n = 511) studies that assessed dietary intake of team sport athletes met the inclusion criteria. Most reported that professional and semi-professional athletes' dietary intakes met or exceeded recommendations during training and competition for protein and/or fat, but not energy and carbohydrate. Limitations in articles include small sample sizes, heterogeneity of data and existence of underreporting. Conclusions: this review highlights the need for sport-specific dietary recommendations that focus on energy and carbohydrate intake. Further exploration of factors influencing athletes' dietary intakes including why athletes' dietary intakes do not meet energy and/or carbohydrate recommendations is required.

Keywords: sports nutrition; carbohydrate intake; energy; nutritional recommendations

---

1. Introduction

1.1. Nutrition for Team Sport Athletes

Team sports can be defined as field- and court-based sports with intermittent and high-intensity game patterns [1]. Match patterns will vary markedly among different sports and for specific positions within a sport. Team sports are divided into three categories: (1) endurance-based sports including football (i.e., soccer), Australian football, hockey (2) strength and power sports such as rugby union and league, American football and (3) batting sports such as baseball, softball and cricket [1]. Athletes participating in professional team sports are supported by high-performance and medical staff, which aim to monitor and optimise fitness, body composition and performance outcomes. The physiological demands of team sports differ and can include a range of performance modes including: running moderate to long distances, high intensity bouts of movement, variable activity patterns and small bouts of rest periods [1–3]. The variable nature of team sport exercise requires use both anaerobic and aerobic systems to fuel performance [1]. Therefore, each team sport and position within the sport, depending on the nature of training and competition, will have unique energy demands and nutrient requirements. To optimise performance and enhance recovery, international sporting committees (i.e., International Olympic Committee (IOC), American College of Sports Medicine (ACSM), International Society of Sports Nutrition (ISSN)) have provided nutrition recommendations to support dietitians working with athletes to meet their individual nutrition needs [4–9].

Dietitians must consider a range of sport-specific factors including the rules, arena size, timing of competition, frequency of matches and length of seasons (including macrocycles: preseason, competition season, off-season) when assessing an athlete's nutrition requirements and goals. Additionally, the physique characteristics and position-specific tasks of the sport will further influence the nutritional requirements of athletes. For example, the sport of rugby union will require forwards to be heavier and stronger in comparison to backs who need to be leaner and faster [10]. Due to the sport-specific factors, physique and position differences, dietary advice for team sport athletes should be individualised.

Recommendations that support athletes to consume sufficient energy and the correct balance of macronutrients and micronutrients, with appropriate timing to enhance performance and recovery, will enable athletes to train and perform optimally [11]. An earlier review by Holway and Spriet [1] found that athletes competing in team sports commonly do not meet recommended dietary intake needs [1,12]. Those that fail to consume energy and/or maintain a diet that encompasses the appropriate balance of macronutrients may find that this impedes on training adaptations and recovery [11,12]. Deficiencies in energy can have implications for an athlete's performance including a loss of fat free mass, disturbances to immune function, decreased bone mineral density, increased susceptibility to injury and increased prevalence of symptoms of overtraining [11].

1.2. Objectives

In the past decade, thousands of new research papers have been published in sports nutrition and 17 new consensus statements and recommendation papers have been released by authoritative organisations such as the IOC, ACSM, ISSN [4–9,11,13–22]. There have also been a large number of published studies on the dietary intake of professional and semi-professional team sport athletes during this time [2,3,10,23–39]. With new sports nutrition recommendations [5–8,11,13–21] and updated literature reporting the dietary intake of team sport athletes, it is now timely to review the literature to determine whether team sport athletes consume diets that align with the sports nutrition recommendations [2,3,10,23–39]. This paper aims to review the literature on dietary intakes of professional and semi-professional team sport athletes systematically with the aim of identifying priority areas for dietetic intervention.

2. Materials and Methods

2.1. Protocol Registration

All methods and search strategies were aligned with Preferred Reporting Items for Systematic Review (PRISMA) guidelines. This review was registered with International Prospective Register of Systematic Reviews (registration number: CRD42018105168) [40,41]. A PICOS criteria (i.e., Participants, Intervention, Comparison, Outcome and Study design) for review is defined in Table 1. A systematic search using terms such as sport or team sport or dietary intake or food intake was conducted by one researcher (SJ). All keywords used in search are listed in Table 2.

Table 1. Participants, Intervention, Comparison, Outcome and Study (PICOS) criteria for inclusion and exclusion of studies.

Parameter	Description
Population	Professional and semi-professional team sport athletes
Intervention OR exposure	Baseline dietary intake
Comparison	Dietary intake in comparison to sports nutrition guidelines and recommendations.
Outcomes	Meeting/not meeting sports nutrition guidelines and recommendations
Study design	RCT (where baseline dietary intake data available), cross-sectional, longitudinal, thesis (unpublished and published)

Abbreviations: RCT Randomised Control Trial.

Table 2. Table of keywords.

Concept	Keywords
Sport OR team sport	"sport*" OR "team sport*" OR "football" OR "soccer" OR "football" OR "netball" OR "AFL" OR "Aussie rules" OR "rugby" OR "basketball" OR "grid iron" OR "American football" OR "hockey"
Dietary intake OR food intake	"nutrient requirement*" OR "dietary intake" OR "daily food intake" OR "food intake"

2.2. Search Strategy

Five electronic databases including MEDLINE (Medlars International Literature Online), Sports DISCUS, CINAHL (Cumulative Index of Nursing and Allied Health Literature), Web of Science (WOS), and Scopus (World's largest abstract and citation database of peer-reviewed literature) were searched to investigate the dietary intake of professional and semi-professional team sport athletes by one researcher (SJ). The timeframe designated for the search included studies published from 2011 to present (i.e., after the 2011 review by Holway and Spriet) [1]. An additional limit regarding age (i.e., >18 years) was included to limit results to adult athletes only. In order to identify any further relevant publications, the reference lists of the studies included were hand searched and other manual searches were conducted (i.e., Google Scholar).

2.3. Eligibility Criteria

All original research (i.e., cross-sectional, longitudinal, published and unpublished thesis) conducted in adult team sport athletes (i.e., 18 years and older) and published since 2011 was considered for inclusion (Table 3). Randomised control trials were additionally included in the review if baseline dietary intake data was available. Randomised control trials where only post intervention dietary intakes were available, conference posters, abstracts and web-based articles were not included for review. Only professional and semi-professional athletes were included in the review; amateur and recreational athletes were not included. Only English-language studies were included for this review. Included studies were required to provide baseline or habitual dietary intake data that quantified energy, macronutrients and micronutrients to allow for the specified conversions made and displayed in the data extraction table i.e., energy (MJ/day), carbohydrate (grams (g) and g·kg^{-1}·day^{-1}), protein (g and g·kg^{-1}·day^{-1}), fat (g and % total energy), calcium (mg/day) and iron (mg/day). Studies that reported dietary habits, dietary knowledge, attitudes, and education strategies where dietary intake was not quantified, were excluded from the review.

Table 3. Eligibility criteria.

Inclusion	Exclusion
1. Studies that include only team sport athletes.	1. Studies that include only individual athletes or sports.
2. Studies published since 2012.	2. Studies published up to 2011.
3. Studies that include only professional or semi-professional team sport athletes.	3. Studies that include only non-professional or amateur team sport athletes.
4. Studies that include only adult team sport athletes (i.e., >18 years of age).	4. Studies that include adolescent and child team sports athletes (i.e., <18 years of age).
5. English language studies.	5. Non-English language studies.
6. Studies that include quantitative measures of dietary intake that can be converted into units of intake per day for each nutrient.	6. Studies that include nutrition habits, attitudes, educational strategies, knowledge, where dietary intakes cannot be compared.
7. Studies that include the dietary assessment of total energy carbohydrate, protein fat, micronutrient intake (i.e., iron (mg/day), calcium (mg/day), folate etc.).	7. Studies where only supplement or antioxidant intake is assessed.
8. Studies that assess dietary intake using a validated method of assessment (i.e., 7 day food diary, 7 day weighed food diary, food records, 3 day food diaries, FFQ, diet histories etc.) and therefore estimates absolute dietary intake.	8. Studies that assess dietary intake, however methods used provide dietary assessments represented in food groups, percentage of total energy etc.
9. Only human studies that include; RCT (where baseline dietary intake data available), cross-sectional, longitudinal, thesis.	9. No animal studies, RCT (where only post intervention dietary intakes available), conference posters, reviews, abstracts and web-based articles.
10. Published and unpublished research (i.e., thesis).	

Abbreviations: FFQ Food Frequency Questionnaire, RCT Randomised Control Trial.

2.4. Study Selection

All studies were screened based on title and abstract by main author (SJ). Articles deemed eligible for full text review were screened against inclusion and exclusion criteria (Table 3) by two authors (SJ and GB). Additional reviewers (AF and RB) provided advice on eligibility if a decision for inclusion and exclusion required feedback. Selection of included studies and reasons for exclusion are reported in Chart 1.

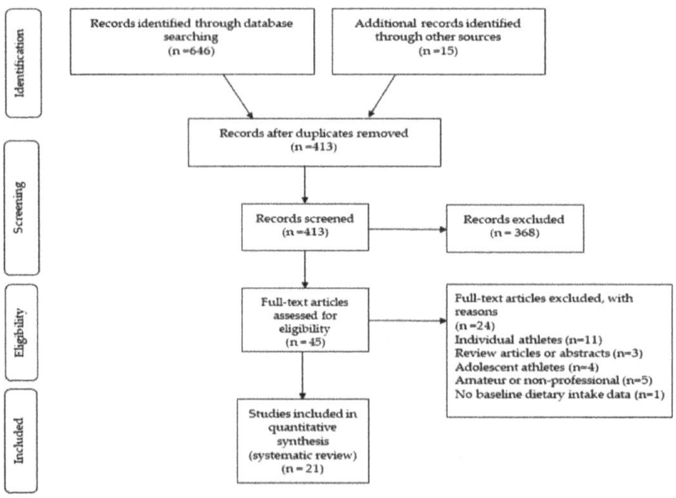

Chart 1. Study section process.

2.5. Data Collection Process

Dietary intake data were extracted from the included studies by two authors (SJ and GB). Data presented in Table 4 include participant demographics including sport, anthropometry measures (total mass (kg), body fat (%), fat free mass (kg)) and athletic level (professional or semi-professional)); details regarding the study background and methods; country of origin and survey method (i.e., 7-day food diary) and dietary intake results including total energy/calories (i.e., MJ), carbohydrate intake (i.e., g and $g \cdot kg^{-1} \cdot day^{-1}$), protein intake (i.e., g and $g \cdot kg^{-1} \cdot day^{-1}$), fat intake (i.e., g and % total energy), calcium intake (i.e., mg) and iron intake (mg). Where total energy intake was reported in calories, this was converted to MJ to enable comparison across studies.

2.6. Study Quality: Risk of Bias

The quality of studies was examined by two authors (SJ and GB) using the Academy of Nutrition and Dietetics Quality Criteria Checklist from the Academy of Nutrition and Dietetics Evidence Analysis Manual [42]. The quality criteria checklist provides an assessment based on relevance and validity criteria questions, ranking studies as either positive, neutral or negative. A third reviewer (AF) reviewed any discrepancies that occurred during the quality analysis. Studies with positive ratings needed to describe study selection adequately (including inclusion and exclusion criteria), methods of comparing groups and the study setting, and include measurements that were valid and reliable.

3. Results

3.1. Study Selection

The original search retrieved 646 studies that fit the search criteria with an additional 15 studies identified by hand searches (Chart 1). After duplicates were removed, a title and abstract exclusion was undertaken and 45 studies were retained for full text assessment. After completion of full text assessment 21 studies were included in this review for data extraction, quality assessment and analysis. All studies included in the review had a positive or neutral quality rating [41].

3.2. Study Characteristics

The majority of studies included in this review included team sport athletes competing professionally and semi-professionally in Australia ($n = 255$) [3,25,26,33,43] and Spain ($n = 81$) [28–30,36], with the remaining studies including athletes from Europe (not-specified) ($n = 34$) [10,27], England ($n = 30$) [23,34], America ($n = 26$) [32,38], Canada ($n = 25$) [39], Brazil ($n = 19$) [37], Netherlands ($n = 14$) [24], South Africa ($n = 11$) [35], United Kingdom ($n = 10$) [2], and Mexico ($n = 6$) [31,37]. The majority of studies included in this review reported the dietary intakes of professional team sport athletes [2,3,10,23,24,26–29,31,33,34,36,37], with additional studies exploring dietary intake of semi-professional team sport athletes [32,35,38,39] and studies exploring the dietary intakes of a combination of sports [25,30,43]. Studies included a range of team sport athletes with the majority of studies reporting on the dietary intakes of football athletes ($n = 210$) [23–25,28,30,31,34,37], followed by Australian football ($n = 139$) [3,26,43]. Across the remaining studies, other team sport athletes represented in this review include; rugby union ($n = 70$) [10,27,33,35], ice-hockey ($n = 25$) [39], wheelchair basketball ($n = 17$) [29], American football ($n = 15$) [32], handball ($n = 14$) [36], volleyball ($n = 11$) [38], rugby league ($n = 10$) [2].

The majority of studies included in this review used a cross-sectional study design ($n = 14$), with the remaining studies using pre-post-test [32,38], case-study [27,29], case control [30] and longitudinal [26,36] designs to assess dietary intake. Dietary intake data were collected most frequently using food diaries/records (weighed and not weighed). Studies used 7-day food diaries [2,3,23,28,33,35,39], 3-day food diaries [29,32,37,38] and 24 hr recalls [10,24,25,43]. Other studies used food diaries of different duration (i.e., 4-day, 6-day, and 8-day) [27,30,34], dietary recalls (i.e., 72-h) [26,36] and a combination of 4-day weighed food diary in addition to a food frequency questionnaire (FFQ) to assess dietary intake [31].

Table 4. Reported energy, macronutrient and micronutrients intakes of male and female professional and semi-professional team sport athletes.

References	Participant Characteristics								Dietary Intake Data								
Author, Year	Sport	Country	Level	N (Gender)	Total Mass (kg)	Lean Mass (kg)	BF%	Energy Intake Reported (Estimated MJ Were Available)	CHO (g)	CHO (g·kg^{-1}·day^{-1})	PRO (g)	PRO (g·kg^{-1}·day^{-1})	Fat (g)	Fat (% TE)	Calcium (mg·day^{-1})	Iron (mg·day^{-1})	Quality Rating
Anderson et al. [23], (2017)	Football (soccer)	England	P	n = 6 (male)	80.5 ± 8.7	11.9 ± 1.2	65.0 ± 6.7	3186 ± 585 kcal·day^{-1} (13.3)	330 ± 98	4.2 ± 1.4	205 ± 30						+
Andrews and Itsiopoulus [25] (2016)	Football (soccer)	Australia	P, SP	n = 73 (male)	P 79.6 ± 7.7 SP 75.6 ± 7.6			P 11,525 ± 1987 kJ·day^{-1} SP 10,831 ± 3842 kJ·day^{-1} (P 11.5 ± 2.0, SP 10.8 ± 3.8)	P 302.4 ± 72.3 SP 298.7 ± 148.5	P 3.5 ± 0.8 SP 3.9 ± 1.8	P 152.3 ± 27.7 SP 149.1 ± 46.8	P 1.9 ± 0.3 SP 2.0 ± 0.6	P 95.9 ±31.7 SP 85.8 ±37.8	P 30.4 ± 7.3 SP 29.5 ± 7.4			Ø
Bettonviel et al. [24] (2016)	Football (soccer)	Netherlands	P	n = 14 (male)	77.0 ± 8.6			2988 ± 583 kcal·day^{-1} (12.5)	365 ± 76	4.7 ± 0.7	145 ± 24	1.9 ± 0.3	97 ± 26	29.0 ± 3.6			Ø
Bilsborough et al. [26] (2016)	Australian Football	Australia	P	n = 45 (male)	86.8 ± 7.9	[7.9 ± 1.8–10.5 ± 2.7]	[71.2 ± 6.8–76.8 ± 6.4]	[11.1–13.9]	[321 ± 142–379 ± 66]	4.1 ± 1.6	[118 ± 67–215 ± 60]	1.9 ± 0.9	[61 ± 29–110 ± 40]	[19.0 ± 5.0–33.1 ±6.7]			Ø
Bradley et al. [27] (2015)	Rugby Union	Europe (non-specified)	P	n = 14 (male)	F 110 ± 6.2 B 93.6 ± 5.9			F 16.6 ± 1.25 MJ·day^{-1} B 14.2 ± 1.20 MJ·day^{-1}		F 3.5 ± 0.8 B 3.4 ± 0.7		F 2.7 ± 0.5 B 2.7 ± 0.3		F 32 B 33	1733 ± 694	24 ± 9	Ø
Bradley et al. [10] (2015)	Rugby Union	Europe (non-specified)	P	n = 20 (male)	F 109.3 ± 6.9 B 91.7 ± 6.6	F 13 ± 3 B 9.3 ± 2	F 94.9 ± 4.5, B 83.1 ± 5.4	F 14.8 ± 1.9 MJ·day^{-1} B 13.3 ± 1.9 MJ·day^{-1}		F 3.3 ±0.7 B 4.14 ± 0.4		F 2.52 ± 0.3 B 2.59 ± 0.6					Ø
Conejos et al [28] (2011)	Football (soccer)	Spain	P	n = 22 (male)				Fwd. 12.7 ± 2.9 MJ·day^{-1} M 14.0 ± 6.2 MJ·day^{-1} D 14.8 ± 2.6 MJ·day^{-1} G 12.2 ± 4.6 MJ·day^{-1}	Fwd. 342.5± 92.9 M 382.1 ± 187.2 D 419.1 ± 98.3 G 320.3 ± 11.9		Fwd. 138.7 ± 27.5 M 144.8 ± 56.9 D 144.5 ± 19.9, G 142.8 ± 100.1		Fwd. 120.3 ± 59.6 M 131.6 ± 62.6 D 124.5 ± 36.1 G 109.8 ± 45.3	Fwd. 34.7 M 35.6 D 32.2 G 34.9	Fwd. 1361.5 ± 549.0 M 1592.3 ± 966.1 D 1208.4 ± 457.1 G 1499.7 ± 1035.9	Fwd. 13.4 ± 3.7 M 18.9 ± 9.7 D 22.6 ± 6.8 G 15.5 ± 10.2	Ø
Devlin et al. [43] (2017)	Australian Football (AF) Football (Soccer, F)	Australia	P, SP	n = 66 AF = 48, F = 18 (male)	AF (P) 87.8 ± 9.2 AF (SP) 82.9 ± 9.0 F (P) 75.6 ± 5.6	AF (P) 15.1 ± 2.4, AF (SP) 16.7 ± 2.7 F (P) 12.8 ± 1.9	AF (P) 65.4 ± 7.9 AF (SP) 61.2 ± 3.9 F (P) 56.8 ± 5.2	AF (P) 17.3 ± 4.2 MJ·day^{-1} AF (SP) 13.2 ± 2.5 MJ·day^{-1} F (P) 9.4 ± 2.3 MJ·day^{-1}	AF (P) 406 ± 132 AF (SP) 368 ± 93 F (P) 220 ± 76	AF (P) 4.6 ± 1.5 AF (SP) 4.5 ± 1.2 F (P) 2.9 ± 1.1	AF (P) 295 ± 97 AF (SP) 171 ± 52 F (P) 140 ± 35	AF (P) 3.4 ± 1.1 AF (SP) 2.1 ± 0.7 F (P) 1.9 ± 0.5		AF (P) 29 ± 6 AF (SP) 28 ± 8 F(P) 33 ± 9			Ø
Grams et al. [29] (2016)	Wheelchair basketball	Spain	P	n = 17 (male)	75.5 ± 13.5			2673 ± 485 kcal·day^{-1} (11.2)		3.9 [Range: 1.8–8.1]		1.7 ± 0.6		33.7 ± 5.5			+
Gravina et al. [30] (2012)	Football (soccer)	Spain	P, SP	n = 28 (female)	61 ± 8.4	16.7 ± 3.2		2271 ± 578 MJ·day^{-1} (9.5)						33 ± 7			+
Hidalgo et al. [31] (2015)	Football (soccer)	Mexico	P	n = 6 (male)	68.3 ± 2.0		32.5 ± 1.0	3042 ± 56 kcal·day^{-1} (12.7)	364 ± 17.5	5.4 ± 0.3	145 ± 14	2.2 ± 0.2	113 ± 6.3	33 ± 0.0			Ø
Jenner et al. [3] (2018)	Australian Football	Australia	P	n = 46 (male)	86.3 ± 9.4	10.8 ± 2.3	73.9 ± 9.1	9.1 ± 1.8 MJ·day^{-1}	201 ± 56	2.4 ± 0.8	150 ± 30	1.8 ± 0.4	78.9 ± 20.0	32 ± 4.5	952 ± 287		Ø
Kirwan et al. [32] (2012)	American Football	America	SP	n = 15 (male)	93.8 ± 15.3		70.5 ± 7.7	3518 ± 849 kcal·day^{-1} (14.7)	353 ± 118		169 ± 52		160 ± 45				Ø
MacKenzie et al. [33] (2015)	Rugby Union	Australia	P	n = 25 (male)	100.2 ± 13.3		77.0 ± 7.0	13605 ± 3639 kJ·day^{-1} (13.6)	352 ± 115	3.6 ± 1.3	211 ± 62	2.2 ± 0.7	101 ± 34	28 ± 5.0			Ø

Table 4. *Cont.*

References		Participant Characteristics							Dietary Intake Data								
Author, Year	Sport	Country	Level	N (Gender)	Total Mass (kg)	Lean Mass (kg)	BF%	Energy Intake Reported (Estimated MJ Were Available)	CHO (g)	CHO (g·kg^{-1}·day^{-1})	PRO (g)	PRO (g·kg^{-1}·day^{-1})	Fat (g)	Fat (% TE)	Calcium (mg·day^{-1})	Iron (mg·day^{-1})	Quality Rating
Molina-lopez et al. [36] (2013)	Handball	Spain	P	*n* = 14 (male)	86.7 ± 5.4	11.6 ± 2.5		2974.5 ± 211.1 kcal·day^{-1} (12.4)	360.9 ± 27.6	4.2 ±0.4	133.4 ±14.3	1.5 ± 0.2	118.6 ± 22.5		1251.4 ± 338.2	24.2 ± 8.5	∅
Ono et al. [34] (2011)	Football (soccer)	England	P	*n* = 24 (male)				[2648-4606 kcal·day^{-1}] (11.1–19.3)	505.2 ± 120		141.7 ± 22.8						∅
Potgieter, et al. [35] (2014)	Rugby Union	South Africa	SP	*n* = 11 (male)	95.5 ± 13.6	18.2 ± 5.7	79.7 ± 9.0	45.4 ± 9.0 kcal·kg^{-1}·day^{-1}		4.3 ± 0.4		2.4 ± 0.7		33.8 ± 4.3	1250 ± 403		∅
Raizel et al. [37] (2017)	Football (soccer)	Brazil	P	*n* = 19 (male)	71.8 ± 8.2	4.9 ± 1.5		40.74 ± 12.8 kcal·kg^{-1}·day^{-1}		5.4 ± 1.9	136.4 ± 57.4	1.9 ± 0.8	91.2 ± 35.9				∅
Tooley et al. [2] (2015)	Rugby League	UK	P	*n* = 10 (male)	97.3 ± 3.1			3731 ± 164 kcal·day^{-1} (15.6)	467 ± 24	4.9 ± 0.3	209 ± 10	2.2 ± 0.2	124 ± 10	30 ± 1.0			∅
Valliant et al. [38] (2012)	Volleyball	America	SP	*n* = 11 (female)	75.4 ± 13.4	24.5 ± 5.9		1756 ± 557.5 kcal·day^{-1} (7.3)	224.3 ± 64.4	3.08 ± 1.1	69.3 ± 26.8	0.9 ± 0.3	67.4 ± 27.8	33.7 ± 6.4			∅
Vermeulen et al. [39] (2017)	Ice-hockey	Canada	SP	*n* = 25 (female)	67.0 ± 1.7			2354 ± 74 kcal·day^{-1} (9.8)	305 ± 15	4.6 ± 0.2	91 ± 4	1.4 ± 0.1	82 ± 4	32 ± 1.0	1041 ± 64	19 ± 3	∅

Abbreviations: AF Australian Football, F Football (soccer), BF% Body fat percentage, CHO Carbohydrate, D Defenders, Fwd Forwards, GK Goal-keepers, kcal·day^{-1} Calories per day, Kcal·kg^{-1}·day^{-1} Calories per kg per day, kJ·day^{-1} Kilojoules per day, MJ·day^{-1} Mega joules per day, M Midfielders *PRO* Protein, *P* Professional, *SP* Semi-professional. Quality rating criteria: Positive (+), Neutral (∅) and Negative (–).

3.3. *Dietary Intake of Team Sport Athletes*

3.3.1. Energy Intake of Team Sport Athletes on Training Days

All studies included assessed the energy intake of team sport athletes. The majority of authors assessed the energy intake of athletes against recommendations advocated by IOC, ACSM, ISSN and sports specific research [1,4,12,35,44–55]. Several studies provided evidence that energy intake of team sport athletes assessed was suboptimal and did not meet recommendations [2,3,10,26,28,35,36,38]. Of the 21 studies included, five studies reported that energy intake was adequate according to the respective dietary recommendations used [23,32,33,37,39]. One study by Devlin et al. [43] reported that the Australian football athletes included met energy recommendations, however the football athletes did not. The remaining studies ($n = 7$) did not report on adequacy of energy intake (i.e., recommendations met versus not met) [24,25,27,29–31,34].

3.3.2. Energy Intake of Team Sport Athletes during Competition

The mean energy intake reported in this review ranged from 9.1–16.6 MJ/day and 7.3–9.8 MJ/day for males and females respectively. Seven studies included comparison data of dietary intake on training days and match days [2,23,24,27,31,35,39]. Two studies that explored the dietary intake of rugby union ($n = 10$) and ice hockey ($n = 25$) athletes on match days found that energy intake did not meet increased requirements for the fueling and recovery required on match days [2,39]. However, in comparison, two studies that included professional rugby union ($n = 14$) and football athletes ($n = 6$), found that energy intake was greater on match days in comparison to training days [23,27]. In particular, research by Bradley et al. [27] found that on average professional rugby union athletes increased their energy intake in preparation for game day in comparison to the first four days of training where energy intake was reduced, irrespective of energy expenditure. Anderson et al. [23] additionally found that professional football players ($n = 6$) had a greater absolute and relative energy intake on match days in comparison to training days.

3.3.3. Macronutrient Intake of Team Sport Athletes on Training Days

Overall, the macronutrient composition of the diets of team sport athletes was inadequate to meet the fuel, recovery and performance demands of their sports. All but one study assessed the dietary intake of carbohydrate and protein [30] and all but two assessed the dietary intake of fat [30,34]. Overall, a macronutrient imbalance was found in the majority of studies with most athletes reported consuming diets high in protein and fat, at the expense of carbohydrate. Team sport athletes including athletes from football ($n = 175$), Australian football ($n = 139$), rugby union ($n = 88$), volleyball ($n = 11$) and rugby league ($n = 10$) consumed diets that consistently did not meet carbohydrate recommendations [2,3,10,23–28,30,33,35–38,43]. Out of the 17 studies that provided mean intakes of carbohydrates, 15 reported low carbohydrate intake and fell below ISSN recommended intakes of 5-8 $g{\cdot}kg^{-1}{\cdot}day^{-1}$ (range: 2.4–4.9 $g{\cdot}kg^{-1}{\cdot}day^{-1}$ and 3.08–4.6 $g{\cdot}kg^{-1}{\cdot}day^{-1}$ for male and female athletes respectively). One study that explored the dietary intakes of male professional football players found that carbohydrate intakes consumed by athletes were closer to meeting recommendations for tactical or skill based sports (3–5 $g{\cdot}kg^{-1}{\cdot}day^{-1}$) [12,25].

Conversely, the majority of studies found that dietary intake of protein [2,10,24–26,28,30,31, 33,35–37,43,56] and fat [24,27,28,32,35–37] exceeded recommendations. Eight studies that included athletes competing professionally and semi-professionally in Australian football, rugby league, rugby union and football found protein intakes in excess of 2.0 $g{\cdot}kg^{-1}{\cdot}day^{-1}$ [2,10,25,27,31,33,35,43], with a study reporting that the diets of professional Australian football athletes on average contained 3.4 ± 1.1 $g{\cdot}kg^{-1}{\cdot}day^{-1}$ of protein per day [43]. Studies included in this review reported dietary intakes that were high in protein, however low in carbohydrates and/or total energy (hypocaloric) [2,3,10, 26,28,35,36,38,43]. Nine studies found that dietary intake of fat exceeded recommendations [2,27–29,31,32,35,37,39]. Three studies that included rugby union athletes ($n = 35$) and football athletes

(n = 25) found that while overall total fat intake exceeded recommendations, polyunsaturated fat intake fell below recommended intakes of 10% of total energy [31,35,37]. Six studies explored the intake of cholesterol, finding that dietary intakes of athletes exceeded recommended intakes of <300 mg/day [2,28,31,32,35,37]. Kirwan et al. [32] linked high cholesterol intakes to potential body composition goals of American football athletes (i.e., to put on mass, quickly).

3.3.4. Macronutrient Intake of Team Sport Athletes during Competition

Three of seven studies that assessed intake on competition days found that carbohydrate consumed in preparation for match day, during the match and during the recovery period post game, did not meet recommended intakes for competitions [24,31,39]. One study in female ice-hockey players found that there was no significant difference in carbohydrate, protein and fat intakes between game, training and rest days [39]. In comparison, three studies on rugby union (2) and football (1) athletes found that carbohydrate intake during and post-game day met recommendations [23,27,35]. In particular, Anderson et al. [23] found that athletes practiced a level of periodization, finding that carbohydrate consumed on the two match days were significantly greater than carbohydrate consumed on training days (p = < 0.05; 6.4 $g{\cdot}kg^{-1}{\cdot}day^{-1}$ and 4.2 $g{\cdot}kg^{-1}{\cdot}day^{-1}$ for match and training days respectively). In comparison, research by Bettonviel et al. [24] found that professional football players as a whole failed to meet carbohydrate recommendations on match days (5.3 ± 1.5 $g{\cdot}kg^{-1}{\cdot}day^{-1}$) and one day post-match (4.5 ± 1.0 $g{\cdot}kg^{-1}{\cdot}day^{-1}$); however, protein intakes on match day and post-match were adequate (2.0 ± 0.4 and 1.6 ± 0.3 $g{\cdot}kg^{-1}{\cdot}day^{-1}$ respectively).

3.3.5. Micronutrient Intake

Six studies reported iron and/or calcium intakes [3,27,28,35–37,39]. The majority of these studies found that team sport athletes were meeting or exceeding recommended intakes of calcium and iron, when compared to the general public [27,28,35,36,39]. One study by Raizel et al. [37] found that professional football players were not meeting general (non-sport specific) recommendations (estimated average requirements) for calcium, reporting that athletes had a marginal intake of 83% of EAR.

4. Discussion

4.1. Energy Intake of Team Sport Athletes

In order for athletes to optimise training and performance, they need to consume sufficient energy for the work required and to support physiological adaptions [11,13,57]. A diet that contains insufficient energy (i.e., energy deficit) during periods of training can result in a number of performance detriments including loss of lean muscle mass and bone mineral density, increased prevalence of overtraining and injury, and may contribute to endocrine and reproductive system disturbances [11]. The mean energy intakes of professional male team sport athletes reported in the literature have decreased from those reported by a previous review [1]; however, in comparison female athletes are consuming diets of relatively similar energy density (i.e., 7.3–9.8 MJ/day) [1]. Simply looking at the difference in energy intakes of male team athletes would suggest that they are eating less and potentially not meeting energy recommendations; however, a range of factors may have influenced the dietary intake of these athletes at the time of assessment.

While not identified as an influencing factor previously [1], three studies included in this review that explored the dietary intakes of rugby union, Australian football and football athletes suggested that low energy intakes were related to the presence of team culture surrounding body composition goals (i.e., to decrease body fat and/or increase lean muscle mass) [3,10,25]. In theory, body composition goals should be individualised to the athlete, with the focus to support training adaptions; however, this is not always reflected in practice [8]. Research by Bradley et al. [10] found that during a rugby union preseason, athletes did not meet energy intake recommendations (14.8 ± 1.9 MJ/day) and it was found that the existence of body composition goals (i.e., to reduce body fat) were potentially influencing intake at the expense of fueling for training demands. Research during a preseason in Australian football, hypothesised that athletes intentionally restricted energy and carbohydrate intake surrounding body composition assessments using dual-energy X-ray absorptiometry (DXA), to meet target body composition goals (actual energy intake: 9.1 ± 1.8 MJ/day) [3]. Similarly, Andrews et al. [25] reported professional and semi-professional football athletes that were recognised as under reporters were those athletes that were identified as attempting to maintain body composition or reduce body fat at the time of recording (11.5 ± 2.0 and 10.8 ± 3.8 MJ/day). Realistic body composition goals must be promoted to prevent under fueling and support the training adaptions and recovery of athletes. Furthermore, in light of recent research regarding relative energy deficiency (RED-S) in male athletes, there is a greater need for education for coaches and support staff regarding the importance of an individualised approach when tailoring body composition goals [8].

4.2. Macronutrient Intake of Team Sport Athletes

4.2.1. Carbohydrate Intake of Team Sport Athletes

Carbohydrate intake is important for optimising performance and recovery. Team sports have varied training and physiological demands, therefore advice must be tailored to match the training demands as well as the demands of specific positions within the sport. Team sport athletes included in this review continue to consume diets that do not align with carbohydrate recommendations, intakes on average insufficient when compared to recommendations [1,11,12,52]. Research included has suggested that carbohydrate recommendations need to be better suited to the demands of the sport, individualising nutrition based on positions [10,23,28,58]. Research by Bradley et al. [27] found that professional rugby union athletes tapered carbohydrate intake across a training week; however, on average intakes fell below recommendations used by authors of 6–10 $g{\cdot}kg^{-1}{\cdot}day^{-1}$ (3.5 $g{\cdot}kg^{-1}{\cdot}day^{-1}$ and 3.4 $g{\cdot}kg^{-1}{\cdot}day^{-1}$ for forwards and backs respectively). Although these intakes did not align with recommendations, Bradley et al. [27] suggested that the tapering of intakes during a training week to match demands of training as well as enhance training adaptions (i.e., alter body fat) may be better suited to this athletic population. The idea of *"fueling for the work required"* is commonly being used by many sports nutrition professionals working in professional sport [59]. The concept of periodising intake is not simple and requires thorough knowledge of the athlete's needs, the sport and the training and competition demands. Anderson et al. [23] found that football athletes were applying the principle of carbohydrate periodization to their daily intakes; consuming significantly greater energy and carbohydrate on game days compared to training days. However, when assessing dietary intakes as a whole; carbohydrate intake the day before a competition was unlikely to maximise glycogen storage and, therefore, meet match demands. Dietitians working with professional team sport athletes need to use an individualised approach when periodising an athlete's carbohydrate intake. Further work is required to support education in this space to optimise glycogen storage and resynthesis and to support athletes' training and match day nutrition goals.

4.2.2. Protein Intake of Team Sport Athletes

Protein is important for muscle protein synthesis, supports recovery processes, promotes satiety and can aid the maintenance of body composition. It also has many other important roles in the body as enzymes, hormones, transporters and antibodies. Athletes with insufficient protein intakes have an increased risk of muscle wasting, illness and injury. ISSN recommendations state that to maintain protein balance athletes should consume 1.4–2.0 $g{\cdot}kg^{-1}{\cdot}day^{-1}$ of high-quality protein [11]. In this review team sport athletes, on average, adequately met recommendations; most athletes adopting a diet high in protein, but low in carbohydrates and/or total energy (hypocaloric) [2,3,10,26,28,35,36,38,43]. Research has suggested that high-protein diets (2.3–3.1 $g{\cdot}kg^{-1}{\cdot}day^{-1}$) may be appropriate for resistance trained athletes who are consuming hypocaloric diets with the aim to maintain lean muscle tissue while reducing fat mass [20,60]. This is supported by research by Bradley et al. [10] who found that although protein intakes of professional rugby athletes (2.5–2.6 $g \cdot kg^{-1} \cdot day^{-1}$) exceeded protein recommendations, since athletes were manipulating carbohydrate intakes during the preseason training week, protein intakes may have been appropriate at the time to optimise body composition. Given the context of the time of season this study was undertaken (i.e., preseason) and the ability for athletes to optimise training adaptions and changes to body composition without any detriment to competition performance, these intakes may be acceptable for this athletic cohort. However, in contrast, research by Potgieter et al. [35] reported that rugby union athletes' intakes in-season did not meet carbohydrate recommendations, and exceeded protein recommendations. Potgieter et al. [35] suggests that greater intakes of protein (i.e., 2.4 $g \cdot kg^{-1} \cdot day^{-1}$) may be suited in times where muscle hypertrophy is required (i.e., offseason); however, in-season where athletes are required to meet training, competition and recovery demands, protein intakes should align with recommendations and not be increased at the expense of carbohydrate intake. Similarly, research by Mackenzie et al. [33] on rugby union athletes reported that there was no compelling evidence to increase the distribution of protein for muscle protein synthesis and that an excess quantity of protein may in fact compromise lean muscle goals by promoting satiety which can result in decreased calorie intake. Taken as a whole, when working with team sport athletes greater emphasis should be placed on the distribution and timing of protein intake across a training day, instead of the total quantity [33]. In addition, it should be highlighted that the need to meet a body composition goal should not come at the expense of meeting nutrient requirements for performance and recovery.

4.2.3. Fat Intake of Team Sport Athletes

Four of the studies that reported athletes' diets exceeding recommended fat intakes (i.e., >30% of total energy) included the dietary intakes of athletes competing in strength and power sports such as rugby union (2), rugby league (1) and American football (1) [2,27,32,35]. Collectively strength and power sports are characterised as high-intensity and intermittent collision sports and may require a greater total mass to protect athletes against the physical impacts of scrumming, tackling etc. [1,2,27,32,35]. A study that explored the dietary intakes of American football athletes found that athletes consumed high intakes of fat (i.e., 41% of total energy) suggesting these intakes were a result of overfeeding to increase weight [32]. In comparison, research by Bradley et al. [27] in rugby union found that athletes had fat intakes that fell slightly above recommendations (i.e., 32% and 33% for forwards and backs respectively); however, in contrast they had suboptimal total energy intake when compared to energy expenditure. Additionally Potgieter et al. [35] found that competing rugby union athletes were consuming an excess in fat (i.e., 33.8 ± 4.3%), however failed to meet recommendations for total energy and carbohydrate. Taken together, these results indicate a reduction in dietary fat intake for these groups may not be warranted in order to support athletes to meet energy requirements. However, as many athletes did not meet these enhanced energy requirements, the addition of carbohydrate may allow athletes to meet energy balance or surplus, without the need for intakes that are in excess of dietary fat.

Although most team sport athletes included in this review consumed diets that were in line with or exceeded recommendations for dietary fat intake, the composition of saturated to unsaturated fats (i.e., mono and poly unsaturated fats) was suboptimal (i.e., saturated fat >10% total energy). This is supported by Hidalgo et al. [31] who found that football players' total dietary fat intake aligned with recommendations (i.e., 30%–33% of total energy); however, saturated fat and cholesterol intake exceeded recommendations. In addition, it was found that polyunsaturated fat intake fell below recommended intakes. Hidalgo et al. [31] and Raizel et al. [37] together suggested that football athletes' high protein intake, including a large intake of animal proteins, may have contributed to their overall high cholesterol intake. Research suggests diets that are rich in saturated fat (i.e., >10%TE), cholesterol and trans fats are linked to chronic diseases such as cardio-vascular disease (i.e., heart disease and stroke) and type 2 diabetes [61]. For the long term health of athletes, dietary advice should aim to include a varied diet with a focus on total and saturated fat, not exceeding recommendations (i.e., total fat <30% total energy and saturated fat <10% total energy) [11]. Additionally, athletes may benefit from the inclusion of mono- and poly unsaturated fat-based protein foods (i.e., fatty fish, nuts and seeds) to help meet energy and protein requirements and provide additional anti-inflammatory benefits for training and recovery [22].

This review highlights the role of dietitians in providing long-term dietary strategies to increase lean muscle and total body mass, in a manner that does not adversely affect performance and/or lipid profile, which may be evident in short term high energy and high fat diets. Greater education regarding the long-term implications of intakes that are in excess of total fat and saturated fat is required in team sport environments.

4.2.4. Dietary Intake during Competition

Due to the elevated requirements for stored glycogen and glycogen resynthesis during training and competition, athletes are recommended to undertake aggressive carbohydrate feeding prior to these periods. Inconsistencies between energy and carbohydrate intakes on training and match days were observed in team sport athletes. In particular research by Bettonviel et al. [24] found that carbohydrate intakes of football athletes did not meet recommendations (6–10 $g \cdot kg^{-1} \cdot day^{-1}$) for match days; however, in comparison these athletes exceeded recommended protein intakes. Additionally, research by Potgieter et al. [35] found that while rugby union athletes were consuming adequate energy and carbohydrate prior to competition, diets were additionally high in protein and fat. Interestingly, research by Tooley et al. [2] found that rugby league athletes had greater fat intakes on the two days post competition (i.e., "recovery period"). This research suggested that this elevated intake of fat might be considered a 'reward' post competition for these athletes [2,62]. Greater education on match day nutrition strategies are required to optimise energy and carbohydrate intake prior to competition. Additionally, in many sports athletes need to compete multiple times a week therefore it is integral that recovery tactics aim to restore muscle glycogen within 24–48 h post-competition [57]. In these instances, it is essential to consume a carbohydrate and protein-rich meal shortly after the game, followed by another carbohydrate-rich meal two hours later to accelerate glycogen resynthesis [11].

4.3. Limitations

Studies in this systematic review included small numbers of participants and may not be generalisable to team sport disciplines more broadly. In addition, the heterogeneity of the included studies led to an inability to compare results across all studies and as a result a meta-analysis of data was not possible. Underreporting is an important consideration when assessing dietary intake; however, suboptimal intakes should not be attributed solely to underreporting and dietary assessment should encompass a range of influencing factors (i.e., body composition, appetite, nutrition knowledge etc.) [3]. Many studies explored the existence of intentional and unintentional underreporting, thus the findings of these analyses should be interpreted with caution.

4.4. Conclusions

This systematic review found that despite the publication of high-quality research studies, expert consensus statements and recognition of the consequences of inadequate intakes, team sport athletes' total energy and carbohydrate intakes did not meet sports nutrition recommendations (i.e., IOC, ISSN, ASCM and sports specific research) for energy and carbohydrate. In contrast, many athletes met or exceeded recommendations for protein and/or fat. Further research into the development of sport-specific recommendations for energy and macronutrients in particular carbohydrate would be beneficial to further optimise distribution throughout a training week. Furthermore, nutrition in team sport environments requires a knowledge base of the physiological demands of training and competition, and therefore sports dietitians should work collaboratively with sports science teams when tailoring nutrition advice to meet energy and macronutrient needs. Future research is required to explore the factors that influence athletes' dietary intakes.

Author Contributions: S.L.J., R.B., and A.K.F. contributed to the design of the systematic review and the interpretation of data. S.L.J., performed the literature search. S.L.J. and G.L.B. performed the data extraction and quality assessment process using the using the Academy of Nutrition and Dietetics "Quality Criteria Checklist" from the Academy of Nutrition and Dietetics Evidence Analysis Manual. S.L.J., B.L.D., R.B, and A.K.F. contributed to the writing of the manuscript. All authors read, revised and approved the final manuscript.

Acknowledgments: Sarah Jenner is currently undertaking her PhD studies and receives a La Trobe University scholarship. Open Access fees was funded by author's research funds.

References

1. Holway, F.E.; Spriet, L.L. Sport-specific nutrition: Practical strategies for team sports. *J. Sports Sci.* **2011**, *29*, S115–S125. [CrossRef] [PubMed]
2. Tooley, E.; Bitcon, M.; Briggs, M.A.; West, D.J.; Russell, M. Estimates of energy intake and expenditure in professional rugby league players. *Int. J. Sports Sci. Coach.* **2015**, *10*, 551–560. [CrossRef]
3. Jenner, S.L.; Trakman, G.; Coutts, A.; Kempton, T.; Ryan, S.; Forsyth, A.; Belski, R. Dietary intake of professional Australian football athletes surrounding body composition assessment. *J. Int. Soc. Sports Nutr.* **2018**, *15*, 43. [CrossRef] [PubMed]
4. Rodriguez, N.R.; Dimarco, N.M.; Langley, S. Position of the American Dietetic Association, Dietitians of Canada, and the American College of Sports Medicine: Nutrition and athletic performance. *J. Am. Diet. Assoc.* **2009**, *109*, 509–527. [CrossRef] [PubMed]
5. Potgieter, S. Sport nutrition: A review of the latest guidelines for exercise and sport nutrition from the American college of sport nutrition, the International Olympic Committee and the international society for sports nutrition. *S. Afr. J. Clin. Nutr.* **2013**, *26*, 6–16. [CrossRef]
6. Kerksick, C.M.; Arent, S.; Schoenfeld, B.J.; Stout, J.R.; Campbell, B.; Wilborn, C.D.; Taylor, L.; Kalman, D.; Smith-Ryan, A.E.; Kreider, R.B.; et al. International society of sports nutrition position stand: Nutrient timing. *J. Int. Soc. Sports Nutr.* **2017**, *14*, 33. [CrossRef] [PubMed]
7. Aragon, A.A.; Schoenfeld, B.; Wildman, R.; Kleiner, S.; Vandusseldorp, T.; Taylor, L.; Earnest, C.P.; Arciero, P.J.; Wilborn, C.; Kalman, D.S.; et al. International society of sports nutrition position stand: diets and body composition. *J. Int. Soc. Sports Nutr.* **2017**, *14*, 16. [CrossRef]
8. Mountjoy, M.; Sundgot-Borgen, J.; Burke, L.; Ackerman, K.E.; Blauwet, C.; Constantini, N.; Lebrun, C.; Lundy, B.; Melin, A.; Meyer, N.; et al. International Olympic Committee (IOC) consensus statement on relative energy deficiency in sport (RED-S): 2018 update. *Int. J. Sport Nutr. Exerc. Metab.* **2018**, *28*, 316–331. [CrossRef]
9. International Olympic Committee. IOC consensus statement on sports nutrition 2010. *Int. J. Sport Nutr. Exerc. Metab.* **2010**, *1003*. [CrossRef]
10. Bradley, W.J.; Cavanagh, B.P.; Douglas, W.; Donovan, T.F.; Morton, J.P.; Close, G.L. Quantification of training load, energy intake, and physiological adaptations during a rugby preseason: A case study from an elite european rugby union squad. *J. Strength Cond. Res.* **2015**, *29*, 534–544. [CrossRef]
11. Kerksick, C.M.; Wilborn, C.D.; Roberts, M.D.; Smith-Ryan, A.; Kleiner, S.M.; Jäger, R.; Collins, R.; Cooke, M.; Davis, J.N.; Galvan, E.; et al. ISSN exercise & sports nutrition review update: research & recommendations. *J. Int. Soc. Sports Nutr.* **2018**, *15*, 38. [CrossRef] [PubMed]
12. Burke, L.M.; Hawley, J.A.; Wong, S.H.; Jeukendrup, A.E. Carbohydrates for training and competition. *J. Sports Sci.* **2011**, *29*, S17–S27. [CrossRef]
13. Thomas, D.T.; Erdman, K.A.; Burke, L.M. American college of sports medicine joint position statement. nutrition and athletic performance. *Med. Sci. Sports Exerc.* **2016**, *48*, 543–568. [CrossRef] [PubMed]
14. Kreider, R.B.; Kalman, D.S.; Antonio, J.; Ziegenfuss, T.N.; Wildman, R.; Collins, R.; Candow, D.G.; Kleiner, S.M.; Almada, A.L.; Lopez, H.L. International Society of Sports Nutrition position stand: safety and efficacy of creatine supplementation in exercise, sport, and medicine. *J. Int. Soc. Sport Nutr.* **2017**, *14*, 18. [CrossRef] [PubMed]

15. Wilson, J.M.; Fitschen, P.J.; Campbell, B.; Wilson, G.J.; Zanchi, N.; Taylor, L.; Wilborn, C.; Kalman, D.S.; Stout, J.R.; Hoffman, J.R.; et al. International Society of Sports Nutrition Position Stand: beta-hydroxy-beta-methylbutyrate (HMB). *J. Int. Soc. Sport Nutr.* **2013**, *10*, 6. [CrossRef]
16. Campbell, B.; Wilborn, C.; La Bounty, P.; Taylor, L.; Nelson, M.; Greenwood, M.; Ziegenfuss, T.N.; Lopez, H.L.; Hoffman, J.R.; Stout, J.R.; et al. International Society of Sports Nutrition position stand: energy drinks. *J. Int. Soc. Sports Nutr.* **2013**, *10*, 1. [CrossRef]
17. Maughan, R.J.; Burke, L.M.; Dvorak, J.; Larson-Meyer, D.E.; Peeling, P.; Phillips, S.M.; Rawson, E.S.; Walsh, N.P.; Garthe, I.; Geyer, H.; et al. IOC Consensus Statement: Dietary Supplements and the High-Performance Athlete. *Int. J. Sport Nutr. Exerc. Metab.* **2018**, *28*, 104–125. [CrossRef] [PubMed]
18. Bergeron, M.F.; Bahr, R.; Bärtsch, P.; Bourdon, L.; Calbet, J.A.; Carlsen, K.H.; Castagna, O.; González-Alonso, J.; Lundby, C.; Maughan, R.J.; et al. International Olympic Committee consensus statement on thermoregulatory and altitude challenges for high-level athletes. *Br. J. Sports Med.* **2012**, *46*, 770–779. [CrossRef] [PubMed]
19. Trexler, E.T.; Smith-Ryan, A.E.; Stout, J.R.; Hoffman, J.R.; Wilborn, C.D.; Sale, C.; Kreider, R.B.; Jäger, R.; Earnest, C.P.; Bannock, L.; et al. International society of sports nutrition position stand: Beta-Alanine. *J. Int. Soc. Sports Nutr* **2015**, *12*, 30. [CrossRef] [PubMed]
20. Jäger, R.; Kerksick, C.M.; Campbell, B.I.; Cribb, P.J.; Wells, S.D.; Skwiat, T.M.; Purpura, M.; Ziegenfuss, T.N.; Ferrando, A.A.; Arent, S.M.; et al. International Society of Sports Nutrition Position Stand: Protein and exercise. *J. Int. Soc. Sports Nutr.* **2017**, *14*, 20. [CrossRef]
21. Position of the Academy of Nutrition and Dietetics. Dietitians of Canada, and the American College of Sports Medicine: Nutrition and Athletic Performance. *Can. J. Diet. Pract. Res.* **2016**, *77*, 54. [CrossRef] [PubMed]
22. Kreider, R.B.; Wilborn, C.D.; Taylor, L.; Campbell, B.; Almada, A.L.; Collins, R.; Cooke, M.; Earnest, C.P.; Greenwood, M.; Kalman, D.S.; et al. ISSN exercise & sport nutrition review: Research & recommendations. *J. Int. Soc. of Sports Nutr.* **2010**, *7*, 7. [CrossRef]
23. Anderson, L.; Orme, P.; Naughton, R.J.; Close, G.L.; Milsom, J.; Rydings, D.; O'Boyle, A.; Di Michele, R.; Louis, J.; Hambly, C.; et al. Energy Intake and Expenditure of Professional Soccer Players of the English Premier League: Evidence of Carbohydrate Periodization. *Int. J. Sport Nutr. Exerc. Metab.* **2017**, *27*, 228–238. [CrossRef] [PubMed]
24. Bettonviel, A.E.O.; Brinkmans, N.Y.J.; Russcher, K.; Wardenaar, F.C.; Witard, O.C. Nutritional Status and Daytime Pattern of Protein Intake on Match, Post-Match, Rest and Training Days in Senior Professional and Youth Elite Soccer Players. *Int. J. Sport Nutr. Exerc. Metab.* **2016**, *26*, 285–293. [CrossRef]
25. Andrews, M.C.; Itsiopoulos, C. Room for improvement in nutrition knowledge and dietary intake of male football (Soccer) players in Australia. *Int. J. Sport Nutr. Exerc. Metab.* **2016**, *26*, 55–64. [CrossRef]
26. Bilsborough, J.C.; Greenway, K.; Livingston, S.; Cordy, J.; Coutts, A.J. Changes in anthropometry, upper-body strength, and nutrient intake in professional Australian football players during a season. *Int. J. Sports Physiol. Perform.* **2016**, *11*, 290–300. [CrossRef] [PubMed]
27. Bradley, W.J.; Cavanagh, B.; Douglas, W.; Donovan, T.F.; Twist, C.; Morton, J.P.; Close, G.L. Energy intake and expenditure assessed 'in-season' in an elite European rugby union squad. *Eur. J. Sport Sci.* **2015**, *15*, 469–479. [CrossRef]
28. Conejos, C.; Giner, A.; Mañes, J.; Soriano, J.M. Energy and nutritional intakes in training days of soccer players according to their playing positions. *Arch. Med. Deporte* **2011**, *28*, 29–35.
29. Grams, L.; Garrido, G.; Villacieros, J.; Ferro, A. Marginal Micronutrient Intake in High-Performance Male Wheelchair Basketball Players: A Dietary Evaluation and the Effects of Nutritional Advice. *PLoS ONE* **2016**, *11*, e0157931. [CrossRef]
30. Gravina, L.; Ruiz, F.; Diaz, E.; Lekue, J.A.; Badiola, A.; Irazusta, J.; Gil, S.M. Influence of nutrient intake on antioxidant capacity, muscle damage and white blood cell count in female soccer players. *J. Int. Soc. Sports Nutr.* **2012**, *9*, 32. [CrossRef]
31. Hidalgo y Teran Elizondo, R.; Martin Bermudo, F.M.; Penaloza Mendez, R.; Berna Amoros, G.; Lara Padilla, E.; Berral de la Rosa, F.J. Nutritional intake and nutritional status in elite Mexican teenagers soccer players of different ages. *Nutr. Hosp.* **2015**, *32*, 1735–1743. [CrossRef]
32. Kirwan, R.D.; Kordick, L.K.; McFarland, S.; Lancaster, D.; Clark, K.; Miles, M.P. Dietary, anthropometric, blood-lipid, and performance patterns of American college football players during 8 weeks of training. *Int. J. Sport Nutr. Exerc. Metab.* **2012**, *22*, 444–451. [CrossRef]

33. MacKenzie, K.; Slater, G.; King, N.; Byrne, N. The measurement and interpretation of dietary protein distribution during a rugby preseason. *Int. J. Sport Nutr. Exerc. Metab.* **2015**, *25*, 353–358. [CrossRef]
34. Ono, M.; Kennedy, E.; Reeves, S.; Cronin, L. Nutrition and culture in professional football. A mixed method approach. *Appetite* **2012**, *58*, 98–104. [CrossRef]
35. Potgieter, S.; Visser, J.; Croukamp, I.; Markides, M.; Nascimento, J.; Scott, K. Body composition and habitual and match-day dietary intake of the FNB Maties Varsity Cup rugby players.(ORIGINAL RESEARCH). *S. Afr. J. Sports Med.* **2014**, *26*, 35–43. [CrossRef]
36. Molina-López, J.; Molina, J.M.; Chirosa, L.J.; Florea, D.; Sáez, L.; Jiménez, J.; Planells, P.; Perez de la Cruz, A.; Planells, E. Implementation of a nutrition education program in a handball team; consequences on nutritional status. *Nutr. Hosp.* **2013**, *28*, 1065–1076. [CrossRef]
37. Raizel, R.; da Mata Godois, A.; Coqueiro, A.Y.; Voltarelli, F.A.; Fett, C.A.; Tirapegui, J.; de Paula Ravagnani, F.C.; de Faria Coelho-Ravagnani, C. Pre-season dietary intake of professional soccer players. *Nutr. Health* **2017**, *23*, 215–222. [CrossRef]
38. Valliant, M.W.; Pittman Emplaincourt, H.; Wenzel, R.K.; Garner, B.H. Nutrition Education by a Registered Dietitian Improves Dietary Intake and Nutrition Knowledge of a NCAA Female Volleyball Team. *Nutrients* **2012**, *4*, 506–516. [CrossRef] [PubMed]
39. Vermeulen, T. Seven Day Dietary Intakes of Female Varsity Ice Hockey Players. Master's Thesis, The University of Guelph, Guelph, ON, Canada, 2017.
40. International Prospective Register of Systematic Reviews. Available online: https://www.crd.york.ac.uk/prospero/display_record.php?RecordID=105168 (accessed on 24 September 2018).
41. Moher, D.; Liberati, A.; Tetzlaff, J.; Altman, D.G.; PRISMA Group. Preferred Reporting Items for Systematic Reviews and Meta-Analyses: The PRISMA statement. *Ann. Intern. Med.* **2009**, *151*, 264–269. [CrossRef] [PubMed]
42. Academy of Nutrition and Dietetics. Evidence Analysis Manual. Available online: https://www.andeal.org/vault/2440/web/files/2016_April_EA_Manual.pdf (accessed on 18 September 2018).
43. Devlin, B.L.; Leveritt, M.D.; Kingsley, M.; Belski, R. Dietary Intake, Body Composition, and Nutrition Knowledge of Australian Football and Soccer Players: Implications for Sports Nutrition Professionals in Practice. *Int. J. Sport Nutr. Exerc. Metab.* **2017**, *27*, 130–138. [CrossRef]
44. Maughan, R.J.; Burke, L.M. Practical Nutritional Recommendations for the Athlete. *Nestle Nutr. Inst. Workshop Ser.* **2011**, *69*, 131–149. [CrossRef]
45. Lemon, P.W. Protein requirements of soccer. *J. Sports Sci.* **1994**, *12*, S17–S22. [CrossRef] [PubMed]
46. Hernandez, A.J.; Nahas, R.M. Modificações dietéticas, reposição hídrica, suplementos alimentares e drogas: comprovação de ação ergogênica e potenciais riscos para a saúde. *Rev. Bras. Med. Esporte* **2009**, *15*, 1–12.
47. Mettler, S.; Mitchell, N.; Tipton, K.D. Increased Protein Intake Reduces Lean Body Mass Loss during Weight Loss in Athletes. *Med. Sci. Sports Exerc.* **2010**, *42*, 326–337. [CrossRef] [PubMed]
48. Tipton, K.D.; Wolfe, R.R. Protein and amino acids for athletes. *J. Sports Sci.* **2004**, *22*, 65–79. [CrossRef]
49. Bishop, N.C.; Blannin, A.K.; Walsh, N.P.; Robson, P.J.; Gleeson, M. Nutritional Aspects of Immunosuppression in Athletes. *Sports Med.* **1999**, *28*, 151–176. [CrossRef] [PubMed]
50. American College of Sports Medicine author issuing body. *ACSM's Guidelines for Exercise Testing and Prescription*, 10th ed.; Wolters Kluwer Health: Philadelphia, PA, USA, 2018.
51. Phillips, S.M.; Van Loon, L.J. Dietary protein for athletes: From requirements to optimum adaptation. *J. Sports Sci.* **2011**, *29*, S29–S38. [CrossRef] [PubMed]
52. Nutrition for football: The FIFA/F-MARC Consensus Conference. *J. Sports Sci.* **2006**, *24*, 663–664. [CrossRef]
53. Bussau, V.A.; Fairchild, T.J.; Rao, A.; Steele, P.; Fournier, P.A. Carbohydrate loading in human muscle: An improved 1 day protocol. *Eur. J. Appli. Physiol.* **2002**, *87*, 290–295. [CrossRef]
54. Krustrup, P.; Mohr, M.; Steensberg, A.; Bencke, J.; Kjær, M.; Bangsbo, J. Muscle and Blood Metabolites during a Soccer Game: Implications for Sprint Performance. *Med. Sci. Sports Exerc.* **2006**, *38*, 1165–1174. [CrossRef]
55. Hargreaves, M. Carbohydrate and lipid requirements of soccer. *J. Sports Sci.* **1994**, *12*, S13–S16. [CrossRef] [PubMed]
56. Bradley, W.J.; Hannon, M.P.; Benford, V.; Morehen, J.C.; Twist, C.; Shepherd, S.; Cocks, M.; Impey, S.G.; Cooper, R.G.; Morton, J.P.; et al. Metabolic demands and replenishment of muscle glycogen after a rugby league match simulation protocol. *J. Sci. Med. Sport* **2017**, *20*, 878–883. [CrossRef] [PubMed]

2

Change of Direction Performance is Influenced by Asymmetries in Jumping Ability and Hip and Trunk Strength in Elite Basketball Players

Filip Ujaković [1,2] and Nejc Šarabon [3,4,*]

[1] Faculty of Kinesiology, University of Zagreb, 10110 Zagreb, Croatia; fujakovic@gmail.com
[2] Basketball Club Cedevita Olimpija Ljubljana, 1000 Ljubljana, Slovenia
[3] Faculty of Health Sciences, University of Primorska, 6310 Izola, Slovenia
[4] S2P, Science to Practice, Ltd., Laboratory for Motor Control and Motor Behavior, 1000 Ljubljana, Slovenia
* Correspondence: nejc.sarabon@fvz.upr.si

Abstract: Change of direction (COD) ability is essential for sport performance in high level team sports such as basketball, however, the influence of asymmetries on COD ability is relatively unknown. Forty-three junior and senior level elite basketball players performed isometric hip and trunk strength testing, passive hip and trunk range of motion testing, and unilateral horizontal and vertical jumps, as well as the T-test to measure COD performance. Mean asymmetry values ranged from 0.76% for functional leg length up to 40.35% for rate of torque development during hip flexion. A six-variable regression model explained 48% ($R^2 = 0.48$; $p < 0.001$) of variation in COD performance. The model included left hip internal/external rotation strength ratio, and inter-limb asymmetries in hip abduction rate of torque development, hip flexion range of motion, functional leg length, single leg triple jump distance, and peak torque during trunk lateral flexion. Results suggest that the magnitude of asymmetries is dependent of task and parameter, and using universal asymmetry thresholds, such as <10 %, is not optimal. The regression model showed the relationship between asymmetries and COD performance. None of tests were sufficient to explain a complex variable like COD performance.

Keywords: asymmetry; agility; basketball; strength; power; inter-limb asymmetry

---

1. Introduction

Inter-limb asymmetry has been mostly researched from the aspect of sports injury risk, especially in view of athletes returning to sport after anterior cruciate ligament reconstruction [1–4]. Only recently, the relationship between inter-limb asymmetry and sports performance has been a popular topic of investigation [5,6]. Inter-limb asymmetry is found to be a normal adaptation in many sports that involve unilateral movements (e.g., cricket) [7], but further research in team sports is needed to elucidate whether asymmetries influence performance or injury risk [5,6]. Lately researchers are trying to elucidate whether asymmetries (and which particular type of asymmetry) influence performance [8]. Inter-limb asymmetry may present at the level of different motor abilities (e.g., strength, power, and range of motion) and can be measured locally (e.g., one joint) and globally (e.g., within a complex movement, such as vertical jump). Therefore, various methods have been used for its quantification [9], however, many studies used local knee isokinetic dynamometry [10,11], isometric mid-thigh pull (IMTP) [12,13] or vertical jump tests [14–18]. Further, Sheppard and Young´s [19] model of change of direction (COD) determinants showed that asymmetries could negatively affect COD performance. However, supporting evidence is inconsistent.

Two studies investigated the relationship between local inter-limb knee strength asymmetry and performance in COD. Lockie et al. [10] showed mostly positive correlation between different parameters and speed of isokinetic strength asymmetries during knee flexion and extension and T-test performance ($r = 0.638, 0.669, p < 0.01$). Exception was one negative correlation ($r = -568, p < 0.01$) between peak torque during knee extension (240°/s) and T-test performance. Similarly, Coratella et al. [11] observed that the same local asymmetries negatively impact COD performance (T-test and 180° turn test) ($r = 0.397$–0.614, $p < 0.05$). As the mentioned studies measured local strength asymmetries in the knee joint, they demonstrate the need to study proximal body parts like hip and trunk.

When it comes to the relationship between global asymmetries and performance in COD, results are less consistent. Many studies, using different tests for assessing asymmetries and COD performance, did not detect a relationship between global asymmetries and COD performance. Chiang [12] investigated the relationship between peak torque asymmetry during IMTP and COD ability (assessed as 180° turn test) and reported no significant correlation. However, he used bilateral IMTP to quantify asymmetry, which may have influenced methodological validity. While this methodological shortcoming was corrected by Dos Santos et al. [13], who used unilateral IMTP test, they have not found any significant correlation between inter-limb asymmetry in various parameters related to unilateral IMTP and COD performance ($r \leq 0.35, p \geq 0.380$). Hoffman et al. [14] have not found any significant correlation between asymmetry in single-leg countermovement jump (SLCMJ) height and COD ability (three-cone drill). Although reporting high average asymmetry in jump height and length (up to 10.2%), Lockie et al. [15], have not found any significant correlation between these asymmetries and COD (505 and T-test) performance ($r = 0.00$–0.018, $p = 0.31$–0.99). Similarly, Dos Santos et al. [16] found no significant correlations between asymmetries in horizontal jumping tasks and performance in two COD tasks ($r \leq 0.35, p > 0.05$). Furthermore, Fort-Vanmeerhaeghe et al. [20] have not found a relationship between asymmetry in jump height during SLCMJ and V-cut COD test ($r = 0.10, p > 0.05$). Finally, Loturco et al. [18], have found no significant correlation between asymmetries in different parameters during single leg vertical jumps and performance in zig-zag test.

By contrast, few studies have found a significant correlation between global asymmetry in jumping tests and COD performance. Studying female soccer players, Bishop et al. [21] found a significant positive correlation between inter-limb asymmetry in single-leg depth jump height and performance in 505 COD test on left ($r = 0.66, p < 0.01$) and right ($r = 0.52, p < 0.05$) side. Another study that reported a relationship between asymmetry and performance was of Maloney et al. [22], that explained 63% ($p < 0.001$) of variance of COD performance with leg stiffness and height asymmetry during vertical depth jump.

The reason for inconsistent findings could lay in discrepancies among populations, methods of asymmetry calculation, and COD tests, as well as in low asymmetry values, that are not large enough to influence performance. Taking that into consideration, Sarabon et al. [23] found that explosive strength parameters like rate of torque development (RTD) are more sensitive to detect inter-limb asymmetries compared to maximal strength outcomes like peak force or peak torque during maximal voluntary contractions (MVC), which were used in previous research. Also, local inter-limb asymmetries were assessed only for the knee joint, while proximal regions of hip and trunk were overlooked. Moreover, asymmetries in range of motion were not previously researched in relation to performance. A substantial portion of asymmetry studies was done on amateur athletes and soccer players, which does not give enough insight into the functioning of elite athletes and other team sports, such as basketball. Basketball is characterized by many high intensity changes of direction (COD) [24], indicating that COD ability plays a critical role in basketball performance.

Therefore, the aim of this study is two-fold: (a) to profile elite basketball players in different local strength and range of motion asymmetries of hip and trunk region, and global power asymmetries in horizontal and vertical jumping and (b) to quantify the relationship of those asymmetries with COD performance. We hypothesized that these asymmetries could predict COD performance.

2. Materials and Methods

2.1. Subjects

Forty-three (17 senior and 26 junior) male elite basketball players (age = 20.54 ± 6 years; height = 194.48 ± 7.19 cm; body mass = 86.77 ± 10.13 kg) from three different professional basketball clubs (Adriatic basketball association league (all three clubs); Liga Nova KBM, Slovenia (one club), and Premier Croatian basketball league (two clubs)) volunteered to participate in the study. A minimum sample size of 18 participants was determined from an a priori power analysis (G*Power 3.1, Heinrich-Heine-Universität, Düsseldorf, Germany) based upon an estimated squared multiple correlation of 0.45 and a power of 0.8 [25]. Subjects were in training program from 18 to 24 h per week, had at least one-year experience in resistance training and reported no previous (within the last 12 months) or present lower-limb injuries. All subjects provided informed consent to participate in the study. For the underage subjects their parents or guardians signed consent prior to their participation. This study was a part of TELASI–PREVENT (Body asymmetries as a risk factor in musculoskeletal injury development: studying etiological mechanisms and designing corrective interventions for primary and tertiary preventive care—L5-1845) project which was approved by Slovenian Medical Ethics committee.

2.2. Procedures

The study was conducted in February of 2019, in the middle of the 2018/2019 basketball season. Testing was performed in each of the clubs playing/training courts. All tests were performed during a single testing session lasting approximately 180 min per participant. Participants attended the sessions in larger groups and rotated between the testing sessions (see below). The subjects were instructed to refrain from any physical activity for at least 24 hours before testing. Testing started with anthropometric measurements, after which the subjects performed a warm-up (5 min of low intensity running, 8 repetitions of dynamic stretching and body weight activation exercises). After the warm-up, subjects were randomized into 4 groups to complete four testing stations in a random order: (i) jumping, (ii) COD, (iii) hip and trunk dynamometry; and (iv) hip and trunk range of motion (ROM). There was a 5-minute rest between the testing stations. Each test began after the subject reported that they felt comfortable with the task (no more than 3 practice trials were taken by a player).

2.2.1. Functional Leg Length

Functional leg length was defined as the distance between anterior-superior iliac spine (ASIS) and the ground, and was measured with laser distance meter (LD 420, Stabila, Hungary). The subjects were instructed to stand with their bare feet on the ground, heels next to the wall, with feet separated hip distance apart. During left leg measurement subjects were instructed to put their left hand on the right shoulder and vice versa. Three measurements on each leg were performed and the mean from these three repetitions was taken for further analysis.

2.2.2. Single-Leg Countermovement Jump

SLCMJ was performed on a force platform (Type 9260AA, Kistler, Winterthur, Switzerland). Subjects were informed to step on the force platform with their testing leg and hands on their hips. The opposite leg was slightly flexed at the knee, but was not touching the shin of the tested leg. Swinging with the opposite leg during jumping was not allowed. The subjects were instructed to jump as high as possible, with the countermovement depth being self-selected, land on two legs and a hold balanced position for 3 s. The jump would be accepted if all of the above-mentioned instructions were met. Three trials on left and right leg were performed with 30 s of rest between each trial. Peak force (N), peak power (W), and highest jump height (m) for each leg was taken for further analysis.

2.2.3. Single-Leg Horizontal Jump

Tape measure was used to measure Single leg horizontal jump (SLHJ), which was performed on the basketball court sufficing the standards of international basketball federation (FIBA). Subjects were informed to put their testing leg with toe at the starting line and hands on the hips. Subjects performed a countermovement to self-selected depth before pushing themselves into the horizontal jump, landing onto both legs and holding a balanced position for 3 s. Three trials on each leg were performed with 30 s of rest between each trial. The distance (m) was measured to the nearest 0.01 m with a tape measure. The longest jump from each leg was taken for further analysis.

2.2.4. Single-Leg Triple Jump

Single leg triple jump (SLTJ) was measured similarly to SLHJ. Subject performed three consecutive horizontal jumps in which they landed onto both legs and held a balanced position for 3 s. The jump would be accepted for if all of the above-mentioned instructions were met. As with the SLHJ, the longest of the three jumps was taken for further analysis for each leg.

2.2.5. Single-Leg Lateral Jump

Tape measure was used to measure Single leg lateral jump (SLLJ). Subjects were informed to put the inner (i.e., medial) edge of their feet at the starting line and hands on their hips. When a subject was ready, he performed a countermovement to self-selected depth before pushing himself into lateral jump landing onto both legs and holding a balanced position for 3 s. Three trials on left and right leg were performed with 30 s of rest between each trial. Distance (m) was measured to the nearest 0.01 m with a tape measure. Longest jump from each leg was taken for further analysis.

2.2.6. Trunk Strength

Trunk strength assessment was done according to Markovic et al. [26] protocol. A trunk dynamometer (S2P Ltd., Ljubljana, Slovenia) with a bending beam load cell (model 1-Z6FC3/200 kg, HBM, Darmstadt, Germany) was used to measure trunk flexion, extension, and lateral flexion isometric strength. Isometric strength was measured as peak torque (Nm/kg) of the best one second interval during maximal voluntary contraction. All of the output variables were normalized with subject's body mass. During trunk extension measurement, subjects were standing with back turned towards the dynamometer with sensors on level of scapular spine and hands crossed on their shoulders. During trunk flexion measurement, subjects were standing turned face towards dynamometer with sensors on the same level as during extension and arms floating in the air to prevent their contribution. During trunk lateral flexion, subjects were standing sideways to the dynamometer, positioned so that their spine was in neutral position. The hand closer to the sensor was placed on their opposite shoulder and the other one was placed on opposite hip. During all trunk strength measurements, subjects were in their training shoes, standing with feet hip width distance apart, while a rigid strap was tightly fastened across pelvic girdle to achieve good fixation. During every trial subject was verbally encouraged to reach his best performance and hold it for 3–5 s. Each task was done three times with 60 s of rest in between. The best result for each task was taken for further analysis.

2.2.7. Hip Strength

Hip strength assessment was modeled based on Markovic et al. [27] protocol. A multipurpose dynamometer (Muscleboard, S2P Ltd., Ljubljana, Slovenija) was used to measure hip flexion, extension, abduction, adduction, internal and external rotation strength. Peak force values were multiplied by lever arm (leg length, in meter) to calculate hip torque. Isometric strength was measured as peak torque (PT) (Nm/kg) during one second interval of maximal voluntary contraction and rate of torque development (RTD) (Nm/ms) was measured in 100 ms interval as Δ torque/Δ time value. During all of the measurements, the offset of the sensor was performed with the relaxed leg, but with the subject having minimal contact with sensor (~5% MVC). Then, the subject was instructed to reach MVC as fast as possible. During all measured actions (except hip rotations), the distance between the mid-part of the aluminum brace of sensor and medial malleoli was set to 5 cm and a rigid strap was tightly fastened across pelvic girdle to achieve good fixation. Hip flexion and extension were measured unilaterally while the remaining tasks were performed bilaterally. During hip flexion (Figure 1A) subject was sitting on dynamometer with hands on the ground and the tested leg extended in knee with hip flexion (~30°), while the non-tested leg was on the ground with knee flexion of ~90°. During hip extension (Figure 1B) subject was laying prone on elbows on the ground, with the tested leg extended, non-tested leg was in the 90° knee flexion, resting on dynamometer surface. During abduction and adduction (Figure 1C) subject was sitting with legs hip apart, knees fully extended and hip in ~30° flexion. During hip internal and external (Figure 1D) rotation, the subject was kneeling on all fours with knees and hip in 90° flexion with knees hip apart. The best out of three results from each movement was taken for further analysis.

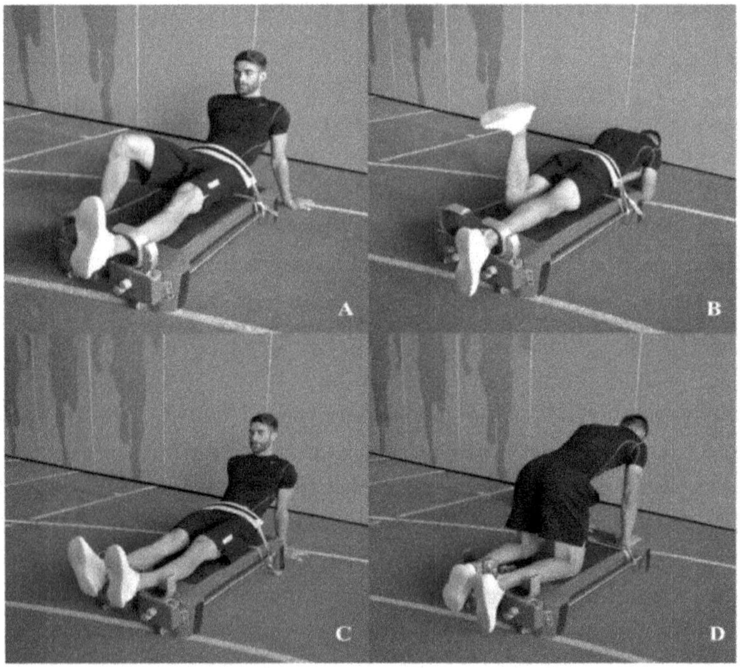

Figure 1. Position of subjects during isometric hip strength testing. (**A**) flexion; (**B**) extension; (**C**) abduction/adduction; and (**D**) internal/external rotation.

2.2.8. Range of Motion

Passive hip range of motion (ROM) during flexion, extension and internal/external rotation was measured with a digital inclinometer (Baseline, Fabrication Enterprises Inc., White Plains, NY, USA) and abduction/adduction with a handheld goniometer (Baseline, Fabrication Enterprises Inc., White Plains, NY, USA). All of the measurements were performed by the same measurer to minimize error. For flexion and extension, the inclinometer was aligned between the tested side femur trochanter major and lateral condyle. Hip flexion ROM was measured with the subject in supine position (the non-tested leg was extended in knee and hip fixated) and the knee of the tested leg in extended position. The tested leg was then moved and kept extended during whole movement until first pelvic movement. During hip extension ROM, subject was in prone position, and tested leg was kept in knee flexion (~90°) during whole movement until first pelvic movement. Hip internal/external rotation ROM was measured with the inclinometer located in the center of vertically positioned (with pendulum) tibia with the subject in pronated position and knee in 90° flexion. Internal and external rotation were performed until the first pelvic movement, with hand-stabilization on the pelvis. Hip abduction and adduction ROM were measured with goniometer with stationary arm pointed toward the opposite anterior superior iliac spine and the movable arm pointed toward the patella of the tested leg. During abduction, the subject was laying supine with both legs in neutral position (start) from which the tested leg was moved into abduction until first pelvic movement (finish). During adduction, the subject was supine with non-tested leg laying from table in ~30° abduction and tested leg in neutral position (start) from which leg was moved into adduction until first pelvic movement (finish). Mean result from three attempts on each leg was taken for further analysis with all of the results expressed in degrees (°).

For the trunk lateral flexion ROM, the subject was standing barefoot with feet hip width distance apart with his back and heels touching the wall. Starting position was measured with a tape as distance between the middle finger (hand on the wall) and the floor. Subjects performed lateral flexion, sliding downwards with the hands without breaking contact with the wall and lifting their heels of the ground. At the end of movement, the end position was measured, and the difference between starting and end position was calculated. Mean result from three attempts on each side was taken for further analysis with all of the results expressed in meters (m).

2.2.9. Change of Direction

For COD performance, the T-test (Figure 2) was used, as outlined by Semenik [28]. All of the COD testing was done on the basketball court sufficing the standards of international basketball federation (FIBA) using photocells timing gates (Brower Timing Systems; Draper, Utah). At the beginning of test, the subject was standing 30 cm behind the start/finish line where photocells were placed. Subject was instructed to sprint (filled line up in Figure 2) from the start to the first cone, touch the tip with one hand, shuffle (dashed lines in Figure 2) to the cone opposite of the touching hand and touch the tip of the lateral cone, then shuffle to the third cone and touch it with the first hand, shuffle back to the middle cone touching the tip with the second hand and then pedal back (filled line down in Figure 2) to the finish line. One-minute recovery was given between each trial. The best out of three trials was taken for further analysis.

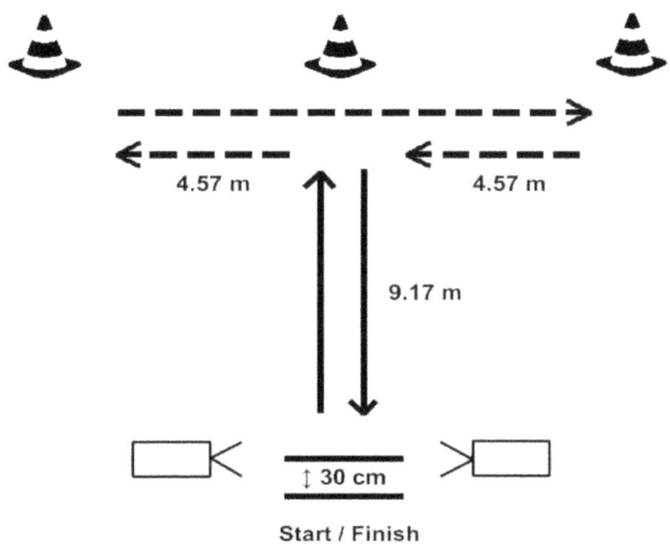

Figure 2. Schematic representation of the T-test.

2.3. Statistical Analyses

Due to the unknown reliability of the strength assessment with a novel MuscleBoard device (S2P Ltd., Ljubljana, Slovenia), particularly in view of RTD, we checked the intra-session reliability of the strength outcome measures that were used as potential predictors for COD performance. We used (a) intra-class coefficient correlation to assess relative reliability, (b) absolute typical error and relative typical error (expressed as coefficient of variation) to assess absolute reliability, and (c) paired-sample two-tailed T-tests to check for systematic bias. We used the data from our larger study involving 115 basketball players, who had completed the exact same protocol for strength assessment, the only difference was the lower number of repetitions (2 compared to 3 in our study) for each task. We used guidelines of Koo and Li [29] for reporting Intraclass Correlation Coefficient (ICC). Based on the 95% confident interval of ICC estimate values < 0.5 = poor, 0.5–0.75 = moderate, 0.75–0.90 = good, and > 0.90 = excellent reliability.

We used multiple regression analysis to model prediction of COD performance (dependent variable) with asymmetries (independent variable). Independent variables were grouped into five categories of asymmetries (anthropometric asymmetries, lateral hip and trunk strength asymmetries, hip and trunk strength ratios, hip and trunk ROM asymmetries and jumping asymmetries)—a total of 33 potential independent variables.

Inter-limb asymmetry was calculated with the following equation [30]:

$$Asymmetry\ (\%) = \left(\frac{stronger - weaker}{stronger}\right) \times 100$$

Shapiro–Wilks tests were performed to assess the normality of distribution of independent variables; only 24 % (8/33) were considered to be normally distributed given an alpha level of $p > 0.05$. Step-wise regression analysis was performed for overall CODS performance using all independent variables. An analysis of standard residuals was carried out, which showed that the data contained no outliers (s standardized residuals minimum: −1.71, standardized residuals maximum: 2.51). A collinearity test indicated that multicollinearity was not a concern (minimum tolerance: 0.75, maximum VIF:1.33). The data met the assumption of independent errors (Durbin–Watson value: 2.26). Also, Breuch–Pagan (10.43, $p > 0.05$) and Koenker (8.32, $p > 0.05$) test indicated the homoscedasticity of the model. Statistical significance was set at alpha level of $p \leq 0.05$ and all statistical procedures were conducted using the Statistical Package for the Social Sciences for Windows (v.26.0; SPSS Inc., Chicago, IL, USA). Mann–Whitney U test was used to for testing statistical significance in difference between hip PT and RTD, and left and right leg strength ratios.

3. Results

The results regarding reliability analyses are summarized in Table 1. No systematic bias was present for any of the outcome measures. Relative reliability was good to excellent for the peak torque measures (ICC > 0.80) and acceptable for RTD measures (ICC = 0.5–0.8). Typical errors, expressed as coefficient of variation were low for peak torque measurements for adduction, abduction, and internal rotation, but higher (>10%) for external rotation, flexion, and extension, and for all RTD outcomes. This suggests that the predictive strength of the parameters related to hip strength in this study can be used on the level of a sample with high confidence, while the generalizability to an individual must be done with high caution.

Inter-limb asymmetry values ranged from 0.76% for functional leg length up to 40.35% for RTD during hip flexion (Table 2). Inter-limb asymmetries of hip peak torque were lower (except for internal rotation) than the rate of torque development (3.68–11.52% vs. 10.72–40.35%, $p < 0.05$) (Table 3). Hip extension/flexion (1.32 ± 0.33; 1.30 ± 0.25), abduction/adduction (1.08 ± 0.19; 1.07 ± 0.20) and internal/external rotation (1.13 ± 0.27; 1.18 ± 0.26) ratios were similar ($p > 0.05$) for the left and right side (Table 4). Mean inter-limb asymmetry in peak torque during trunk lateral flexion exceeded the 10% threshold (12.48 ± 9.61 %). Mean inter-limb asymmetry in hip ROM (5.91–13.54%), was above the 10% threshold for extension and internal/external rotations, while the trunk lateral flexion showed good symmetry (2.01 ± 1.27%). Asymmetries in horizontal jumps showed lower results (3.48–4.60%) than various parameters of SLCMJ (4.77–11.12%).

Table 1. Reliability results for outcome measures.

Outcome/Task		Repetition 1		Repetition 2		Systematic Bias		Relative Reliability			Absolute Reliability			
		Mean	SD	Mean	SD	T	P	ICC	95% CI for ICC		TE	CV	95% CI for CV	
Peak torques at the hip (Nm)	Hip Abduction—Left	73.1	18.8	72.9	19.8	0.908	0.365	0.97	0.96	0.98	3.4	4.65	4.59	4.74
	Hip Abduction—Right	71.9	18.6	71.5	19.4	1.384	0.168	0.97	0.96	0.98	3.3	4.54	4.49	4.63
	Hip Adduction—Left	70.4	19.5	71.2	19.7	−1.695	0.092	0.93	0.91	0.95	5.0	7.09	6.90	7.43
	Hip Adduction—Right	69.0	19.1	69.8	19.3	−1.435	0.153	0.93	0.91	0.95	5.0	7.16	6.96	7.50
	Hip Internal rotation—Left	73.1	21.7	72.6	20.7	0.617	0.538	0.92	0.89	0.94	5.9	8.06	7.82	8.51
	Hip Internal rotation—Right	74.8	20.9	74.6	19.9	−0.592	0.555	0.93	0.90	0.95	5.4	7.26	7.06	7.63
	Hip External rotation—Left	62.5	32.2	64.5	16.8	0.172	0.872	0.85	0.80	0.88	10.2	16.06	15.07	17.69
	Hip External rotation—Right	63.8	16.6	63.7	16.3	−0.263	0.793	0.86	0.81	0.90	11.5	17.99	17.01	19.83
	Hip Flexion—Left	139.8	45.9	138.8	39.8	−0.554	0.712	0.94	0.91	0.96	20.6	14.77	14.33	15.53
	Hip Flexion—Right	146.1	42.7	146.8	42.7	−0.114	0.909	0.96	0.94	0.97	18.2	12.41	12.19	12.79
	Hip Extension—Left	163.3	71.5	160.9	55.2	1.195	0.234	0.84	0.78	0.88	27.8	17.13	15.99	19.30
	Hip Extension—Right	169.4	53.0	169.4	50.6	−0.721	0.472	0.91	0.87	0.93	16.6	9.83	9.45	10.51
Peak force at the trunk (N)	Trunk extension	534.5	199.2	560.3	190.7	−3.506	*0.001*	0.88	0.83	0.91	65.3	11.82	9.64	13.32
	Trunk flexion	415.5	144.2	431.0	144.9	−4.106	*0.000*	0.94	0.91	0.96	33.5	7.91	5.42	9.11
	Trunk lat. flexion—Left	395.4	121.2	393.9	125.3	0.114	0.910	0.88	0.84	0.91	51.8	13.1	10.02	15.89
	Trunk lat. flexion—Right	395.3	129.8	405.5	129.8	−2.474	*0.014*	0.92	0.88	0.94	36.8	9.22	7.88	11.76
Hip RTD (Nm/s)	Hip Abduction—Left	268.2	138.9	278.8	145.1	−0.836	0.404	0.50	0.37	0.61	102.6	37.52	27.61	62.50
	Hip Abduction—Right	257.0	132.8	269.2	136.1	−1.266	0.208	0.51	0.38	0.62	94.4	35.89	26.83	58.25
	Hip Adduction—Left	285.9	157.2	299.2	170.8	−1.375	0.171	0.61	0.50	0.71	101.4	34.67	28.16	49.22
	Hip Adduction—Right	276.6	157.7	285.4	163.4	−1.167	0.245	0.62	0.51	0.71	97.1	34.55	28.19	48.71
	Hip Internal rotation—Left	209.1	117.3	219.7	121.8	−1.441	0.152	0.62	0.51	0.71	72.8	33.95	28.03	47.11
	Hip Internal rotation—Right	215.9	119.5	221.0	119.6	−0.784	0.434	0.56	0.43	0.66	79.2	36.24	28.28	54.91
	Hip External rotation—Left	244.5	257.8	229.8	123.7	1.112	0.264	0.72	0.61	0.79	77.7	32.78	27.78	42.33
	Hip External rotation—Right	236.9	129.1	225.3	122.1	1.425	0.156	0.69	0.60	0.76	79.6	34.46	29.86	44.02
	Hip Flexion—Left	418.9	283.9	427.7	289.9	−0.799	0.426	0.58	0.45	0.69	193.5	45.70	35.38	69.83
	Hip Flexion—Right	444.1	290.6	446.4	283.1	0.343	0.732	0.67	0.56	0.76	170.0	38.18	31.90	51.54
	Hip Extension—Left	460.3	321.9	487.9	289.1	−1.421	0.158	0.53	0.40	0.64	207.0	43.67	33.10	69.40
	Hip Extension—Right	534.9	303.3	518.1	313.4	0.271	0.786	0.63	0.51	0.72	191.4	36.34	29.70	51.05

SD—standard deviation; t—T-test statistics; p—statistical significance; CI—confidence interval; TE—typical error; CV—coefficient of variation; RTD—rate of torque development

Table 2. Descriptive and normality analysis of asymmetry variables.

Asymmetry (%)	Mean	SD	S-W
Functional leg length	0.76	0.62	0.002
Single-leg Countermovement Jump— height	11.12	8.36	0.005
Single-leg Countermovement Jump— PF	4.77	4.40	0.000
Single-leg Countermovement Jump—PP	7.06	5.98	0.001
Single-leg Horizontal Jump—distance	4.60	3.19	0.051
Single-leg Lateral Jump—distance	4.82	3.70	0.001
Single-leg Triple Jump—distance	3.48	2.67	0.005
Hip Abduction—PT	3.68	3.15	0.001
Hip Abduction—RTD	11.23	9.67	0.000
Hip Adduction—PT	5.59	4.77	0.001
Hip Adduction—RTD	10.72	10.34	0.000
Hip External Rotation—PT	7.90	5.82	0.000
Hip External Rotation—RTD	13.18	8.83	0.000
Hip Internal Rotation—PT	11.52	7.17	0.150
Hip Internal Rotation—RTD	13.17	9.55	0.020
Hip Extension—PT	11.01	8.92	0.000
Hip Extension—RTD	30.56	21.79	0.031
Hip Flexion—PT	9.86	8.36	0.000
Hip Flexion—RTD	40.35	20.42	0.619
Trunk Lateral Flexion—PT	12.81	9.61	0.013
Trunk Lateral Flexion—ROM	8.98	5.94	0.054
Hip Abduction—ROM	8.94	5.72	0.165
Hip Adduction—ROM	8.83	6.73	0.002
Hip Flexion—ROM	5.91	6.24	0.000
Hip Extension—ROM	12.80	10.95	0.000
Hip External Rotation—ROM	13.00	14.10	0.000
Hip Internal Rotation—ROM	13.54	10.57	0.002
Hip extension/flexion strength ratio (left leg)	1.32	0.33	0.183
Hip extension/flexion strength ratio (right leg)	1.30	0.25	0.011
Hip abduction/adduction strength ratio (left leg)	1.08	0.19	0.048
Hip abduction/adduction strength ratio (right leg)	1.07	0.20	0.010
Hip internal/external rotation strength ratio (left leg)	1.13	0.27	0.266
Hip internal/external rotation ratio (right leg)	1.18	0.26	0.279
Trunk extension/flexion strength ratio	1.27	0.27	0.331
T-test	9.10	0.50	0.013

SD = standard deviation, S-W = Shapiro–Wilks tests, PF = peak force, PP = peak power, RTD = rate of torque development, ROM = range of motion.

Table 3. Peak torque and Rate of torque development differences (Mann–Whitney U test).

Asymmetry (%)	PT Mean ± SD	RTD Mean ± SD	*p*-Value	Effect Size
Hip abduction	3.68 ± 3.15	11.23 ± 9.67	0.000	0.56
Hip adduction	5.59 ± 4.77	10.72 ± 10.34	0.002	0.23
Hip external rotation	7.90 ± 5.82	13.18 ± 8.83	0.001	0.27
Hip internal rotation	11.52 ± 7.17	13.17 ± 9.55	0.514	0.01
Hip extension	11.01 ± 8.92	30.56 ± 21.79	0.000	0.38
Hip flexion	9.86 ± 8.36	40.35 ± 20.42	0.000	1.00

PT = peak torque, RTD = rate of torque development; SD = standard deviation.

Table 4. Hip strength ratio differences between left and right leg (Mann–Whitney U test).

Hip Strength Ratio	Left Leg Mean ± SD	Right Leg Mean ± SD	*p*-Value	Effect Size
Extension/Flexion	1.32 ± 0.33	1.30 ± 0.25	0.779	0.00
Abduction/Adduction	1.08 ± 0.19	1.07 ± 0.20	0.826	0.00
Internal/External Rotation	1.13 ± 0.27	1.18 ± 0.26	0.218	0.03

SD = standard deviation

A six-variable regression model explained 48% ($R^2 = 0.48$; $p < 0.01$) of the variation in the T-test performance (Table 5). T-test time was predicted by left hip internal/external rotation strength ratio ($\beta = -0.58$; $p < 0.01$) and inter-limb asymmetries in hip abduction RTD ($\beta = -0.38$; $p = 0.01$), hip flexion ROM ($\beta = 0.32$; $p = 0.03$), functional leg length ($\beta = 0.31$; $p = 0.02$), SLTJ distance ($\beta = 0.29$; $p = 0.04$), and peak torque during trunk lateral flexion ($\beta = 0.27$; $p = 0.05$).

Table 5. Final regression model with six independent variables (dependent T-test).

Depended Variable	Independent Variable	B	Beta	R^2	*p*-Value
T-test (s)	-	-	-	0.48	<0.001
-	Left hip internal/external rotation strength ratio	−1.08	−0.58	-	0.00
-	Asymmetry in hip abduction RTD (%)	−0.02	−0.38	-	0.01
-	Asymmetry in hip flexion ROM (%)	0.03	0.32	-	0.03
-	Asymmetry in functional leg length (%)	0.25	0.31	-	0.02
-	Asymmetry in SLTJ (%)	0.06	0.29	-	0.04
-	Asymmetry in peak force during trunk lateral flexion (%)	0.01	0.27	-	0.05

RTD—rate of torque development; ROM—range of motion; SLTJ—single-leg triple jump.

4. Discussion

The aims of the present study were twofold: (a) to profile elite basketball players in different local strength and range of motion asymmetries of hip and trunk region, global power asymmetries in horizontal and vertical jumping and (b) to quantify the relationship of these asymmetries with COD performance. Results showed different magnitudes of asymmetries among tests, body regions, and parameters.

Regarding the magnitude of asymmetry scores reported in this study, largest asymmetries were found in hip RTD (10.72–40.35%), which were significantly larger (except internal rotation) than peak force asymmetries of different hip action (3.68–11.52%) (as shown in Table 2). Compared to local peak torque asymmetries, rate of torque development showed to be a more sensitive parameter for assessment of asymmetries. That is in accordance with findings of Sarabon et al. [23], who reported that the RTD showed larger magnitudes of asymmetries than peak torque during unilateral isometric knee flexion and extension.

To our knowledge, only one study profiled hip strength ratios in professional athletes using fixed point dynamometer [31]. Although study was done on Australian football players, it detected similar results in flexion/extension mean ratio (0.8) as our study (1.3). Moreover, their mean internal/external ratio was 1.15 which is in accordance to our values (1.13 and 1.18 for left and right leg).

They observed a hip adductor/abductor ratio of 1.05 which is much different from our abduction/adduction ratios (1.08 and 1.07), such differences can be attributed to sport specificity of ball kicking in Australian football.

Our results are also showing various magnitudes in hip range of motion asymmetries (5.91–13.54%), with largest being found for extension (12.80 ± 10.95%), internal rotation (13.54 ± 10.57%), and external rotation (13.00 ± 14.10%). Although some research indicates that there are significant differences in hip ROM between the dominant and non-dominant leg in football players [32], a direct comparison of results is limited because authors have not reported asymmetry indexes.

Mean asymmetry in functional leg length was 0.76 ± 0.62%. To our knowledge, studies that assessed asymmetries in anthropometry had not used the functional leg length to investigate the relationship with performance instead, they had utilized other anthropometric measurements, such as knee and ankle joint width [33] or lean mass asymmetry [34]. Although, there is no past research to compare our results with, a review of Knutson et al. [35] set a threshold of normal functional leg length discrepancy at 2 cm. The mean absolute asymmetry in our study was 0.9 cm, which is thus considered as normal leg length variation.

Inter-limb asymmetries in vertical jumping parameters (4.77–11.12%) showed larger values compared to horizontal jumps (3.48–4.60%), which is in accordance with research conducted by Lockie et al. [15], who reported SLCMJ mean inter-limb asymmetries at 10.4 % and only 5.4% and 3.3% for horizontal jumps (SLHJ and SLLJ). Similar results were reported by Bishop et al. [36] who found larger inter-limb asymmetries in SLCMJ (12.5%) compared to SLHJ (6.8%). Both of these studies were conducted on football players, which indicates that the variability between the testing methods might be substantially higher than the variability between the athletic populations. With that in mind, it can be suggested that vertical jumping is more sensitive for detecting asymmetries than horizontal jumping.

While all of our maximal strength measures showed an excellent reliability (displayed in Table 1), the explosive strength (rate of torque development) were only moderately reliable. As the structured strength and conditioning training as well as the experience level contribute to reliability of data [37], our data can be interpreted with confidence. In the past years, there has been a lot of debate about defining normal asymmetry threshold, most common one being 10%, but different authors suggested values from 5% to 20% [6]. Taking all that into consideration, variability of asymmetry results in our data shows that asymmetry magnitude is dependent on the specific movement, test and parameter which indicates that a unifying asymmetry threshold cannot be established.

Regression analysis revealed a relationship between asymmetries and performance: six variable model explained 49% of T-test performance variance. Independent variable Beta scores (0.27–0.58) show a small to medium individual relationship between different type of asymmetry and COD performance. Although several studies (including the present study) observed negative influence of asymmetries on COD performance, a number of studies identified contradicting evidence. Lockie et al. [10] showed negative influence ($r = 0.638, 0.669, p < 0.01$) of isokinetic concentric (60°/s, 180°/s, 240°/s) and eccentric (30°/s) knee strength asymmetries and COD performance (assessed with T-test). The study of Coratella et al. [11] reported similar results of association between knee strength asymmetries in slow (30°/s) and fast (300°/s) contractions and COD performance (T-test and 180° turn test). On the other hand, the relationship between COD performance (180° turn test) and strength asymmetries tested with the whole kinetic chain movements (e.g., IMTP) has not been detected [12,13]. This observation could be explained by local strength asymmetries show higher magnitudes. Negative influence of asymmetry in vertical drop jump height and COD performance (180° turn test) ($r = 0.66, p < 0.01$ and $0.52, p < 0.05$; depending on the side of the turn) was found by Bishop et al. [21]. Also, using horizontal jumps to assess asymmetries, Madruga-Parera et al. [38] found much lower correlations ($r = 0.32$ and 0.31, $p < 0.05$) between asymmetry in horizontal jumping length (SLLJ) and COD performance (V-cut and 180° turn test). Such a relationship was not found by Lockie et al. [15], who did not observe significant correlations between asymmetry in vertical (SLCMJ height) and horizontal (SLHJ and SLLJ distance) jumping and COD performance (T-test and 180° turn test). Similarly, Loturco et al. [18] suggested that asymmetry in various parameters during single-leg squat jump and CMJ do not influence COD performance (zig-zag test). The study conducted by Maloney et al. [22] is probably the most comparable to ours, it showed that stiffness and asymmetry in single-leg drop jump explained 63% variance of COD performance (2 × 90°cut test). However, they used just one type of asymmetry as the secondary predictor, while the stiffness during drop jump was main predictor in the model.

Our model consists of several independent variables, each representing a different type of asymmetry and together showing a significant relationship with COD performance. This is important because findings indicated an independent nature of asymmetry [39]. The most important finding of this study is the connection between asymmetry and COD performance, but also that testing large variety of asymmetry types is needed to gain a more complete understanding of athlete asymmetry and its relationship to performance.

Certain limitations of this study should be noted. The main limitation is the modest reliability of hip explosive strength measure, however, we find this acceptable as RTD is a highly variable parameter. Moreover, a slightly larger sample size would have been useful in the linear regression analyses, as the best model included a relatively large number of predictor variables.

5. Conclusions

This study was conducted to explore asymmetries in local strength, vertical jumping and ROM, and to investigate whether these asymmetries are related to COD performance in healthy elite-basketball players. A substantial variability among asymmetries in different tests was noted. This implies that coaches and physiotherapists should not rely exclusively on the <10 % threshold when they are deciding on the athletes return to play, or planning interventions for reducing asymmetries. In particular, it is expected for RTD asymmetries to be larger than maximal strength (i.e., peak torque) asymmetries. In the attempt to elucidate which asymmetries are more relevant for performance, specifically to the COD ability, we performed linear regressions which showed more than one type of asymmetry is should be considered in the analyses to sufficiently explain the COD performance. Notably, the best model for predicting COD performance included both maximal strength and RTD asymmetry, both hip and trunk asymmetry, one vertical jump asymmetry, one ROM asymmetry, as well as asymmetry in functional leg length. Therefore, interventions should likely target multiple types of asymmetries when trying to improve COD performance. We encourage practitioners to use a wide testing battery to test different aspects on local and global level of the body to obtain a clearer picture of athletes' asymmetries.

Author Contributions: Conceptualization, F.U. and N.Š.; Data curation, F.U.; Formal analysis, F.U.; Funding acquisition, N.Š.; Investigation, F.U.; Methodology, N.Š.; Project administration, N.Š.; Resources, N.Š.; Software, N.Š.; Supervision, N.Š.; Validation, F.U. and N.Š.; Writing—original draft, F.U. All authors have read and agreed to the published version of the manuscript.

Acknowledgments: The authors would like to thank the athletes and management from the basketball clubs participating in this study. Additionally, many thanks to the research assistants who helped at testing.

References

1. Bates, N.A.; Ford, K.R.; Myer, G.D.; Hewett, T.E. Impact differences in ground reaction force and center of mass between the first and second landing phases of a drop vertical jump and their implications for injury risk assessment. *J. Biomech.* **2013**, *46*, 1237–1241. [CrossRef]
2. Zwolski, C.; Thomas, S.; Schmitt, L.C.; Hewett, T.E.; Paterno, M.V. The Utility of Limb Symmetry Indices in Return-to-Sport Assessment in Patients With Bilateral Anterior Cruciate Ligament Reconstruction. *Am. J. Sports Med.* **2016**, *44*, 2030–2038. [CrossRef]
3. Mayer, S.W.; Queen, R.; Taylor, D.; Moorman, I.C.T.; Toth, A.P.; Garrett, J.W.E.; Butler, R. Functional Testing Differences in Anterior Cruciate Ligament Reconstruction Patients Released Versus Not Released to Return to Sport. *Am. J. Sports Med.* **2015**, *43*, 1648–1655. [CrossRef]
4. Paterno, M.V.; Ford, K.R.; Myer, G.D.; Heyl, R.; E Hewett, T. Limb Asymmetries in Landing and Jumping 2 Years Following Anterior Cruciate Ligament Reconstruction. *Clin. J. Sport Med.* **2007**, *17*, 258–262. [CrossRef] [PubMed]
5. Bishop, C.; Turner, A.; Read, P. Effects of inter-limb asymmetries on physical and sports performance: A systematic review. *J. Sports Sci.* **2017**, *36*, 1135–10144. [CrossRef] [PubMed]

6. McGrath, T.M.; Waddington, G.; Scarvell, J.M.; Ball, N.; Creer, R.; Woods, K.; Smith, D. The effect of limb dominance on lower limb functional performance – a systematic review. *J. Sports Sci.* **2015**, *34*, 289–302. [CrossRef] [PubMed]
7. Engstrom, C.M.; Walker, D.G.; Kippers, V.; Mehnert, A. Quadratus Lumborum Asymmetry and L4 Pars Injury in Fast Bowlers. *Med. Sci. Sports Exerc.* **2007**, *39*, 910–917. [CrossRef] [PubMed]
8. Bishop, C.; Read, P.; Bromley, T.; Brazier, J.; Jarvis, P.; Chavda, S.; Turner, A. The Association Between Interlimb Asymmetry and Athletic Performance Tasks. *J. Strength Cond. Res.* **2020**. [CrossRef]
9. Bishop, C.; Read, P.; Chavda, S.; Turner, A. Asymmetries of the Lower Limb. *Strength Cond. J.* **2016**, *38*, 27–32. [CrossRef]
10. Lockie, R.G.; Schultz, A.B.; Jeffriess, M.D.; Callaghan, S.J. The relationship between bilateral differences of knee flexor and extensor isokinetic strength and multi-directional speed. *Isokinet. Exerc. Sci.* **2012**, *20*, 211–219. [CrossRef]
11. Coratella, G.; Beato, M.; Schena, F. Correlation between quadriceps and hamstrings inter-limb strength asymmetry with change of direction and sprint in U21 elite soccer-players. *Hum. Mov. Sci.* **2018**, *59*, 81–87. [CrossRef] [PubMed]
12. Chiang, C.-Y. Lower Body Strength and Power Characteristics Influencing Change of Direction and Straight-Line Sprinting Performance in Division I Soccer Players: An Exploratory Study. Ph.D. Thesis, East Tennessee State University, Johnson City, TN USA, July 2014.
13. Dos'Santos, T.; Thomas, C.; Jones, P.A.; Comfort, P. Asymmetries in Isometric Force-Time Characteristics Are Not Detrimental to Change of Direction Speed. *J. Strength Cond. Res.* **2018**, *32*, 520–527. [CrossRef] [PubMed]
14. Hoffman, J.R.; Ratamess, N.A.; Klatt, M.; Faigenbaum, A.D.; Kang, J. Do Bilateral Power Deficits Influence Direction-Specific Movement Patterns? *Sport. Med.* **2007**, *15*(2), 125–132. [CrossRef] [PubMed]
15. Lockie, R.G.; Callaghan, S.J.; Berry, S.P.; Cooke, E.R.A.; Jordan, C.A.; Luczo, T.M.; Jeffriess, M.D. Relationship Between Unilateral Jumping Ability and Asymmetry on Multidirectional Speed in Team-Sport Athletes. *J. Strength Cond. Res.* **2014**, *28*, 3557–3566. [CrossRef] [PubMed]
16. Dos'Santos, T.; Thomas, C.; Jones, P.A.; Comfort, P. Asymmetries in single and triple hop are not detrimental to change of direction speed. *J. Trainology* **2017**, *6*, 35–41. [CrossRef]
17. Fort-Vanmeerhaeghe, A.; Montalvo, A.; Sitjà-Rabert, M.; Kiefer, A.W.; Myer, G.D.; Fort-Vanmeerhaeghe, A. Neuromuscular asymmetries in the lower limbs of elite female youth basketball players and the application of the skillful limb model of comparison. *Phys. Ther. Sport* **2015**, *16*, 317–323. [CrossRef]
18. Loturco, I.; Pereira, L.A.; Kobal, R.; Abad, C.C.C.; Rosseti, M.; Carpes, F.P.; Bishop, C. Do Asymmetry Scores Influence Speed and Power Performance in Elite Female Soccer Players? *Biol. Sport* **2019**, *36*, 209–216. [CrossRef]
19. Sheppard, J.M.; Young, W.B. Agility literature review: Classifications, training and testing. *J. Sports Sci.* **2006**, *24*, 919–932. [CrossRef]
20. Fort-Vanmeerhaeghe, A.; Bishop, C.; Buscà, B.; Aguilera-Castells, J.; Vicens-Bordas, J.; Gonzalo-Skok, O. Inter-limb asymmetries are associated with decrements in physical performance in youth elite team sports athletes. *PLoS ONE* **2020**, *15*, e0229440. [CrossRef]
21. Bishop, C.; Turner, A.; Maloney, S.J.; Lake, J.P.; LoTurco, I.; Bromley, T.; Read, P. Drop Jump Asymmetry is Associated with Reduced Sprint and Change-of-Direction Speed Performance in Adult Female Soccer Players. *Sports* **2019**, *7*, 29. [CrossRef]
22. Maloney, S.J.; Richards, J.; Nixon, D.G.D.; Harvey, L.J.; Fletcher, I.M. Do stiffness and asymmetries predict change of direction performance? *Sports Sci.* **2017**, *35*, 547–556. [CrossRef] [PubMed]
23. Sarabon, N.; Kozinc, Z.; Bishop, C.; Maffiuletti, N.A. Factors influencing bilateral deficit and inter-limb asymmetry of maximal and explosive strength: Motor task, outcome measure and muscle group. *Graefe's Arch. Clin. Exp. Ophthalmol.* **2020**, *120*, 1681–1688. [CrossRef] [PubMed]
24. Ben Abdelkrim, N.; Castagna, C.; Jabri, I.; Battikh, T.; El Fazaa, S.; El Ati, J. Activity Profile and Physiological Requirements of Junior Elite Basketball Players in Relation to Aerobic-Anaerobic Fitness. *J. Strength Cond. Res.* **2010**, *24*, 2330–2342. [CrossRef] [PubMed]
25. Beck, T.W. The Importance of A Priori Sample Size Estimation in Strength and Conditioning Research. *J. Strength Cond. Res.* **2013**, *27*, 2323–2337. [CrossRef] [PubMed]

26. Markovic, G.; Šarabon, N.; Greblo, Z.; Križanić, V. Effects of feedback-based balance and core resistance training vs. Pilates training on balance and muscle function in older women: A randomized-controlled trial. *Arch. Gerontol. Geriatr.* **2015**, *61*, 117–123. [CrossRef]
27. Markovic, G.; Šarabon, N.; Pausic, J.; Hadžić, V. Adductor Muscles Strength and Strength Asymmetry as Risk Factors for Groin Injuries among Professional Soccer Players: A Prospective Study. *Int. J. Environ. Res. Public Health* **2020**, *17*, 4946. [CrossRef]
28. Semenick, D. The T-Test. *NSCA J.* **1990**, *12*, 36–37.
29. Koo, T.K.; Li, M.Y. A Guideline of Selecting and Reporting Intraclass Correlation Coefficients for Reliability Research. *J. Chiropr. Med.* **2016**, *15*, 155–163. [CrossRef]
30. Bishop, C.; Read, P.; Lake, J.P.; Chavda, S.; Turner, A. Inter-Limb Asymmetries. *Strength Cond. J.* **2018**, *40*, 1. [CrossRef]
31. Althorpe, T.; Beales, D.; Skinner, A.; Caputi, N.; Mullings, G.; Stockden, M.; Boyle, J. Isometric hip strength and strength ratios in elite adolescent and senior Australian Rules Football players: An initial exploration using fixed-point dynamometry. *J. Sci. Med. Sport* **2018**, *21*, S81. [CrossRef]
32. Oliveira, A.; Barbieri, F.A.; Goncalves, M. Flexibility, torque and kick performance in soccer: Effect of dominance. *Sci. Sports* **2013**, *28*, e67–e70. [CrossRef]
33. Trivers, R.; Palestis, B.G.; Manning, J.T. The Symmetry of Children's Knees Is Linked to Their Adult Sprinting Speed and Their Willingness to Sprint in a Long-Term Jamaican Study. *PLoS ONE* **2013**, *8*, e72244. [CrossRef] [PubMed]
34. Bell, D.R.; Sanfilippo, J.L.; Binkley, N.; Heiderscheit, B.C. Lean Mass Asymmetry Influences Force and Power Asymmetry During Jumping in Collegiate Athletes. *J. Strength Cond. Res.* **2014**, *28*, 884–891. [CrossRef] [PubMed]
35. Knutson, G.A. Anatomic and functional leg-length inequality: A review and recommendation for clinical decision-making. Part I, anatomic leg-length inequality: Prevalence, magnitude, effects and clinical significance. *Chiropr. Osteopat.* **2005**, *13*, 11. [CrossRef]
36. Bishop, C.; Read, P.; McCubbine, J.; Turner, A. Vertical and Horizontal Asymmetries are Related to Slower Sprinting and Jump Performance in Elite Youth Female Soccer Players. *J. Strength Cond. Res.* **2018**. Available online: http://eprints.mdx.ac.uk/23569/ (accessed on 23 September 2020). [CrossRef]
37. Bishop, C.; Berney, J.; Lake, J.; LoTurco, I.; Blagrove, R.; Turner, A.; Read, P. Bilateral Deficit During Jumping Tasks. *J. Strength Cond. Res.* **2019**. Available online: http://eprints.chi.ac.uk/id/eprint/4183/ (accessed on 23 September 2020). [CrossRef]
38. Madruga-Parera, M.; Bishop, C.; Read, P.; Lake, J.; Brazier, J.; Romero-Rodriguez, D. Jumping-based Asymmetries are Negatively Associated with Jump, Change of Direction, and Repeated Sprint Performance, but not Linear Speed, in Adolescent Handball Athletes. *J. Hum. Kinet.* **2020**, *71*, 47–58. [CrossRef]
39. Raya-González, J.; Bishop, C.; Gómez-Piqueras, P.; Veiga, S.; Viejo-Romero, D.; Navandar, A. Strength, Jumping, and Change of Direction Speed Asymmetries Are Not Associated With Athletic Performance in Elite Academy Soccer Players. *Front. Psychol.* **2020**, *11*, 1. [CrossRef]

3

Influence of Equimolar Doses of Beetroot Juice and Sodium Nitrate on Time Trial Performance in Handcycling

Joelle Leonie Flueck [1,*], Alessandro Gallo [2], Nynke Moelijker [3], Nikolay Bogdanov [3], Anna Bogdanova [3] and Claudio Perret [1]

1 Institute of Sports Medicine, Swiss Paraplegic Centre Nottwil, CH-6207 Nottwil, Switzerland
2 Department of Health and Technology, ETH Zurich (Swiss Federal Institute of Technology Zurich), CH-8003 Zurich, Switzerland
3 Institute of Veterinary Physiology, Vetsuisse Faculty and the Zurich Center for Integrative Human Physiology (ZIHP), University of Zurich, CH-8057 Zurich, Switzerland
* Correspondence: joelle.flueck@paraplegie.ch

Abstract: This study aimed to investigate the influence of a single dose of either beetroot juice (BR) or sodium nitrate (NIT) on performance in a 10 km handcycling time trial (TT) in able-bodied individuals and paracyclists. In total, 14 able-bodied individuals [mean ± SD; age: 28 ± 7 years, height: 183 ± 5 cm, body mass (BM): 82 ± 9 kg, peak oxygen consumption (VO_{2peak}): 33.9 ± 4.2 mL/min/kg] and eight paracyclists (age: 40 ± 11 years, height: 176 ± 9cm, BM: 65 ± 9 kg, VO_{2peak}: 38.6 ± 10.5 mL/min/kg) participated in the study. All participants had to perform three TT on different days, receiving either 6 mmol nitrate as BR or NIT or water as a placebo. Time-to-complete the TT, power output (PO), as well as oxygen uptake (VO_2) were measured. No significant differences in time-to-complete the TT were found between the three interventions in able-bodied individuals ($p = 0.80$) or in paracyclists ($p = 0.61$). Furthermore, VO_2 was not significantly changed after the ingestion of BR or NIT in either group ($p < 0.05$). The PO to VO_2 ratio was significantly higher in some kilometers of the TT in able-bodied individuals ($p < 0.05$). The ingestion of BR or NIT did not increase handcycling performance in able-bodied individuals or in paracyclists.

Keywords: Paralympic; sports nutrition; supplementation

---

1. Introduction

Sports nutrition and performance enhancing supplements are prominently discussed topics in today's sports science. Currently, dietary nitrate is one of the latest trends in sports nutrition [1]. The main sources of dietary nitrate are green leafy and root vegetables, including beetroot, spinach, and rocket [2]. After ingestion, nitrate (NO_3^-) is reduced to nitrite (NO_2^-) and then to nitric oxide (NO), leading to a temporary increase in plasma and muscle NO [3]. Production of NO from nitrate and nitrite is enhanced under hypoxic and acidic conditions [4]. The role of NO as a signaling molecule is that it interacts with multiple targets (e.g., heme and thiol groups of proteins), triggering numerous downstream events, among which stimulation of protein kinase G and control over mitochondrial function are just a few [5]. At the organism level, NO controls heart and muscle function [6,7], vascular tone [7,8], O_2 transport by red blood cells, and other processes important for sports performance [4]. It has been proven that dietary nitrate supplementation reduces blood pressure in healthy individuals as well as in patients suffering from hypertension, diabetes, or ischemia [9–11]. Besides its beneficial therapeutic application, dietary nitrate supplementation, either as nitrate-rich beetroot juice (BR) or as sodium nitrate (NIT), has become a popular sport supplement based on its ergogenic effects (for review, see [12–14]).

Several studies have investigated the use of dietary nitrate for athletes in different disciplines, predominantly focusing on lower-body or whole-body exercises, including cycling [15,16] and running [17,18]. It has been demonstrated that dietary nitrate supplementation can improve both exercise capacity (e.g., time-to-exhaustion) [19,20] as well as exercise performance (e.g., time-to-completion) [16,21]. In addition, nitrate supplementation has been shown to reduce the oxygen cost (VO_2) of exercise [19,22]. It is assumed that these observed effects of nitrate supplementation are a consequence of an improved mitochondrial efficiency (reduced oxygen cost of ATP production) [23] and/or due to enhanced muscle contractile functions [24,25]. Complementary nitrate supplementation might promote vasorelaxation and elevate skeletal muscle oxygen delivery during exercise, as shown in rodents [26]. However, it seems unclear whether vasodilatation might improve performance [27,28]. Noteworthy targeted effects of nitrate supplementation on fast-twitch muscle fibers have been demonstrated previously [29,30].

Fat-twitch muscle fibers are more abundant in the upper body compared to the lower body muscles [31,32], and they exhibit different cardiovascular regulation mechanisms during exercise [33]. Furthermore, previous investigations reported that the cardiovascular strain in arm cranking was much higher compared to leg pedaling [34], and that arm cranking relies more on glycolytic metabolism [35]. All these physiological features of the upper body suggest that it should be sensitive to nitrate supplementation. However, the effects of dietary nitrate on upper body exercise performance have never been investigated in detail.

To date, only few studies have examined the effect of dietary nitrate supplementation on upper body exercise performance such as kayaking [36,37] or rowing [38,39]. These studies reported inconsistent results. Some investigations reported that BR supplementation improved repeated sprint and 2 km rowing performance in well trained athletes [38,39]. Furthermore, Peeling et al. [37] demonstrated that 500 m kayaking performance was significantly improved after the intake of BR. On the other hand, Muggeridge et al. [36] could not observe any ergogenic effects of BR supplementation on repeated sprint or 1 km time trial (TT) performance in trained kayakers.

To our knowledge, the effects of dietary nitrate supplementation on handcycling performance were never examined. Therefore, we aimed to investigate whether a single dose of 6 mmol nitrate as BR or NIT supplement improved 10 km handcycling TT performance in recreationally active individuals compared to paracycling athletes. Furthermore, we aimed to assess the effects of dietary nitrate supplementation on VO_2 during the TT. We hypothesized that, compared to placebo (PLA), a single intake of dietary nitrate would either (1) improve 10 km TT performance with similar VO_2 or (2) reduce VO_2 (whereas TT performance would remain unchanged).

2. Materials and Methods

2.1. Participants

Upper body trained able-bodied individuals as well as paracyclists with a spinal cord injury were recruited for this study. Athletes with a minimal training duration of 3 h per week and 3 sessions per week were admitted into the study. All participants were non-smokers. Participants using medication that might influence performance were excluded from the study. Furthermore, participants with nitrate hypersensitivity, diabetes, cardiovascular disease, pulmonary disease, or any other disease were not allowed to participate. Participants were aware of the study aim and the effects of nitrate. Before the start of the study, all participants provided written informed consent. The study was approved by the local ethical committee (EC-No. 2015-209, SNCTP-No. NCT02454049, Ethikkomission Nordwest- und Zentralschweiz, EKNZ, Basel, Switzerland) and met all ethical standards of the institutional and national research committee and the 1964 Helsinki Declaration [40].

2.2. Study Design

A randomized, placebo-controlled, single-blind, and cross-over study was performed at the Institute of Sports Medicine Nottwil, Switzerland. Each participant visited the exercise lab on five separate occasions. On the first visit, medical history was checked to fulfill all inclusion criteria, and participants were asked to carefully read and sign the written informed consent. On the second visit, a screening questionnaire was completed, and a subsequent incremental exercise test was performed to determine peak oxygen consumption (VO_{2peak}) and maximal power output (PO_{max}). Shortly after, a familiarization TT was performed. On the following three occasions, the participants performed a 10 km handcycling TT after the ingestion of BR, NIT, or PLA. Diet, sleep, training load, and acute sickness were recorded by a questionnaire before each trial to ensure equal testing conditions. All experimental trials were conducted within a maximum of six weeks, and TTs were at minimum 48 h apart for recovery purposes.

For the three experimental trials, participants arrived at the laboratory at approximately the same time of day (± 2 h). After a 5 min resting period and the completion of the questionnaire, resting blood pressure and heart rate were measured in triplets in a sitting position at the wrist using an automated cuff (Boso medistars, Bosch + Sohn GmbH, Jungingen, Germany). The forearm was placed at heart level. Subsequently, participants received a non-transparent flask containing the supplement, which they ingested immediately. Afterwards, a 3 h resting period followed, where participants could leave the laboratory but were asked to refrain from any strenuous physical activity. During this time, participants were allowed to drink water ad libitum but were not allowed to eat. Following the 3 h resting period, blood pressure and heart rate were measured again. Thereafter, participants started with the 10 km TT.

2.3. Physical Activity and Dietary Standardization

Participants were asked to maintain their regular training schedule as consistent as possible over the time course of the study and were instructed to avoid high-intensity training the last two days before each experimental trial. They were allowed to maintain their habitual diet but were requested to abstain from nitrate-enriched foods (e.g., beetroot, spinach, rocket, lettuce, etc.) the last two days before each test. Furthermore, participants were requested to abstain from caffeine and alcohol the last 12 h before each test and were advised to eat a standardized meal 1 h before the arrival at the laboratory. They were instructed to maintain their sleep constant at a minimum of 7 h. To prevent any modification in the degradation process of nitrate by commensal bacteria in the oral cavity, participants were instructed to abstain from anti-bacterial mouthwash on all testing days [41].

2.4. Supplementation

Supplements were ingested in a fluid form. The supplements were either BR (6 mmol nitrate), water with sodium nitrate (NIT) (6 mmol nitrate), or plain water (PLA). The BR was a special production by an external company and was delivered in the form of a standardized shot (Biotta AG, Tägerwilen, Switzerland). For the preparation of the 6 mmol NIT supplements, the amount of 510 mg of sodium nitrate (Pure sodium nitrate, POCH S.A., supplier: Pharmaserv LTD, Stansstad, Switzerland) was weighted and dissolved in 85 mL of plain water. All supplements were bottled in 85 mL non-transparent flasks. Shortly after each exercise test, participants were asked about the supplement they received. Optically, they could not distinguish between NIT and PLA but could set PLA/NIT apart from BR because of taste and color. Only 60% of the athletes chose the right supplement after the NIT and PLA test. All athletes were able to distinguish BR apart from the other supplements.

2.5. Exercise Testing

2.5.1. Maximal Oxygen Uptake and Familiarization

Participants performed an incremental exercise ramp test on the handcycle ergometer Cyclus 2 (Avantronic, Leipzig, Germany) to detect VO_{2peak} and PO_{max}. After a baseline measurement of 1 min at rest, a standardized warm-up of 2 min cycling at 20 W was performed. Subsequently, the test started at 20 W. The workload increased continuously by 10 W per minute. Participants cycled until exhaustion and were verbally encouraged. Participants cycled at a self-selected pedal rate (60–100 rpm) and were instructed to keep this frequency constant during the test. Pedal rates < 50 rpm were regarded as test termination. During the test, heart rate was monitored (S610i, Polar Electro Oy, Kempele, Finland). These data were analyzed with the Polar Pro Trainer 5 software (Polar Electro Oy, Kempele, Finland). The breath-by-breath pulmonary gas exchange data were continuously measured during the test and averaged over 15 s periods (Oxycon Pro, Jaeger GmbH, Würzburg, Germany). VO_{2peak} was determined as the highest 15 s VO_2 value during the test. Ergometer configurations were recorded and maintained equally for all following exercise tests. After a 20 to 30 min break, participants performed a 10 km familiarization TT identical to the following experimental TT.

2.5.2. Time Trial

Three hours after the ingestion of the supplement, participants performed a simulated 10 km TT (0.5% incline) on the Cyclus 2 with a provided handbike (able-bodied individuals) or with their own handbike (paracyclists). All TTs were performed with the same fixed gearing. Participants performed a 5 min warm-up at self-selected pedal rate and with the fixed gearing. After a 1 min measurement at rest for baseline parameters, the 10 km TT began. After the warm-up and at the end of the TT, a capillary blood sample was taken from the earlobe and analyzed for blood lactate concentrations ([Lac]) using an enzymatic amperometric chip sensor system (Biosen C-Line Clinic, EKF diagnostic GmbH, Cardiff, UK), and rating of perceived exertion (RPE) was recorded using a Borg scale ranging from 6–20 [42]. During the test, a computer screen was placed in front of participants, which displayed the distance they had already cycled. No information was given about completion time, and participants received no feedback on performance during or after the TT. Furthermore, no verbal encouragement was provided during the TT. Heart rate was monitored during the warm-up and the TT. Respiratory gas exchange parameters were measured continuously during the TT using the above mentioned metabolic cart. Shortly before each measurement, the metabolic cart was calibrated by automatic volume calibration and by gas calibration using a standardized gas containing 16% O_2 and 5% CO_2 (Pangas, Dagmarsellen, Switzerland).

2.6. Plasma Nitrate and Nitrite Measurements

Venous blood samples were drawn into lithium-heparin tubes (2.7 mL Monovette Lithium Heparin; Sarstedt, Sevelen, Switzerland). All samples were immediately centrifuged at 3000 $r \cdot min^{-1}$ (1549 g) and 4 °C for 10 min within 1 min of collection. Blood plasma was harvested and stored at −80 °C in 1.5 mL tubes (Eppendorf, Wesseling–Berzdorf, Germany). Plasma nitrate ($[NO_3^-]$) and nitrite ($[NO_2^-]$) concentrations were assessed by chemiluminescence NO analyzer (CLD 88 sp NO Analyzer, ECO Medics AG, Duernten, Switzerland). $[NO_2^-]$ was reduced to NO in Brown's solution (0.57 g 99.99% iodine; 1.62 g KI, 15 mL bi-distilled water, 200 mL acetic acid), and subsequent photons produced as NO interacted with O_3 were detected. Detection of $[NO_3^-]$ included one more step in which $[NO_3^-]$ was quantitatively reduced to $[NO_2^-]$ using World Precisions Instrument's Nitralyzer kit (World Precision Instruments, Sarasota, FL, USA). Reduction of $[NO_3^-]$ to $[NO_2^-]$ was performed on copper-coated cadmium beads. Thereafter, total NO metabolites level (NO_x) = ($[NO_2^-]$ + $[NO_3^-]$) was measured, and $[NO_3^-]$ concentrations were calculated as a difference between $[NO_2^-]$ levels before and after the reduction step. Calibration solutions of sodium nitrite ($NaNO_2^-$) (50, 100, 150, and 200 $nmol \cdot L^{-1}$) and sodium nitrate ($NaNO_3^-$) (20, 40, 60, 80, and 100 μmol·L^{-1}) were prepared in bi-distilled water to produce calibration plots.

2.7. Data Analysis and Statistics

The statistical analysis was performed using the IBM SPSS Statistics software for Windows (Version 24, IBM Corp., Armonk, NY, USA). Statistical significance was set at an α-level of 0.05. The analysis with the Q-Q plot and the Shapiro-Wilk test showed that data for the able-bodied individuals were normally distributed, and data from paracycling athletes were not normally distributed. The data were presented as mean ± standard deviation (SD). The data of the able-bodied participants were analyzed using parametric testing. To analyze changes in blood pressure and heart rate from pre- to post-ingestion between NIT, BR, and PLA, a one-way repeated-measures ANOVA was performed. Differences in completion time, mean PO, mean VO_2, mean PO/VO_2 ratio, and other cardiorespiratory parameters were assessed using a one-way repeated-measures ANOVA. Pairwise t-tests were used for post hoc analysis, and Bonferroni corrections were applied for multiple testing. The PO and PO/VO_2 ratio data were graphed for the 10 km distance and analyzed using a two-way (supplement x distance) repeated-measures ANOVA with Bonferroni correction. In case of violation of sphericity, Greenhouse–Geisser correction was applied. The effect of order on TT performance was analyzed using a one-way repeated-measures ANOVA and pairwise t-tests with Bonferroni correction.

The data from paracyclists were analyzed using non-parametric testing. The Friedman test was applied to detect differences between the three groups for all parameters. If significant differences occurred, the Wilcoxon post-hoc test was applied with Bonferroni correction. For comparison between able-bodied individuals and paracyclists, the Mann-Whitney-U test was used to detect any differences.

3. Results

Fourteen healthy, recreationally active men [mean ± SD; age: 28 ± 7 years, height: 183 ± 5 cm, body mass (BM): 82 ± 9 kg, VO_{2peak}: 33.9 ± 4.2 mL/min/kg, PO_{max}: 152 ± 20 W] who were used to upper body exercises volunteered to participate in this study. They trained 4 ± 2 times per week with a total weekly duration of 6 ± 3 h. Additionally, eight paracyclists from the national team (data presented in Table 1) participated in this study. They trained 11 ± 4 h and 7 ± 2 times per week.

Table 1. Characteristics of the eight paracyclists.

ID	Age [year]	Height [cm]	Body Mass [kg]	VO_{2peak} [ml/min/kg]	PO_{max} [W]	Lesion Level	Category
1	42	188	66	41.5	200	Th5	MH3
2	34	169	72	29.7	144	L4	MH4
3	29	170	47	42.8	151	C4	MH2
4	54	178	75	49.7	222	Th12	MH5
5	32	173	60	36.9	180	Th3	MH3
6	61	178	61	45.9	208	Th4	MH3
7	40	165	64	44.8	220	Th10	MH4
8	35	190	76	17.3	98	C6	MH1
	40 ± 11	176 ± 9	65 ± 9	38.6 ± 10.5	178 ± 44		

Note: Data presented as mean ± standard deviation, PO_{max} = maximal power output in the ramp test, VO_{2peak} = peak oxygen uptake measured during the ramp test.

3.1. Blood Pressure and Heart Rate at Rest

No significant differences ($p > 0.05$) in systolic and diastolic blood pressure pre and post ingestion of the supplements between the interventions were found in able-bodied participants or paracyclists. Neither in able-bodied individuals nor in paracyclists did the change in blood pressure from pre to post ingestion significantly differ ($p > 0.05$) in all three interventions. No significant difference in systolic and diastolic blood pressure was found between able-bodied individuals and paracyclists ($p >$

0.05). No significant differences between the three interventions in able-bodied individuals and in paracyclists were observed for the change of heart rate from pre to post ingestion of the supplement ($p < 0.05$). No significant difference between able-bodied individuals and paracyclists was found ($p < 0.05$). Data are presented in Table 2.

Table 2. Blood pressure and heart rate before and after ingestion of the supplements.

	Able-Bodied Individuals			Paracyclists		
	PLA	NIT	BR	PLA	NIT	BR
Systolic BP [mmHg]						
Pre	124 ± 9	125 ± 9	124 ± 10	129 ± 16	130 ± 19	128 ± 17
Post	125 ± 9	125 ± 13	125 ± 10	134 ± 14	131 ± 18	135 ± 17
Diastolic BP [mmHg]						
Pre	77 ± 7	78 ± 10	79 ± 9	79 ± 15	78 ± 18	79 ± 15
Post	80 ± 8	80 ± 9	82 ± 9	84 ± 13	83 ± 16	84 ± 14
HR [bpm]						
Pre	61 ± 6	62 ± 6	61 ±7	70 ± 17	70 ± 14	67 ± 17
Post	56 ± 7	55 ± 7	55 ± 9	61 ± 10	62 ± 10	59 ± 12

Note: data presented as mean ± SD, HR = heart rate, BP = blood pressure, PLA = placebo, NIT = sodium nitrate, BR = beetroot juice, bpm = beats per minute.

3.2. *Plasma Nitrate and Nitrite Concentrations Pre and Post Supplement Ingestion*

Plasma [NO_2^-] and [NO_3^-] concentrations before and after the ingestion of NIT, BR, or PLA are illustrated in Table 3. No significant difference was found in plasma [NO_2^-] and [NO_3^-] pre supplement ingestion in able-bodied individuals ($p = 0.99$) or in paracyclists ($p = 0.19$). A significantly higher [NO_2^-] and [NO_3^-] concentration was found in able-bodied individuals (NO_2^-: $p = 0.011$; NO_3^-: $p = 0.001$) and in paracyclists (NO_2^-: $p = 0.002$; NO_3^-: $p = 0.001$) in the BR intervention compared to PLA. No significant difference was found post ingestion between plasma [NO_3^-] and [NO_2^-] concentration in BR and NIT in either group ($p > 0.05$). Able-bodied individuals showed significantly higher [NO_2^-] concentrations after BR consumption compared to paracyclists ($p < 0.05$). Paracyclists showed significantly higher [NO_3^-] concentrations after BR and NIT consumption compared to able-bodied individuals ($p < 0.05$).

Table 3. Plasma [NO_3^-] and [NO_2^-] in able-bodied individuals and paracycling pre and post ingestion of BR, NIT, and PLA.

		Able-Bodied Individuals		Paracyclists	
		Pre	Post	Pre	Post
Plasma [NO_3^-] in uM	PLA	68.5 ± 8.4	67.9 ± 8.6	37.9 ± 18.8	38.1 ±18.9
	NIT	64.8 ±10.9	278.7 ± 154.9 *†	36.8 ± 19.9	85.9 ± 73.2 *†
	BR	63.5 ± 8.9	273.7 ± 82.8 *†	38.8 ± 17.9	125.8 ± 99.3 *†
Plasma [NO_2^-] in nM	PLA	44.7 ± 21.5	41.2 ± 28.7	66.9 ± 27.9	92.3 ± 109.9
	NIT	56.7 ± 22.6	141.2 ± 75.7 *†	57.7 ± 11.6	136.7 ± 69.6 *†
	BR	61.5 ± 53.8	121.2 ± 57.3 *†	108.7 ± 134.3 †	263.3 ± 159.2 *†

Note: PLA = placebo, NIT = sodium nitrate, BR = beetroot juice, * significant difference ($p < 0.05$) compared to pre ingestion, † = significant difference ($p < 0.05$) to PLA, pre = before ingestion of the supplement, post = 3 h after ingestion of the supplement.

3.3. *Performance Parameters during Warm-up and TT*

The warm-up parameters were not significantly different in the three intervention groups in paracyclists or in able-bodied individuals ($p < 0.05$). [Lac] in the warm-up was significantly lower in paracyclists compared to able-bodied individuals ($p = 0.029$). Maximal and average heart rate (HR) as well as PO during the warm-up were all significantly different between the two groups of participants ($p < 0.05$). Data are presented in Table 4.

Table 4. Warm-up data for the two groups.

	Able-Bodied Individuals			Paracyclists		
	PLA	**NIT**	**BR**	**PLA**	**NIT**	**BR**
$PO_{average}$ [W]	55 ± 19	58 ± 16	55 ± 18	90 ± 31 *	95 ± 31 *	88 ± 29 *
$HR_{average}$ [bpm]	93 ± 19	95 ± 15	94 ± 16	119 ± 20 *	115 ± 18 *	111 ± 19 *
HR_{max} [bpm]	105 ± 21	107 ± 15	107 ± 16	140 ± 25 *	137 ± 23 *	137 ± 26 *
RPE [6; 20]	11 [7; 13]	11 [7; 12]	11 [7; 13]	12 [8; 14]	11 [7; 12]	12 [8; 13]
[Lac] [mmol/L]	2.57 ± 1.43	2.67 ± 1.34	2.68 ± 1.13	1.89 ± 0.86 *	1.74 ± 0.77 *	1.87 ± 0.73 *

Note: Data presented as mean ± standard deviation and mean [min; max] for RPE, PLA = placebo, NIT = sodium nitrate, BR = beetroot juice, [Lac] = plasma lactate concentration after the time trial, RPE = rated perceived exertion, HR = heart rate, PO = power output, * = significant difference ($p < 0.05$) compared to able-bodied individuals.

No significant difference in time to complete the 10 km handcycling TT (Table 5) was found between the three interventions in able-bodied individuals ($p = 0.61$). Furthermore, no significantly different time to complete the TT in paracyclists was found ($p = 0.80$). Paracyclists completed the 10 km TT significantly faster in all three trials compared to able-bodied individuals ($p < 0.05$) and therefore showed a significantly higher $PO_{average}$ compared to able-bodied individuals ($p < 0.05$).

Table 5. Data from the 10 km time trail (TT) performance in both groups of participants.

	Able-Bodied Individuals			Paracyclists		
	PLA	**NIT**	**BR**	**PLA**	**NIT**	**BR**
Time to complete [s]	1182 ± 84	1194 ± 102	1195 ± 94	1106 ± 247 *	1091 ± 235 *	1071 ± 199 *
$PO_{average}$ [W]	114 ± 16	113 ± 20	112 ± 17	142 ± 49	144 ± 44	145 ± 42
$HR_{average}$ [bpm]	152 ± 13	153 ± 9	150 ± 11	162 ± 27 *	158± 30 *	158 ± 31 *
HR_{max} [bpm]	174 ± 10	175± 8	175 ± 9	176 ± 24	170 ± 31	173 ± 28
RPE [6; 20]	18 [16; 20]	19 [17; 20]	18.5 [17; 20]	19 [17; 20]	19 [17; 20]	19 [17; 20]
[Lac] [mmol/L]	11.94 ± 2.40	12.28 ± 2.84	11.66 ± 2.15	10.13 ± 5.98	10.05 ± 6.37	9.92 ± 5.99

Note: Data presented as mean ± standard deviation and mean [min; max] for RPE, RPE = rated perceived exertion, $HR_{average}$ = average heart rate during the test, HR_{max} = maximal heart rate during the test, $PO_{average}$ = average power output during the test, [Lac] = lactate concentration after the test, NIT = sodium nitrate, BR = beetroot juice, PLA = placebo, * = significant ($p < 0.05$) difference between the two groups of participants.

Neither [Lac] ($p = 0.31$) after the time trial nor rated perceived exertion (RPE) ($p = 0.41$) for the trials were significantly different between the three interventions in able-bodied individuals. The same was true in paracyclists between the three interventions (RPE: $p = 0.43$; [Lac]: $p = 0.68$). No significant differences were found in RPE ($p = 0.08$) and [Lac] ($p = 0.86$) concentration between able-bodied individuals and paracyclists. No significant differences between the three interventions were found in $HF_{average}$ in able-bodied individuals ($p = 0.25$) or in paracyclists ($p = 0.69$) during the TT, and there was no difference between the two groups of participants ($p = 0.11$). Data are presented in Table 5.

Out of all 22 participants, only one suffered from gastrointestinal side effects. The participant reported nausea. No significant order effect was found comparing time to complete the first, the second, and the third TT regardless of the supplement in able-bodied individuals ($p = 0.07$) and in paracyclists ($p = 0.14$). $PO_{average}$ was significantly greater in the third TT compared to the second in able-bodied individuals ($p = 0.039$, mean difference + 4.4 W, 95%-CI [0.2; 8.85]) but not in paracycling athletes ($p = 0.11$).

3.4. Oxygen Uptake and PO to VO_2 Ratio

No significant difference was found in $VO_{2average}$ between the three interventions in able-bodied individuals ($p = 0.15$) or in paracyclists ($p = 0.07$). $VO_{2average}$ was found to be significantly higher in paracyclists ($VO_{2average}$: NIT = 35.4 ± 9.5 min/kg, BR = 34.7 ± 10.3 mL/min/kg, PLA = 35.2 ± 9.9 mL/min/kg) compared to able-bodied ($VO_{2average}$: NIT = 29.0 ± 4.2 mL/min/kg,

BR = 27.8 ± 4.6 mL/min/kg, PLA = 29.3 ± 4.4 mL/min/kg) individuals ($p = 0.042$). Furthermore, no significant difference was found in PO to VO_2 ratio between the three interventions in able-bodied individuals ($p = 0.62$) or in paracyclists ($p = 0.88$). PO to VO_2 ratio was significantly different in some kilometers over the course of the TT in able-bodied individuals ($p < 0.05$). No significant differences in the same parameter were found in the paracyclists ($p > 0.05$) during the TT (Figure 1).

(a)

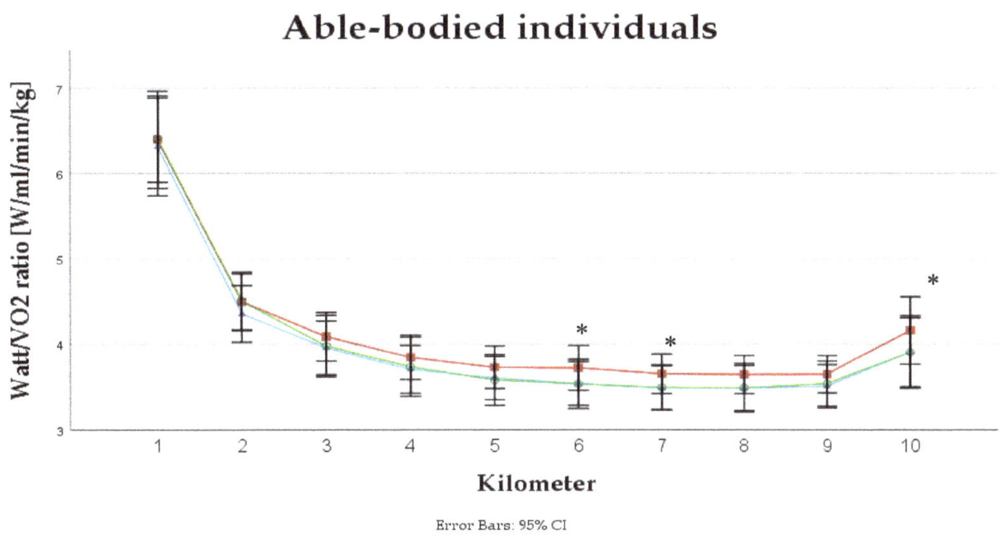

(b)

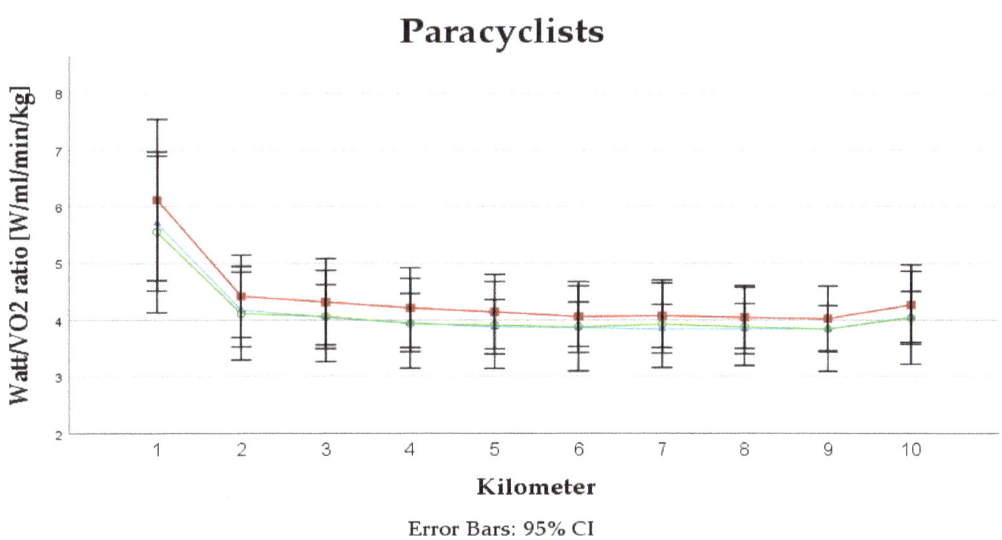

Figure 1. PO to VO_2 ratio in (**a**) able-bodied individuals and (**b**) in paracyclists during a 10 km handcycling TT. Note: * = significant difference ($p < 0.05$), red squares (■) = beetroot juice intervention, blue triangles (▲) = sodium nitrate intervention and green circles (○) = placebo intervention.

4. Discussion

To our knowledge, this is the first study examining the effects of acute nitrate supplementation on 10 km handcycling TT performance. The principal finding of the current investigation was that acute nitrate supplementation did not improve 10 km handcycling TT performance in recreationally active men or in trained paracyclists by BR or by NIT ingestion.

4.1. Performance

A single dose of 6 mmol nitrate (BR or NIT) did not improve 10 km handcycling TT performance in able-bodied, upper body trained individuals or in trained paracyclists with a spinal cord injury (Table 5). To date, only a few studies examined the effects of nitrate supplementation on upper body exercise performance [36–39,43,44]. It is worth mentioning that rowing is a whole body exercise; most of its performance is produced by the lower extremities. Furthermore, these studies focused on short-term exercises, including 4 min maximal effort exercises [37], single [43] or repeated sprint tests [36,38], and 500 m to 2 km TT [36–38]. In the study of Peeling et al. [37], the ingestion of 9.6 mmol BR significantly enhanced 500 m kayaking TT performance by 1.7%. However, in the same study, a 4 min TT performance remained unchanged after the intake of 4.8 mmol BR. Comparable results were shown by Hoon et al. [39], where the authors concluded that the ingestion of 8.4 mmol but not 4.2 mmol BR may improve 2 km rowing TT performance [39]. Furthermore, Bond et al. [38] reported improved repeated sprint rowing performance after six days of BR supplementation. The fact that these studies did not reveal any ergogenic effects after the ingestion of a small nitrate dose (e.g., 4.2 to 5 mmol BR) may lead to the assumption that the dose used in the present study (6 mmol BR or NIT) was insufficient to induce any significant effects specifically on upper body exercise performance. Therefore, we hypothesize that a higher dosage of BR or NIT is needed for an acute supplementation protocol to improve 10 km handcycling TT performance. However, of course, a lack of effect of BR supplementation on performance cannot be ruled out.

In the review of Jones [45], it was concluded that nitrate supplementation appears to be more effective in exercises within the duration from 5 to 30 min compared to exercises lasting more than 40 min. Short duration exercises are typically performed at high intensity with predominant fast-twitch muscle fiber contribution and are likely to result in hypoxic and acidic skeletal muscle state. Recalling that the reduction from [NO_3^-] to NO is enhanced in hypoxic and acidic conditions [4] and that nitrate has targeted effects on fast-twitch muscle fibers [29,30], it becomes clear that short duration exercises may benefit more from nitrate supplementation. Nevertheless, type II muscle fibers are also recruited during prolonged low-intensity exercise. In the present study, the exercise duration was around 20 min, and the mean intensity was about 85% of VO_{2peak}, which indicates that the 10 km handcycling TT would provide optimal conditions for effective nitrate supplementation, particularly in view of the fact that upper body muscles possess a higher contribution of fast-twitch muscle fibers compared to the muscles of the lower body in healthy humans [31,32]. Furthermore, individuals with a spinal cord injury, M. deltoideus, seem to have a higher portion of type I muscle fibers [46]. Thus, nitrate would be expected to be less beneficial in those individuals compared to healthy, able-bodied controls. However, our study showed no improvement in performance in either group of athletes.

To date, only one study examined the effect of chronic nitrate supplementation on whole body exercise performance [38]. They reported an improved repeated 500 m sprint rowing performance after six days of BR supplementation (5.5 mmol per day). The dosage was therefore very similar to the 6 mmol used in our study but, interestingly, the authors revealed beneficial effects on performance. Therefore, it may be suggested that a chronic supplementation protocol may be more beneficial in terms of improving exercise performance compared to an acute supplementation protocol. This assumption is in line with the findings of Vanhatalo et al. [47], who reported that a chronic 15 day BR supplementation (5.2 mmol per day) resulted in a greater effect on incremental cycling exercise performance compared to a single dose of BR [47]. These findings are supported by the two studies of Cermak et al. [15], [48]. In the first study, the authors reported significant improvements in 10 km cycling TT performance after six days of BR supplementation (8 mmol per day) [15]. Conversely, in the second study, acute BR ingestion (8.7 mmol) did not show any positive effects on 1 h cycling performance [48]. The authors assumed that a longer supplementation period (chronic) is necessary to potentiate any ergogenic effects of BR. It is worth noting that, in these two studies, exercise duration and participant characteristics were different; therefore, comparison of the two studies should be taken with caution. A recent investigation by Jo et al. [49] compared the effects of acute (i.e., 2.5 h before exercise) and chronic (i.e., 15 days) nitrate supplementation (8 mmol per day) on 8 km cycling TT performance. The authors reported significant improvements in TT performance after chronic supplementation, whereas acute nitrate ingestion was unable to induce any ergogenic effects. Taking all these findings into account, we assume that the missing ergogenic effect of nitrate supplementation in the present study is partly attributable to the acute supplementation regimen. To date, no study investigated the effect of chronic BR supplementation on upper body exercise performance.

Recent studies reporting no improvement of performance after nitrate supplementation concluded that the fitness level of their participants (VO_{2peak} > 6 min/kg) might play an important role [36,50–53]. It has been shown that highly trained athletes exhibit increased NO synthase activity (NOS) and a better muscle capillarization compared to untrained individuals [54]. Furthermore, highly trained endurance athletes showed higher plasma nitrite levels [55] and fewer type II muscle fibers compared to recreationally active individuals [56]. All these adaptations to training may result in limited or attenuated effects of nitrate supplementation on performance in trained individuals [45]. In the study of Porcelli et al. [21], nitrate supplementation improved 3 km running TT performance in low to moderate trained participants but not in highly trained athletes (VO_{2peak} > 63 mL/min/kg). Therefore, it was concluded that highly trained athletes are less likely to benefit from nitrate supplementation [21]. In the present study, we tested recreationally active participants (VO_{2peak} = 33.7 ± 4 mL/min/kg) and paracyclists (VO_{2peak} = 38.6 ± 10.5 mL/min/kg). To note, the recorded VO_{2peak} may not reflect the true VO_{2max} value, as during our specific test, only upper body muscles were active. According to the literature [57], we expect the real VO_{2peak} values to be in a range of 45 to 55 mL/min/kg for the able-bodied individuals. Calculating the according value for the paracyclists produces a range between 50 to 60 mL/min/kg, but of course those athletes have secondary conditions such as a limited heart rate [58] or a reduced muscle mass in the core and the upper body [59]. Therefore, we assume that their VO_{2peak} would be even higher, as in able-bodied cyclists. Nevertheless, our able-bodied participants did not fall in the category of highly trained individuals. It seems that the fitness level of those participants would not be a major reason for missing performance enhancing effects.

It is possible that some of our athletes could have been identified as a so-called "responder" with a beneficial effect of either BR or NIT supplementation. Several studies have identified responders and non-responders in their participant samples [51,60–62]. The physiological background of these individual responses to nitrate supplementation is presently unknown and requires further investigation. It is suggested that habitual nitrate intake, baseline [NO_2^-] concentrations, activity of oral and gut bacteria, training status, and fiber type distribution may play a major role in the appearance of responders and non-responders [45]. Although the present study did not report an ergogenic effect of nitrate supplementation, some participants improved their 10 km TT performance after the ingestion of both BR and NIT. Therefore, we would recommend athletes trialing whether they benefit from nitrate ingestion or not. As long as it is well tolerated, we would not advise athletes against the use of nitrate supplementation. Furthermore, it might possibly be an advantage to follow a chronic supplementation protocol over several days or to use a higher dosage than 6 mmol nitrate.

4.2. Oxygen Consumption and PO to VO_2 Ratio

It is assumed that the ergogenic effect of nitrate supplementation is due to a reduction in VO_2, as a consequence of enhanced mitochondrial efficiency [23] and/or improved muscle contractile functions [24,25,29]. Larsen et al. [23] demonstrated that following three days of nitrate supplementation VO_2 at a given workload was significantly reduced by 3% during submaximal cycling exercise. This reduction in VO_2 was predominately related to the increased mitochondrial P/O ratio (ATP produced by O_2 consumed) [23]. Further investigations revealed that, after chronic nitrate supplementation, the expression of adenine nucleotide translocase (ANT) was reduced, a protein that is responsible for a substantial part of mitochondrial proton leakage, thus improving mitochondrial efficiency [23]. On the other hand, Bailey et al. [24] demonstrated that the reduction in VO_2 after six days of BR ingestion was related to a reduced ATP cost of muscle force production (i.e., higher muscle efficiency). However, the exact mechanisms remained unsolved. Furthermore, Hernandez et al. [29] reported that after seven days of nitrate supplementation in mice, force production of fast-twitch muscle fibers was increased. The authors suggested that the result was due to an increased expression of muscle Ca^{2+}-handling proteins in fast-twitch muscle fibers after nitrate supplementation [28]. In addition to these findings, Haider et al. [25] revealed that seven days of BR ingestion enhanced excitation–contraction coupling in human skeletal muscles. Thus, upper body muscles in general would benefit more, as they tend to have more type II muscle fibers [32]. However, a lesion of the spinal cord (and therefore a predominant use of upper body muscle) seems to lead to an increase in muscle type I fibers [46]. Therefore, we expected an increase in performance following nitrate ingestion in able-bodied individuals but possibly not in paracyclists with a spinal cord injury.

To date, it was shown that dietary nitrate supplementation either by BR or NIT reduces steady-state VO_2 (3 to 14%) for a given PO during submaximal exercises irrespective of exercise modality (cycling, running, kayaking, etc.) [20,47,63,64]. However, not all studies were able to detect such a reduction of VO_2 [65,66]. Our study (Figure 1) showed that PO to VO_2 ratio tended to be higher in the BR trial compared to NIT and PLA in able-bodied individuals with a significant difference in some km during the TT. However, VO_2 alone was not significantly lower in the BR trial. To summarize the most recent literature, it was noticed that the PO/VO_2 ratio increased to a larger extent during cycling (i.e., lower body: 7 to 11%) compared to handcycling and kayaking (i.e., upper body: 2 to 3%) [16,37]. It could be hypothesized that the smaller increase in the PO/VO_2 ratio is simply a consequence of a smaller active muscle mass during upper body exercise compared to cycling. On the other hand, upper body exercises rely largely on fast-twitch muscle fibers [67,68], and therefore it would be expected that upper body exercises may show greater benefits compared to cycling or running. However, the results of the present study do not support this assumption.

In the present study, we found an increase in PO/VO_2 ratio in some km of the TT after BR ingestion but not after NIT despite the same dosages (6 mmol) of the supplements (Figure 1a). This observation is contradictory, since several studies reported a reduced VO_2 during exercise following NIT supplementation [23,63]. In contrast to our study, these investigations used a chronic supplementation protocol. Thus far, few studies examined the effects of acute NIT ingestion on VO_2 [65,66]. Bescos et al. [66] reported that 10 mg/kg BM nitrate (~11 mmol) did not reduce VO_2 during submaximal cycling in trained endurance athletes. These results are in close agreement with those obtained by Flueck et al. [65], where different dosages of NIT (3, 6, and 12 mmol) did not reduce VO_2 response of moderate- and severe-intensity cycling. On the other hand, BR supplementation appeared to elicit greater effects on VO_2 due to the additional antioxidants, which facilitate nitrate reduction. Additionally, BR contains polyphenols with a potential for ergogenic effects in performance [69]. It is possible that BR might be more beneficial in reducing VO_2 compared to NIT, but more research is needed to confirm those assumptions.

4.3. Other Parameters

In the present study, neither BR nor NIT had any significant influence on systolic or diastolic blood pressure at rest (Table 2). Similar findings were shown in a similar study [65], whereas only the ingestion of a higher BR dosage seemed to result in a significantly lower blood pressure at rest. It seems that a dose-dependent decrease in blood pressure occurs after the ingestion of nitrate supplementation [10]. The mechanism by which dietary nitrate supplementation lowers blood pressure may be explained by the increased bioavailability of NO via the nitrate-nitrite-NO-pathway [70,71]. NO is known as a potent vasodilator that governs systemic blood pressure by reducing arterial pressure and peripheral resistance [4]. Therefore, a sufficient amount of nitrate needs to be ingested to increase the concentration of NO, thus inducing a reduction in blood pressure. Previous studies concluded that, compared to nitrate salts, BR has a greater potential to reduce systolic blood pressure due to the additional antioxidants in BR that facilitate the reduction of nitrite to NO [65]. However, the findings of the present study did not confirm this assumption.

Resting levels of [NO_3^-] seemed to be lower in the paracyclists (~38 uM) compared to able-bodied individuals (~66 uM). To our knowledge, no other study measured resting [NO_3^-] concentration in participants with a spinal cord injury. Therefore, we might only speculate about the reason for such a difference. Possible reasons might be the lower energy or the nitrate intake in general due to lower active muscle mass resulting in lower energy expenditure. Another explanation might involve the slower gastrointestinal transition time in those participants due to the impaired nervous system [72]. This might also affect the absorption of nutrients. Significant increases in [NO_2^-] and [NO_3^-] concentrations after NIT and BR were found in both groups of athletes. Interestingly, able-bodied individuals showed significantly higher [NO_2^-] concentrations after BR consumption compared to paracyclists, whereas paracyclists showed significantly higher [NO_3^-] concentrations after BR and NIT ingestion compared to able-bodied individuals. It seems possible that reduction from [NO_3^-] to [NO_2^-] was reduced in the paracyclists and therefore a higher [NO_3^-] was present 3 h after the ingestion. Such a hypothesis needs to be confirmed in future studies. No significant differences were found in [NO_2^-] and [NO_3^-] concentrations between NIT and BR ingestion in the same group. These findings seemed to be very similar to the previous study with a 6 mmol NIT and BR intervention in able-bodied individuals [65]. Thus, the results for [NO_2^-] and [NO_3^-] concentrations in this study seem to be consistent with the literature.

4.4. Limitations

One major limitation of this study was that we did not use a nitrate-depleted BR as a placebo supplement. The participants were possibly able to distinguish between BR and NIT or between BR and PLA. Therefore, we cannot exclude the possibility that our findings were influenced by a potential placebo effect in the BR group. However, the participants were not able to distinguish between PLA and NIT because of similar taste, smell, and appearance.

Additionally, there was a significant difference between the two groups. Able-bodied individuals showed a significantly higher body mass compared to paracyclists. This fact evolved mainly from the loss of muscle mass in the legs of athletes with a spinal cord injury due to immobilization. Furthermore, the age was significantly different between the two groups, as paracyclists were older. This is a known phenomenon in Paralympic sports, as most athletes start their career after the incident of the injury. Last but not least, both groups showed a different fitness level, as paracyclists appeared to be more highly trained than able-bodied individuals. All these issues might have influenced the outcome of the study and therefore needed to be acknowledged.

Finally, although our able-bodied participants were used to upper body exercise, we still reported a significant order effect on 10 km handcycling TT performance in this group of participants. Therefore, we assume that only one familiarization trial was insufficient in the present study. We cannot exclude the possibility that the effects of dietary nitrate on exercise performance and VO_2 in the present study were masked or blunted by the observed order effect.

5. Conclusions

Our study demonstrated that acute nitrate supplementation either by BR or NIT (6 mmol) did not improve 10 km handcycling TT performance in recreationally active men or in paracyclists. BR ingestion seemed to increase PO to VO_2 ratio in some km of the TT compared to PLA in able-bodied individuals but not in paracyclists. Overall, the present results do not support previous findings where acute nitrate supplementation enhanced short-term, high-intensity TT performance [36–38] in upper body exercise. Further research is required to examine optimal supplementation strategies and effects of nitrate supplementation on upper body exercise performance, especially in wheelchair athletes with physiological adaptations following the incident of the spinal cord injury.

Author Contributions: Individual contributions were as following: conceptualization, J.L.F. and C.P.; methodology, J.L.F., A.B., C.P.; validation, J.L.F., A.B. and C.P.; formal analysis, J.L.F., A.G., A.B.; investigation, A.G., J.L.F., N.M. and N.B.; resources, J.L.F.; data curation, J.L.F., A.G., A.B.; writing—original draft preparation, J.L.F. and A.G.; writing—review and editing, C.P. and A.B.; visualization, J.L.F. and A.G.; supervision, J.L.F.; project administration, J.L.F.

Acknowledgments: We are grateful for the participation of all athletes in this study. Furthermore, we would like to thank the medical staff, Eliane Arnold, Melanie Müller and Ruth Heller, for helping with the blood withdrawal. This may include administrative and technical support, or donations in kind (e.g., materials used for experiments).

References

1. Ahrendt, D.M. Ergogenic aids: Counseling the athlete. *Am. Fam. Physician* **2001**, *63*, 913–922. [PubMed]
2. Santamaria, P. Nitrate in vegetables: Toxicity, content, intake and ec regulation. *J. Sci. Food Agric.* **2006**, *86*, 10–17. [CrossRef]
3. Nyakayiru, J.; Kouw, I.W.K.; Cermak, N.M.; Senden, J.M.; van Loon, L.J.C.; Verdijk, L.B. Sodium nitrate ingestion increases skeletal muscle nitrate content in humans. *J. Appl. Physiol.* **2017**, *123*, 637–644. [CrossRef] [PubMed]
4. Lundberg, J.O.; Weitzberg, E.; Gladwin, M.T. The nitrate-nitrite-nitric oxide pathway in physiology and therapeutics. *Nat. Rev. Drug Discov.* **2008**, *7*, 156–167. [CrossRef] [PubMed]
5. Pacher, P.; Beckman, J.S.; Liaudet, L. Nitric oxide and peroxynitrite in health and disease. *Physiol. Rev.* **2007**, *87*, 315–424. [CrossRef] [PubMed]
6. Reid, M.B. Role of nitric oxide in skeletal muscle: Synthesis, distribution and functional importance. *Acta Physiol. Scand.* **1998**, *162*, 401–409. [CrossRef]
7. Stamler, J.S.; Meissner, G. Physiology of nitric oxide in skeletal muscle. *Physiol. Rev.* **2001**, *81*, 209–237. [CrossRef]
8. Moncada, S.; Palmer, R.M.; Higgs, E.A. Nitric oxide: Physiology, pathophysiology, and pharmacology. *Pharmacol. Rev.* **1991**, *43*, 109–142.
9. Gilchrist, M.; Shore, A.C.; Benjamin, N. Inorganic nitrate and nitrite and control of blood pressure. *Cardiovasc. Res. Cent. Bull.* **2011**, *89*, 492–498. [CrossRef]
10. Kapil, V.; Milsom, A.B.; Okorie, M.; Maleki-Toyserkani, S.; Akram, F.; Rehman, F.; Arghandawi, S.; Pearl, V.; Benjamin, N.; Loukogeorgakis, S.; et al. Inorganic nitrate supplementation lowers blood pressure in humans: Role for nitrite-derived no. *Hypertension* **2010**, *56*, 274–281. [CrossRef]
11. Kapil, V.; Weitzberg, E.; Lundberg, J.O.; Ahluwalia, A. Clinical evidence demonstrating the utility of inorganic nitrate in cardiovascular health. *Nitric Oxide* **2014**, *38*, 45–57. [CrossRef] [PubMed]
12. Hoon, M.W.; Johnson, N.A.; Chapman, P.G.; Burke, L.M. The effect of nitrate supplementation on exercise performance in healthy individuals: A systematic review and meta-analysis. *Int. J. Sport Nutr. Exerc. Metab.* **2013**, *23*, 522–532. [CrossRef] [PubMed]
13. Jones, A.M. Dietary nitrate supplementation and exercise performance. *Sports Med.* **2014**, *44* (Suppl. 1), S35–S45. [CrossRef]
14. McMahon, N.F.; Leveritt, M.D.; Pavey, T.G. The effect of dietary nitrate supplementation on endurance exercise performance in healthy adults: A systematic review and meta-analysis. *Sports Med.* **2017**, *47*, 735–756. [CrossRef] [PubMed]
15. Cermak, N.M.; Gibala, M.J.; van Loon, L.J. Nitrate supplementation's improvement of 10-km time-trial performance in trained cyclists. *Int. J. Sport Nutr. Exerc. Metab.* **2012**, *22*, 64–71. [CrossRef] [PubMed]
16. Lansley, K.E.; Winyard, P.G.; Bailey, S.J.; Vanhatalo, A.; Wilkerson, D.P.; Blackwell, J.R.; Gilchrist, M.; Benjamin, N.; Jones, A.M. Acute dietary nitrate supplementation improves cycling time trial performance. *Med. Sci. Sports Exerc.* **2011**, *43*, 1125–1131. [CrossRef] [PubMed]
17. Vasconcellos, J.; Henrique Silvestre, D.; Dos Santos Baiao, D.; Werneck-de-Castro, J.P.; Silveira Alvares, T.; Paschoalin, V.M. A single dose of beetroot gel rich in nitrate does not improve performance but lowers blood glucose in physically active individuals. *J. Nutr. Metab.* **2017**, *2017*, 7853034. [CrossRef]

18. Shannon, O.M.; Barlow, M.J.; Duckworth, L.; Williams, E.; Wort, G.; Woods, D.; Siervo, M.; O'Hara, J.P. Dietary nitrate supplementation enhances short but not longer duration running time-trial performance. *Eur. J. Appl. Physiol.* **2017**, *117*, 775–785. [CrossRef]
19. Bailey, S.J.; Winyard, P.; Vanhatalo, A.; Blackwell, J.R.; Dimenna, F.J.; Wilkerson, D.P.; Tarr, J.; Benjamin, N.; Jones, A.M. Dietary nitrate supplementation reduces the o2 cost of low-intensity exercise and enhances tolerance to high-intensity exercise in humans. *J. Appl. Physiol.* **2009**, *107*, 1144–1155. [CrossRef]
20. Lansley, K.E.; Winyard, P.G.; Fulford, J.; Vanhatalo, A.; Bailey, S.J.; Blackwell, J.R.; DiMenna, F.J.; Gilchrist, M.; Benjamin, N.; Jones, A.M. Dietary nitrate supplementation reduces the o2 cost of walking and running: A placebo-controlled study. *J. Appl. Physiol.* **2011**, *110*, 591–600. [CrossRef]
21. Porcelli, S.; Ramaglia, M.; Bellistri, G.; Pavei, G.; Pugliese, L.; Montorsi, M.; Rasica, L.; Marzorati, M. Aerobic fitness affects the exercise performance responses to nitrate supplementation. *Med. Sci. Sports Exerc.* **2015**, *47*, 1643–1651. [CrossRef] [PubMed]
22. Wylie, L.J.; Kelly, J.; Bailey, S.J.; Blackwell, J.R.; Skiba, P.F.; Winyard, P.G.; Jeukendrup, A.E.; Vanhatalo, A.; Jones, A.M. Beetroot juice and exercise: Pharmacodynamic and dose-response relationships. *J. Appl. Physiol.* **2013**, *115*, 325–336. [CrossRef] [PubMed]
23. Larsen, F.J.; Schiffer, T.A.; Borniquel, S.; Sahlin, K.; Ekblom, B.; Lundberg, J.O.; Weitzberg, E. Dietary inorganic nitrate improves mitochondrial efficiency in humans. *Cell Metab.* **2011**, *13*, 149–159. [CrossRef] [PubMed]
24. Bailey, S.J.; Fulford, J.; Vanhatalo, A.; Winyard, P.G.; Blackwell, J.R.; DiMenna, F.J.; Wilkerson, D.P.; Benjamin, N.; Jones, A.M. Dietary nitrate supplementation enhances muscle contractile efficiency during knee-extensor exercise in humans. *J. Appl. Physiol.* **2010**, *109*, 135–148. [CrossRef] [PubMed]
25. Haider, G.; Folland, J.P. Nitrate supplementation enhances the contractile properties of human skeletal muscle. *Med. Sci. Sports Exerc.* **2014**, *46*, 2234–2243. [CrossRef]
26. Ferguson, S.K.; Hirai, D.M.; Copp, S.W.; Holdsworth, C.T.; Allen, J.D.; Jones, A.M.; Musch, T.I.; Poole, D.C. Impact of dietary nitrate supplementation via beetroot juice on exercising muscle vascular control in rats. *J. Physiol.* **2013**, *591*, 547–557. [CrossRef] [PubMed]
27. Lundby, C.; Boushel, R.; Robach, P.; Moller, K.; Saltin, B.; Calbet, J.A. During hypoxic exercise some vasoconstriction is needed to match o2 delivery with o2 demand at the microcirculatory level. *J. Physiol.* **2008**, *586*, 123–130. [CrossRef] [PubMed]
28. Calbet, J.A.; Lundby, C.; Sander, M.; Robach, P.; Saltin, B.; Boushel, R. Effects of atp-induced leg vasodilation on vo2 peak and leg o2 extraction during maximal exercise in humans. *Am. J. Physiol. Regul. Integr. Comp. Physiol.* **2006**, *291*, R447–R453. [CrossRef]
29. Hernandez, A.; Schiffer, T.A.; Ivarsson, N.; Cheng, A.J.; Bruton, J.D.; Lundberg, J.O.; Weitzberg, E.; Westerblad, H. Dietary nitrate increases tetanic [ca2+]i and contractile force in mouse fast-twitch muscle. *J. Physiol.* **2012**, *590 Pt 15*, 3575–3583. [CrossRef]
30. Jones, A.M.; Ferguson, S.K.; Bailey, S.J.; Vanhatalo, A.; Poole, D.C. Fiber type-specific effects of dietary nitrate. *Exerc. Sport Sci. Rev.* **2016**, *44*, 53–60. [CrossRef]
31. Kiilerich, K.; Birk, J.B.; Damsgaard, R.; Wojtaszewski, J.F.; Pilegaard, H. Regulation of pdh in human arm and leg muscles at rest and during intense exercise. *Am. J. Physiol. Endocrinol. Metab.* **2008**, *294*, E36–E42. [CrossRef] [PubMed]
32. Schantz, P.; Randall-Fox, E.; Hutchison, W.; Tyden, A.; Astrand, P.O. Muscle fibre type distribution, muscle cross-sectional area and maximal voluntary strength in humans. *Acta Physiol. Scand.* **1983**, *117*, 219–226. [CrossRef] [PubMed]
33. Calbet, J.A.; Holmberg, H.C.; Rosdahl, H.; van Hall, G.; Jensen-Urstad, M.; Saltin, B. Why do arms extract less oxygen than legs during exercise? *Am. J. Physiol. Regul. Integr. Comp. Physiol.* **2005**, *289*, R1448–R1458. [CrossRef] [PubMed]
34. Calbet, J.A.; Gonzalez-Alonso, J.; Helge, J.W.; Sondergaard, H.; Munch-Andersen, T.; Saltin, B.; Boushel, R. Central and peripheral hemodynamics in exercising humans: Leg vs arm exercise. *Scand J. Med. Sci. Sports.* **2015**, *25* (Suppl. 4), 144–157. [CrossRef] [PubMed]
35. Van Hall, G.; Jensen-Urstad, M.; Rosdahl, H.; Holmberg, H.C.; Saltin, B.; Calbet, J.A. Leg and arm lactate and substrate kinetics during exercise. *Am. J. Physiol. Endocrinol. Metab.* **2003**, *284*, E193–E205. [CrossRef] [PubMed]

36. Muggeridge, D.J.; Howe, C.C.; Spendiff, O.; Pedlar, C.; James, P.E.; Easton, C. The effects of a single dose of concentrated beetroot juice on performance in trained flatwater kayakers. *Int. J. Sport Nutr. Exerc. Metab.* **2013**, *23*, 498–506. [CrossRef] [PubMed]
37. Peeling, P.; Cox, G.R.; Bullock, N.; Burke, L.M. Beetroot juice improves on-water 500 m time-trial performance, and laboratory-based paddling economy in national and international-level kayak athletes. *Int. J. Sport Nutr. Exerc. Metab.* **2015**, *25*, 278–284. [CrossRef]
38. Bond, H.; Morton, L.; Braakhuis, A.J. Dietary nitrate supplementation improves rowing performance in well-trained rowers. *Int. J. Sport Nutr. Exerc. Metab.* **2012**, *22*, 251–256. [CrossRef]
39. Hoon, M.W.; Jones, A.M.; Johnson, N.A.; Blackwell, J.R.; Broad, E.M.; Lundy, B.; Rice, A.J.; Burke, L.M. The effect of variable doses of inorganic nitrate-rich beetroot juice on simulated 2,000-m rowing performance in trained athletes. *Int. J. Sports Physiol. Perform.* **2014**, *9*, 615–620. [CrossRef]
40. World Medical Association. Declaration of Helsinki—Ethical principles for medical research involving human subjects. *J. Indian Med. Assoc.* **2009**, *107*, 403–405.
41. Govoni, M.; Jansson, E.A.; Weitzberg, E.; Lundberg, J.O. The increase in plasma nitrite after a dietary nitrate load is markedly attenuated by an antibacterial mouthwash. *Nitric Oxide* **2008**, *19*, 333–337. [CrossRef] [PubMed]
42. Borg, G.A. Psychophysical bases of perceived exertion. *Med. Sci. Sports Exerc.* **1982**, *14*, 377–381. [CrossRef] [PubMed]
43. Esen, O.; Nicholas, C.; Morris, M.; Bailey, S.J. No effect of beetroot juice supplementation on 100-m and 200-m swimming performance in moderately trained swimmers. *Int. J. Sports Physiol. Perform.* **2019**. [CrossRef] [PubMed]
44. Bruce, C.R.; Anderson, M.E.; Fraser, S.F.; Stepto, N.K.; Klein, R.; Hopkins, W.G.; Hawley, J.A. Enhancement of 2000-m rowing performance after caffeine ingestion. *Med. Sci. Sports Exerc.* **2000**, *32*, 1958–1963. [CrossRef] [PubMed]
45. Jones, A.M. Influence of dietary nitrate on the physiological determinants of exercise performance: A critical review. *Appl. Physiol. Nutr. Metab.* **2014**, *39*, 1019–1028. [CrossRef]
46. Schantz, P.; Sjoberg, B.; Widebeck, A.M.; Ekblom, B. Skeletal muscle of trained and untrained paraplegics and tetraplegics. *Acta Physiol. Scand.* **1997**, *161*, 31–39. [CrossRef]
47. Vanhatalo, A.; Bailey, S.J.; Blackwell, J.R.; DiMenna, F.J.; Pavey, T.G.; Wilkerson, D.P.; Benjamin, N.; Winyard, P.G.; Jones, A.M. Acute and chronic effects of dietary nitrate supplementation on blood pressure and the physiological responses to moderate-intensity and incremental exercise. *Am. J. Physiol. Regul. Integr. Comp. Physiol.* **2010**, *299*, R1121–R1131. [CrossRef] [PubMed]
48. Cermak, N.M.; Res, P.; Stinkens, R.; Lundberg, J.O.; Gibala, M.J.; van Loon, L.J. No improvement in endurance performance after a single dose of beetroot juice. *Int. J. Sport Nutr. Exerc. Metab.* **2012**, *22*, 470–478. [CrossRef]
49. Jo, E.; Fischer, M.; Auslander, A.T.; Beigarten, A.; Daggy, B.; Hansen, K.; Kessler, L.; Osmond, A.; Wang, H.; Wes, R. The effects of multi-day vs. Single pre-exercise nitrate supplement dosing on simulated cycling time trial performance and skeletal muscle oxygenation. *J. Strength Cond. Res.* **2019**, *33*, 217–224. [CrossRef]
50. Bescos, R.; Ferrer-Roca, V.; Galilea, P.A.; Roig, A.; Drobnic, F.; Sureda, A.; Martorell, M.; Cordova, A.; Tur, J.A.; Pons, A. Sodium nitrate supplementation does not enhance performance of endurance athletes. *Med. Sci. Sports Exerc.* **2012**, *44*, 2400–2409. [CrossRef]
51. Christensen, P.M.; Nyberg, M.; Bangsbo, J. Influence of nitrate supplementation on vo(2) kinetics and endurance of elite cyclists. *Scand. J. Med. Sci. Sports* **2013**, *23*, e21–e31. [CrossRef] [PubMed]
52. Peacock, O.; Tjonna, A.E.; James, P.; Wisloff, U.; Welde, B.; Bohlke, N.; Smith, A.; Stokes, K.; Cook, C.; Sandbakk, O. Dietary nitrate does not enhance running performance in elite cross-country skiers. *Med. Sci. Sports Exerc.* **2012**, *44*, 2213–2219. [CrossRef] [PubMed]
53. Lane, S.C.; Hawley, J.A.; Desbrow, B.; Jones, A.M.; Blackwell, J.R.; Ross, M.L.; Zemski, A.J.; Burke, L.M. Single and combined effects of beetroot juice and caffeine supplementation on cycling time trial performance. *Appl. Physiol. Nutr. Metab.* **2014**, *39*, 1050–1057. [CrossRef] [PubMed]
54. Cocks, M.; Shaw, C.S.; Shepherd, S.O.; Fisher, J.P.; Ranasinghe, A.M.; Barker, T.A.; Tipton, K.D.; Wagenmakers, A.J. Sprint interval and endurance training are equally effective in increasing muscle microvascular density and enos content in sedentary males. *J. Physiol.* **2013**, *591*, 641–656. [CrossRef] [PubMed]

55. Totzeck, M.; Hendgen-Cotta, U.B.; Rammos, C.; Frommke, L.M.; Knackstedt, C.; Predel, H.G.; Kelm, M.; Rassaf, T. Higher endogenous nitrite levels are associated with superior exercise capacity in highly trained athletes. *Nitric Oxide* **2012**, *27*, 75–81. [CrossRef] [PubMed]
56. Gollnick, P.D.; Matoba, H. The muscle fiber composition of skeletal muscle as a predictor of athletic success. An overview. *Am. J. Sports Med.* **1984**, *12*, 212–217. [CrossRef] [PubMed]
57. Ade, C.J.; Broxterman, R.M.; Craig, J.C.; Schlup, S.J.; Wilcox, S.L.; Barstow, T.J. Upper body aerobic exercise as a possible predictor of lower body performance. *Aerosp. Med. Hum. Perform.* **2015**, *86*, 599–605. [CrossRef]
58. Bhambhani, Y. Physiology of wheelchair racing in athletes with spinal cord injury. *Sports Med.* **2002**, *32*, 23–51. [CrossRef]
59. Keil, M.; Totosy de Zepetnek, J.O.; Brooke-Wavell, K.; Goosey-Tolfrey, V.L. Measurement precision of body composition variables in elite wheelchair athletes, using dual-energy x-ray absorptiometry. *Eur. J. Sport Sci.* **2016**, *16*, 65–71. [CrossRef]
60. Boorsma, R.K.; Whitfield, J.; Spriet, L.L. Beetroot juice supplementation does not improve performance of elite 1500-m runners. *Med. Sci. Sports Exerc.* **2014**, *46*, 2326–2334. [CrossRef]
61. Wilkerson, D.P.; Hayward, G.M.; Bailey, S.J.; Vanhatalo, A.; Blackwell, J.R.; Jones, A.M. Influence of acute dietary nitrate supplementation on 50 mile time trial performance in well-trained cyclists. *Eur. J. Appl. Physiol.* **2012**, *112*, 4127–4134. [CrossRef] [PubMed]
62. Bourdillon, N.; Fan, J.L.; Uva, B.; Muller, H.; Meyer, P.; Kayser, B. Effect of oral nitrate supplementation on pulmonary hemodynamics during exercise and time trial performance in normoxia and hypoxia: A randomized controlled trial. *Front. Physiol.* **2015**, *6*, 288. [CrossRef] [PubMed]
63. Larsen, F.J.; Weitzberg, E.; Lundberg, J.O.; Ekblom, B. Effects of dietary nitrate on oxygen cost during exercise. *Acta Physiol.* **2007**, *191*, 59–66. [CrossRef] [PubMed]
64. Pawlak-Chaouch, M.; Boissiere, J.; Gamelin, F.X.; Cuvelier, G.; Berthoin, S.; Aucouturier, J. Effect of dietary nitrate supplementation on metabolic rate during rest and exercise in human: A systematic review and a meta-analysis. *Nitric Oxide* **2016**, *53*, 65–76. [CrossRef] [PubMed]
65. Flueck, J.L.; Bogdanova, A.; Mettler, S.; Perret, C. Is beetroot juice more effective than sodium nitrate? The effects of equimolar nitrate dosages of nitrate-rich beetroot juice and sodium nitrate on oxygen consumption during exercise. *Appl. Physiol. Nutr. Metab.* **2016**, *41*, 421–429. [CrossRef] [PubMed]
66. Bescos, R.; Rodriguez, F.A.; Iglesias, X.; Ferrer, M.D.; Iborra, E.; Pons, A. Acute administration of inorganic nitrate reduces vo(2peak) in endurance athletes. *Med. Sci. Sports Exerc.* **2011**, *43*, 1979–1986. [CrossRef] [PubMed]
67. Pimental, N.A.; Sawka, M.N.; Billings, D.S.; Trad, L.A. Physiological responses to prolonged upper-body exercise. *Med. Sci. Sports Exerc.* **1984**, *16*, 360–365. [CrossRef]
68. Pendergast, D.R. Cardiovascular, respiratory, and metabolic responses to upper body exercise. *Med. Sci. Sports Exerc.* **1989**, *21* (Suppl. 5), S121–S125. [CrossRef]
69. Braakhuis, A.J.; Hopkins, W.G. Impact of dietary antioxidants on sport performance: A review. *Sports Med.* **2015**, *45*, 939–955. [CrossRef]
70. Webb, A.J.; Patel, N.; Loukogeorgakis, S.; Okorie, M.; Aboud, Z.; Misra, S.; Rashid, R.; Miall, P.; Deanfield, J.; Benjamin, N.; et al. Acute blood pressure lowering, vasoprotective, and antiplatelet properties of dietary nitrate via bioconversion to nitrite. *Hypertension* **2008**, *51*, 784–790. [CrossRef]
71. Siervo, M.; Lara, J.; Ogbonmwan, I.; Mathers, J.C. Inorganic nitrate and beetroot juice supplementation reduces blood pressure in adults: A systematic review and meta-analysis. *J. Nutr.* **2013**, *143*, 818–826. [CrossRef] [PubMed]
72. Krogh, K.; Mosdal, C.; Laurberg, S. Gastrointestinal and segmental colonic transit times in patients with acute and chronic spinal cord lesions. *Spinal Cord* **2000**, *38*, 615–621. [CrossRef] [PubMed]

4

Asymmetries in the Technique and Ground Reaction Forces of Elite Alpine Skiers Influence their Slalom Performance

Matej Supej [1,*], Jan Ogrin [1], Nejc Šarabon [2] and Hans-Christer Holmberg [3,4]

1 Faculty of Sport, University of Ljubljana, 1000 Ljubljana, Slovenia; jan.ogrin@fsp.uni-lj.si
2 Faculty of Health Sciences, University of Primorska, Polje 42, 6310 Izola, Slovenia; nejc.sarabon@fvz.upr.si
3 Department of Physiology and Pharmacology, Biomedicum C5, Karolinska Institute, 171 77 Stockholm, Sweden; integrativephysiobiomech@gmail.com
4 China Institute of Sport and Health Science, Beijing Sport University, Beijing 100084, China
* Correspondence: matej.supej@fsp.uni-lj.si

Abstract: Background: Although many of the movements of skiers are asymmetric, little is presently known about how such asymmetry influences performance. Here, our aim was to examine whether asymmetries in technique and the ground reaction forces associated with left and right turns influence the asymmetries in the performance of elite slalom skiers. Methods: As nine elite skiers completed a 20-gate slalom course, their three-dimensional full-body kinematics and ground reaction forces (GRF) were monitored with a global navigation satellite and inertial motion capture systems, in combination with pressure insoles. For multivariable regression models, 26 predictor skiing techniques and GRF variables and 8 predicted skiing performance variables were assessed, all of them determining asymmetries in terms of symmetry and Jaccard indices. Results: Asymmetries in instantaneous and sectional performance were found to have the largest predictor coefficients associated with asymmetries in shank angle and hip flexion of the outside leg. Asymmetry for turn radius had the largest predictor coefficients associated with asymmetries in shank angle and GRF on the entire outside foot. Conclusions: Although slalom skiers were found to move their bodies in a quite symmetrical fashion, asymmetry in their skiing technique and GRF influenced variables related to asymmetries in performance.

Keywords: biomechanics; kinematics; kinetics; global navigation satellite system; GPS; IMU; inertial motion capture; pressure insoles; ski racing

---

1. Introduction

In connection with highly competitive elite alpine skiing, differences in finishing time are often very small [1]. Indeed, the overall finishing time is a major factor in determining a skier's FIS (International Ski Federation) ranking and it is therefore hardly surprising that analysis of gate-to-gate times has focused on determining where a skier loses or gains time in as much detail as possible [2,3]. However, although easy for coaches and athletes to understand [4], times on short sections of a course, such as from gate-to-gate, are not good direct indicators of either instantaneous or turning performance [5]. In this context, variables related to the dissipation of mechanical energy reflect kinetic performance more closely [5–7] and kinematic parameters related to the trajectory of the skis are also more reliable [8,9].

Although numerous descriptions of alpine skiing technique have been published, relatively little is yet known about the biomechanical factors that influence competitive performance [6]. One such factor is the start strategy, including the technique utilized and number of start-pushes [10]. Furthermore, the slalom skiing technique chosen exerts an impact on both ground reaction forces (GRF) and performance [11–13].

Thus, in the case of slalom, the larger the "attack angle" (i.e., the angle between the orientation of the skis and direction of skiing) when entering a turn, the more energy is dissipated [14], whereas with giant slalom, the choice of trajectory and smoothness of skiing during a turn are also major influences on energy loss and performance [7–9]. Furthermore, use of a more "dynamic" body posture reduces energy loss due to aerodynamic drag [15], although this is not a major determinant of the performance of elite giant slalom skiers [16]. Air drag is more important in super-G skiing and even more so when skiing downhill [17]. When skiing straight, the movement of the center of mass forwards and backwards does not affect skiing time, whereas the edge angle does [18].

Although the body movements of athletes, and especially those of left and right turns by elite alpine skiers, are often asymmetric, little is presently known about how these asymmetries influence performance [19]. Bell [20] and Hoffman [21] and co-workers have shown that asymmetries affect jump height, while Beck and colleagues [22] found that asymmetries in stride while running result in more consumption of energy. Although ski coaches are often concerned with eliminating such asymmetries (i.e., correcting "mistakes" made when performing the "worse" turn), to our knowledge, with respect to alpine skiing, only preferential usage of one of the legs is known to affect turning and the potential impact of asymmetry on overall performance remains to be determined [23].

Accordingly, our aim here was to examine whether asymmetries in technique and in the ground reaction forces associated with left and right turns influence the competitive performance of elite slalom skiers. Our hypothesis was that asymmetries in the performance of elite slalom skiers are influenced by asymmetries in their technique and in ground reaction forces.

2. Materials and Methods

2.1. Participants

Nine male slalom skiers, all members of the Swedish National Ski Team (age: 22.7 ± 3.4 y; height: 181.8 ± 6.9 cm; weight: 82.2 ± 5.6 kg; current SL FIS points: 24.9 ± 18.6 (means ± SD)), provided their written informed consent before participating in this study, which was conducted in accordance with the Declaration of Helsinki and pre-approved by the National Medical Ethics Committee (Approval ID: 0120-99/2018/5, Project ID: L5-1845).

2.2. Experimental Setup

Starting twice from the left and twice from the right side, in randomized order, each skier performed four runs on a corridor-shaped slalom course with 20 gates placed symmetrically at 12-m intervals and with a displacement of 4 m (Figure 1). To ensure that this course was set precisely, the gates were positioned using the Leica Geodetic Global Satellite Navigation System (GNSS) 1200 with its built-in Stake-Out application (Leica Geosystems AG, Heerbrugg, Switzerland). The terrain selected had an average incline of 16°, with a maximal tilt to either side of <1°, and was groomed on each day of testing. In light of the hard, icy snow and temperatures between −2 and 0 °C, the coaches and experimental team smoothed the course prior to each and every run in an attempt to standardize conditions for side-skidding.

As described previously [24,25], three-dimensional whole-body kinematics were monitored utilizing the MVN Biomech V2018 inertial system (Xsens Technologies B.V., Enschede, The Netherlands) and Leica Zeno GG04 plus Real-Time Kinematics RTK GNSS (Leica Geosystems AG, Heerbrugg, Switzerland). The inertial system (calibrated twice prior to each run) was worn under the skier's racing suit and the smart antenna (RTK GNSS) was integrated into the back protector and positioned at shoulder height to allow unobstructed satellite reception (Figure 2). Data collected by the inertial system were recorded on a memory card, while data from the GNSS RTK system were transmitted wirelessly to a handheld device (Conker NS6, Conker, Takeley, England). In connection with each measurement, the precise position of the smart antenna relative to the thoracic (T12) and cervical vertebrae (C7) was determined to allow reliable integration of these two sets of data.

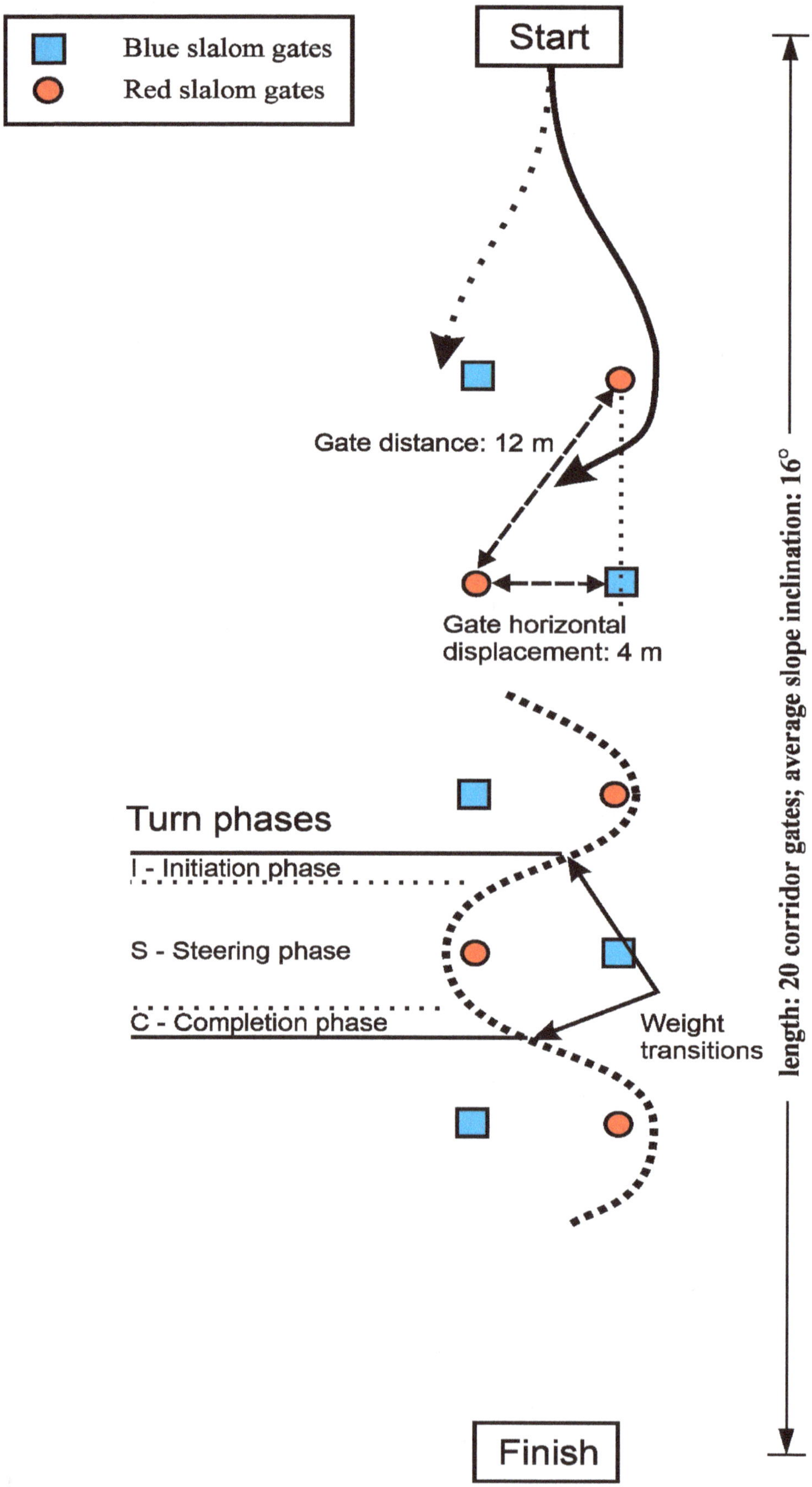

Figure 1. Schematic illustration of the corridor-shaped slalom course.

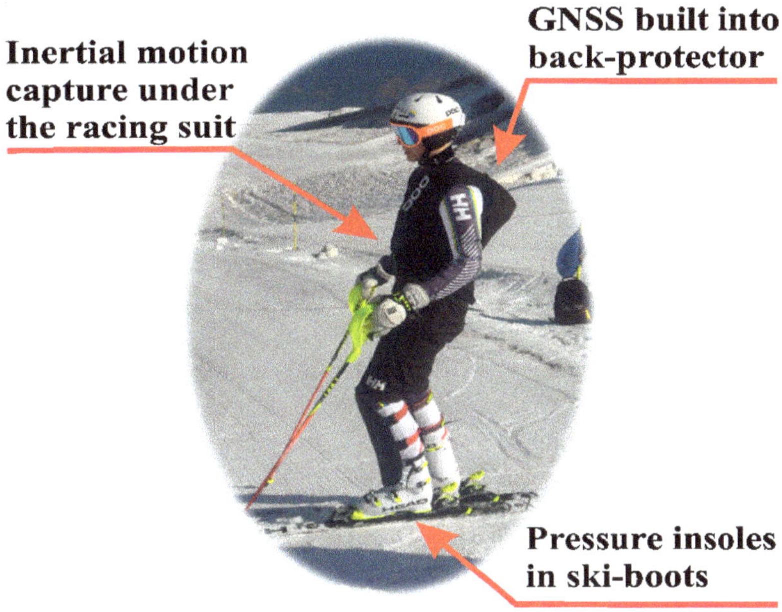

Figure 2. Equipment of the slalom skier with the global navigation satellite and inertial motion capture systems and pressure insoles.

In addition, the skier's boots were equipped with pressure insoles (Loadsol, Novel GmbH, Munich, Germany) that assessed the total ground reaction force acting perpendicular to the sole of the ski boot, the individual forces acting on the entire inside and outside foot and the distribution of force between the fore and rear foot. To assist analysis, all runs were also filmed at 50 Hz with a high-resolution camera (GC-PX100, The Japan Victor Company Ltd., Yokohama, Japan). To allow synchronization of all measurements, each skier performed three active squats and three hits with one of his skis on the ground before each start.

2.3. Computation

To match the frequency of the inertial system, the RTK GNSS system's captured trajectories at 20 Hz and the force measurements at 100 Hz were interpolated with cubic splines to 240 Hz. Following synchronization of the data collected by these three systems, these data were smoothed with the Rauch–Tung–Striebel algorithm [26], which utilizes a zero-lag two-way Kalman filter, in a manner similar to an earlier study [24]. The local coordinates provided by the inertial system were thereafter transformed into the global coordinates employed for RTK GNSS measurements by adding an extra node to the position of the RTK GNSS smart antenna. The data were subsequently transferred from Matlab R2016b (Mathworks, Natick, MA, USA) to the Visual 3D v6 software (C-Motion, Germantown, MD, USA), where the skier's center of mass (CoM) and the trajectory of the skis were calculated. The CoM was calculated utilizing Demster's regression equations [27], with inclusion of the mass of both the skiing and measuring equipment. The trajectory of the skis was defined as the arithmetic mean of the trajectories of the ankle joints [11].

The distance travelled and turn radius [7] were determined from the trajectory of the skis. From the trajectory of the CoM, the differential specific mechanical energy (i.e., the change in mechanical energy per unit change in altitude, normalized to the mass of the skier) [7] and mechanical energy for each specific section (normalized to the entrance speed) [5], which reflect instantaneous and sectional performance, respectively, were calculated. The definitions of both of these performance parameters mean that their values are negative when energy is dissipated. The flexion angles of the knee and hip joints on the left and right legs were provided directly by the inertial system. The angles of the inside and outside shanks, defined as the minimal tilt of the shank around the axis defined by the ski in relationship to the surface of the slope (Figure 3), were also calculated. Each turn was divided into initiation, steering and completion phases, as described previously [11] (Figure 1). To examine for temporal asymmetries, the left and right turning times were compared.

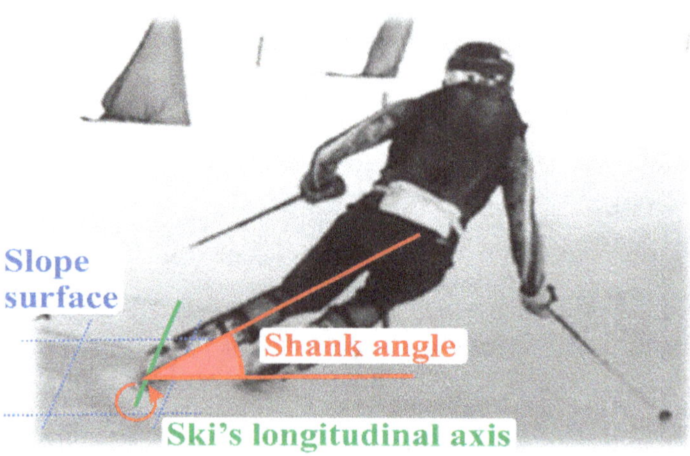

Figure 3. Photograph of a skier illustrating the angle of the shank.

Asymmetry between the left (L) and right (R) sides was expressed as the index SI = 1 − (|L − R|)/(L + R), where L and D represent the average values of parameters during the steering phase of the turn, with the exceptions of turn length, time, speed and sectional energy loss, which were determined for the entire turn. As an indicator of overall (as opposed to average) asymmetries throughout the entire turn, the Jaccard index (JI) [28] was also calculated. To obtain this index, the mean value and standard deviation of each parameter at each % of the turn were calculated. Then, the two curves obtained by adding or subtracting the standard deviation to the mean value were taken to represent the upper and lower boundaries, respectively, of the polygon delineating the turn. Thereafter, the overall JI was calculated as (A∩B)/(A∪B), where A and B represent the polygons associated with the left and right turns, respectively. In practice, when JI is equal to 1, the areas defined by the mean ± standard deviation boundaries for the left and right turns overlap entirely, whereas when JI is equal to zero, there is no overlap at all.

2.4. Statistical Analyses

All data are presented as mean values and standard deviations. The Shapiro–Wilk test was used to assess normality. Outliers detected employing standard Tukey's fences (1.5 interquartile range) were excluded from further analysis. A paired sample t-test was used for post hoc analysis of potential differences. In connection with the multivariable linear regression models, no more than two predictive (independent) variables were allowed. The dependent (predicted) variables were based on the objectives of the study related to performance (SI for turn time, turn length and average speed, and SI and JI for energy losses), while the independent (predictor) variables were related to skiing technique (SI and JI for the angles of flexion and inclination) and load (SI and JI for ground reaction forces). In connection with the multivariable linear regression models, no more than two predictive (independent) variables related to skiing technique (SI and JI for the angles of flexion and inclination) and load (SI and JI for ground reaction forces) were allowed, while the dependent (predicted) variables were related to performance (SI for turn time, turn length and average speed, and SI and JI for energy losses). All predictions in which G * Power (Faul et al., 2009, Heinrich University Heine Düsseldorf, Germany) was less than 0.8 were excluded. The level of statistical significance was set at $p < 0.05$. All statistical analyses were performed in the Matlab software.

3. Results

3.1. Descriptive Statistics, Symmetry and Jaccard Indices (SI and JI)

The descriptive statistics and symmetry indices for the independent variables (skiing technique and ground reaction forces) and dependent variables (skiing performance) during skiing are presented in Tables 1 and 2, respectively. In most cases, the differences in the independent variables during left and right turns were statistically insignificant (Table 1), the exception being GRF on the entire inside foot ($p < 0.05$). The mean symmetry indices (SI) for the independent variables related to skiing technique ranged from approximately 92 to 98%, with associated Jaccard indices (JI) during the steering phase ranging from approximately 29 to 53%. The corresponding values for the independent variables related to GRF ranged from approximately 85 to 98% and approximately 42 to 71%, respectively.

Table 1. The inclination, flexion of the joints and ground reaction forces (GRF) acting on various parts of the legs during the steering phase of left and right turns by elite slalom skiers, together with the corresponding symmetry (SI) and Jaccard (JI) indices (independent variables). All values presented are means ± standard deviations.

Variable	Left Turn	Right Turn	*p*-Value	SI [%]	JI [%]
Shank angle [°]					
Outside leg	30.8 ± 4.5	29.4 ± 4.6	0.49	93.8 ± 5.4	52.2 ± 19.5
Inside leg	33.2 ± 3.8	34.2 ± 2.4	0.84	92.8 ± 4.0	41.5 ± 16.2
Knee flexion [°]					
Outside leg	46.99 ± 8.9	52.20 ± 7.2	0.11	92.5 ± 4.4	28.7 ± 24.3
Inside leg	85.73 ± 9.3	81.25 ± 9.9	0.34	96.1 ± 2.2	39.1 ± 21.7
Hip flexion [°]					
Outside leg	37.4 ± 3.3	28.02 ± 3.0	0.70	95.71 ± 2.2	53.35 ± 14.9
Inside leg	71.8 ± 4.4	68.79 ± 5.5	0.22	97.52 ± 1.7	50.64 ± 15.5
GRF (pressure insoles) [% BW]					
On the entire foot					
Outside leg	126.2 ± 19.2	113.6 ± 21.6	0.21	92.9 ± 4.7	56.1 ± 18.9
Inside leg	66.8 ± 7.4	76.0 ± 10.0	0.04	91.4 ± 5.7	56.0 ± 19.6
On the fore foot [% BW]					
Outside leg	62.5 ± 20.6	58.7 ± 26.85	0.75	88.4 ± 8.4	47.2 ± 21.6
Inside leg	27.4 ± 9.2	37.8 ± 17.6	0.14	85.1 ± 10.1	42.7 ± 23.2
On the rear foot [% BW]					
Outside leg	63.8 ± 7.7	54.9 ± 16.6	0.17	87.8 ± 7.3	51.6 ± 14.4
Inside leg	39.4 ± 9.13	38.6 ± 15.8	0.85	85.8 ± 15.2	52.9 ± 23.2
GRF *					
Overall [% BW]	287.5 ± 26.3	283.7 ± 17.5	0.72	98.2 ± 1.1	71.3 ± 2.7

BW—body weight; SI—symmetry index; JI—Jaccard index; * approximated on the basis of the movement of the center of mass.

Moreover, none of the values for the dependent variables reflecting skiing performance differed significantly between the left and the right turns (Table 2). The mean SI for the dependent variables ranged from approximately 71% (in the case of instantaneous performance) to approximately 100% (average velocity). The nature of the parameters involved allowed the JI values to be calculated only for the turning radius and instantaneous performance during the steering phase as approximately 56% and 47%, respectively.

The patterns of the angle of the outside shank of all nine skiers during left and right turns, together with the corresponding JI during the steering phase (ranging from 14% for Skier I to 87% for Skier G), are shown in Figure 4. As depicted in the diagram, the mean angle of the outside shank during left and right turns differed during the entire steering phase for Skiers H and I, during the second half of the steering phase for Skiers B, D and E and during the first half of this phase in the case of Skier A. In contrast, the mean angle of the outside shank of Skier G was largely the same throughout the entire steering phase. With respect to the mean turning radius of left and right turns, most of the skiers demonstrated visible differences during the second half of the steering phase, with Skier G again being the exception (Figure 5). Moreover, the JI of 81% for the turning radius of Skier G was the largest observed, while the smallest JI of 56% in this regard was demonstrated by Skier C. Visually larger differences were observed between left and right turn instantaneous performance (Figure 6) with the JI ranging from 31% (Skier I) to 78% (Skier G).

Table 2. The time, trajectory, velocity and energy dissipation during left and right turns by elite slalom skiers, together with the corresponding symmetry (SI) and Jaccard indices (JI) (dependent variables). All values presented are means ± standard deviations.

Dependent Variable	Left Turn	Right Turn	*p*-Value	SI [%]	JI [%]
Time					
Turning time [s]	0.87 ± 0.03	0.87 ± 0.03	0.68	97.5 ± 1.7	*n*/a
Trajectory					
Turning length [m]	12.61 ± 0.30	12.51 ± 0.39	0.59	97.9 ± 1.5	*n*/a
Turningradius[m]	9.34 ± 0.44	9.32 ± 0.52	0.95	97.6 ± 1.5	56.1 ± 18.9
Velocity					
Average velocity [m/s]	14.5 ± 0.42	14.5 ± 0.37	0.97	99.6 ± 0.00	*n*/a
Energy associated with					
Instantaneous performance [J/kg/m]	−10.69 ± 4.67	−10.51 ± 2.98	0.92	70.6 ± 23.0	47.3 ± 14.1
Sectional performance [Js/kg/m]	−1.90 ± 0.39	−1.87 ± 0.50	0.91	84.2 ± 13.7	*n*/a

n/a—not applicable; SI—symmetry index; JI—Jaccard index.

3.2. *Multivariable Regression Models*

Altogether, our multivariable linear regression models, each involving no more than two predictor (independent) variables, included a total of 26 predictor and 8 predicted (dependent) variables. Models were discarded if the *p*-value was >0.05, $R^2 < 0.7$ or when the model's predictor coefficients did not differ significantly from 0 (t-statistic, $p < 0.05$). In addition, to restrict our analysis to results that could be meaningful, only the 13 models for which at least one of the predictor coefficient values was >0.1 are shown in Table 3. Of these, all included two independent variables, with the exception of Model #10, which only included one.

The largest predictor coefficients were associated with the SI values for instantaneous (differential specific mechanical energy) and sectional performance (mechanical energy for each specific section/turn normalized to the entrance speed) (Models #10–13, Table 3). The independent variables in Models #10 and 12 were related only to skiing technique, while those in Models #11 and 13 were related to skiing technique in combination with GRF. The remainder of the models had smaller predictive coefficients of 0.46 (Model #5) or lower, among which the coefficients for SI and JI for turning radius were largest (Models #4 and 5). Interestingly, the largest predictive coefficients obtained with Models #6–9, designed to predict the SI for average velocity, all corresponded to the SI for overall GRF.

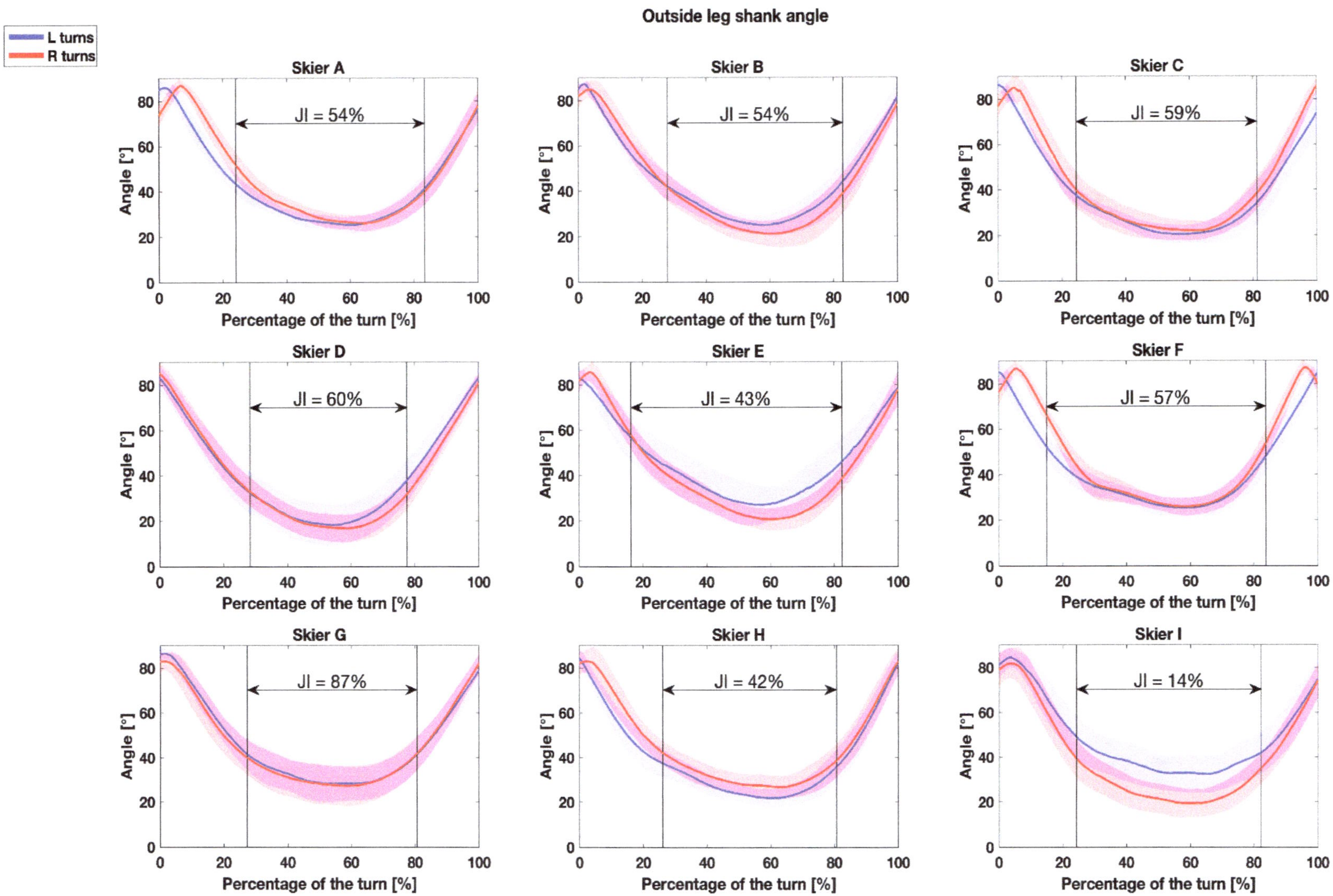

Figure 4. The angle of the outside shank of the 9 elite slalom skiers (**A–I**) during the steering phase of left and right turns, together with the corresponding Jaccard indices (JI). The two vertical lines indicate the beginning and end of the steering phase.

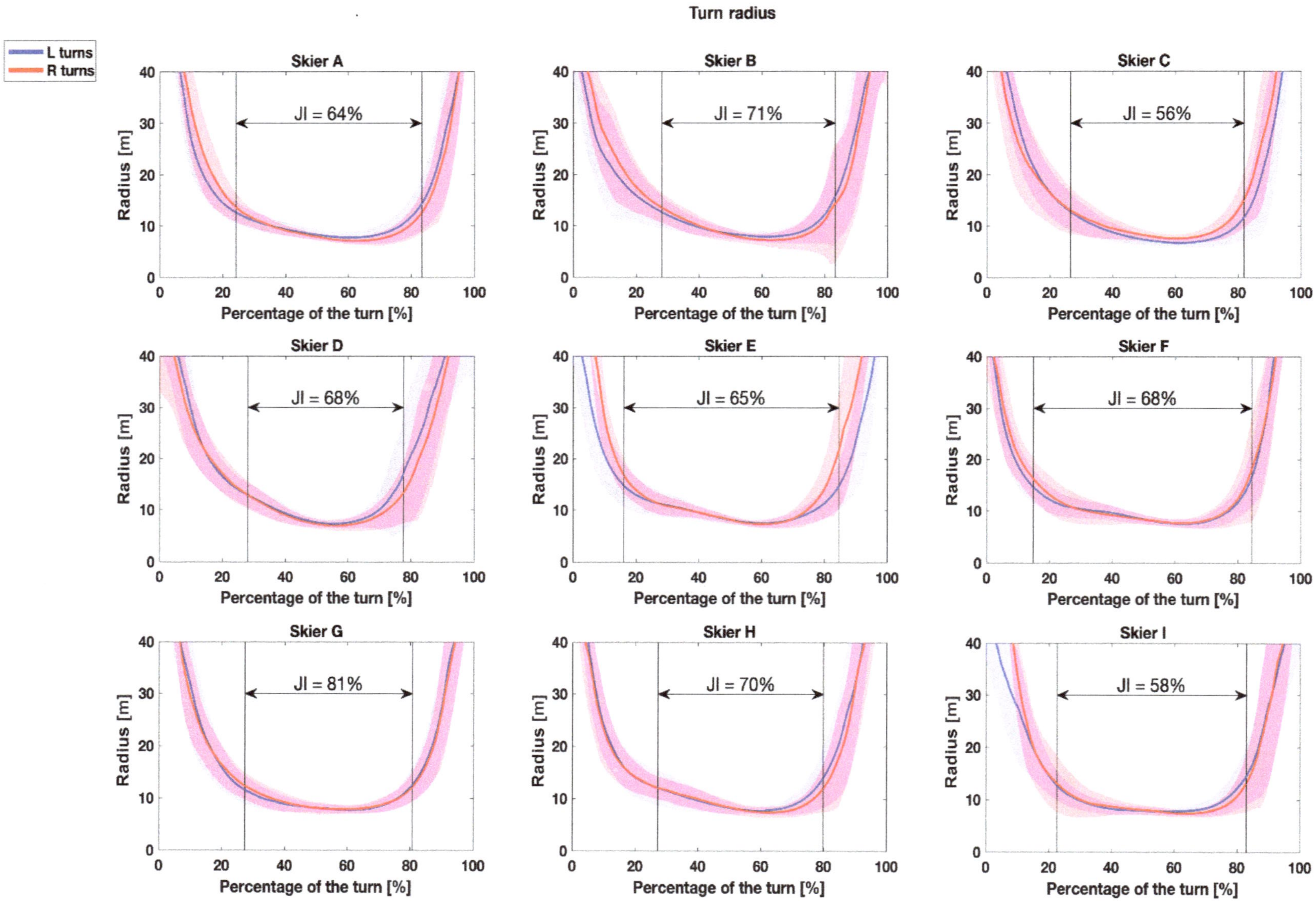

Figure 5. The turn radii during the steering phase of left and right turns by 9 elite slalom skiers (**A–I**) and corresponding Jaccard indices (JI). The two vertical lines indicate the beginning and end of the steering phase.

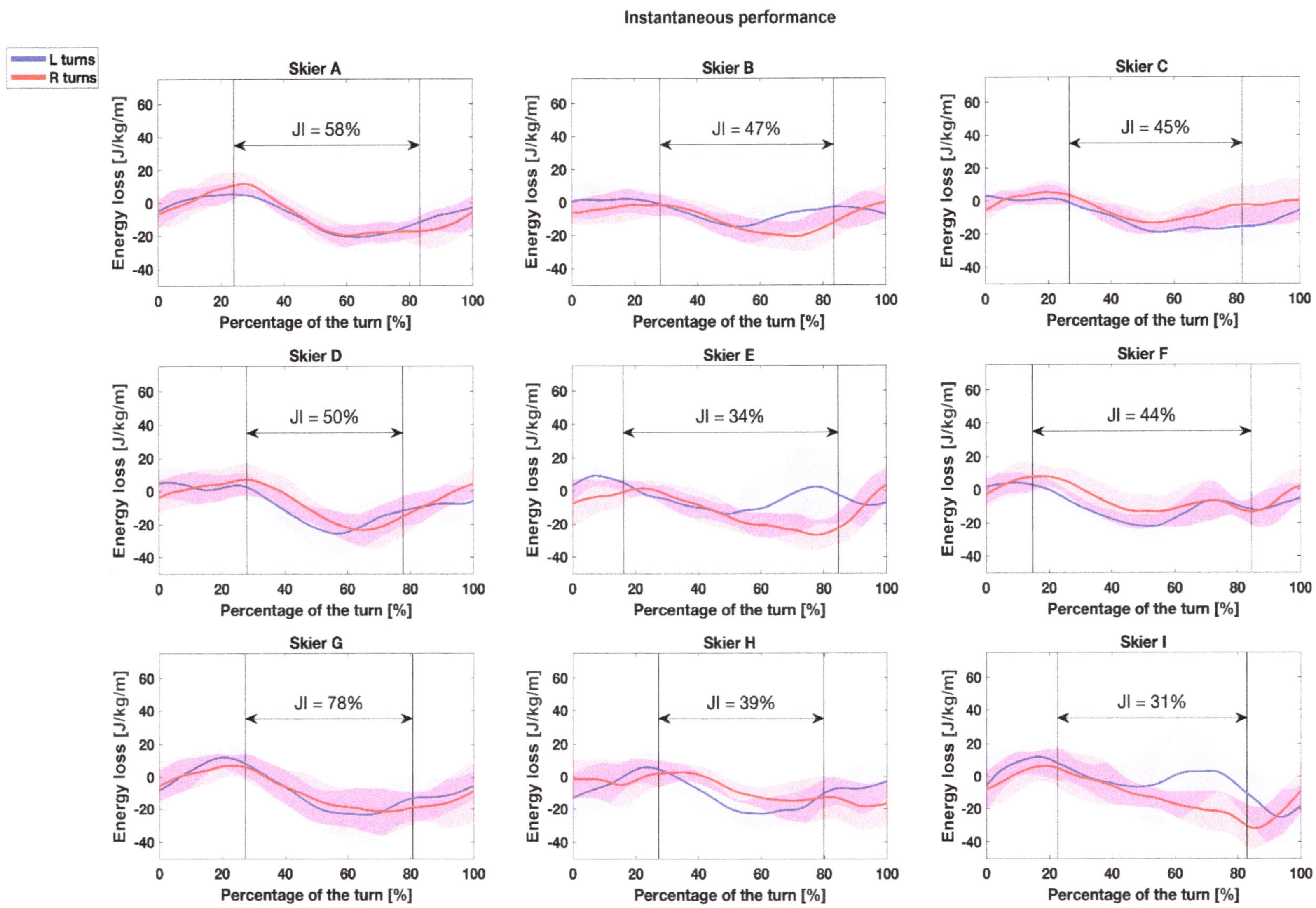

Figure 6. The instantaneous performance during the steering phase of left and right turns by 9 elite slalom skiers (**A–I**) and corresponding Jaccard indices (JI). The two vertical lines indicate the beginning and end of the steering phase. Instantaneous performance is defined as energy dissipation per change in altitude normalized relative to the mass of the skier and his equipment.

Table 3. Multivariable linear regression analysis of the relationships between the predicted (dependent, columns) and predictor (independent, rows) variables. The values in each column represent the coefficients of predictor variables.

Dependent Variables → Independent Variables ↓	SI for Turning Time	SI for Turning Length	JI for Turning *n* Radius	SI for Turning Radius	SI for Average Velocity	SI for Instantaneous Performance	SI for Sectional Performance
Shank angle							
JI for outside leg	-	-	$0.33^{**,\#4}$	-	-	-	-
SI for outside leg	-	-	-	-	-	$3.97^{***,\#10}$	$3.01^{**,\#13}$
JI for inside leg	$0.08^{*,\#1}$	$0.07^{**,\#2}$	-	-	-	-	-
SI for inside leg	-	-	-	-	-	$5.77^{**,\#11}$, $7.16^{**,\#12}$	-
Hip flexion							
JI for outside leg	-	-	-	$-0.10^{*,\#5}$	$0.01^{*,\#6}$	-	-
SI for outside leg	-	-	-	-	$0.09^{*,\#7}$	$8.33^{*,\#12}$	-
GRF on entire foot [a]							
JI for GRF outside leg	-	-	$0.25^{*,\#4}$	-	-	-	-
SI for GRF outside leg	-	-	-	$0.46^{**,\#5}$	-	-	-
SI for GRF inside leg	$0.14^{*,\#1}$	$0.13^{**,\#2}$, $0.11^{*,\#3}$	-	-	-	-	-
JI for GRF inside leg	-	-	-	-	-	-	$0.56^{*,\#13}$
GRF on rear foot [a]							
JI for outside leg	-	-	-	-	$-0.02^{**,\#8}$	$-1.03^{**,\#11}$	-
SI for GRF outside leg	-	-	-	-	$-0.03^{**,\#9}$	-	-
Overall GRF [b]							
JI	-	$0.16^{*,\#3}$	-	-	-	-	-
SI	-	-	-	-	$0.10^{*,\#6}$, $0.12^{**,\#7}$, $0.15^{**,\#8}$, $0.16^{**,\#9}$	-	-
R^2	$0.72^{*,\#1}$	$0.80^{**,\#2}$, $0.75^{*,\#3}$	$0.80^{**,\#4}$	$0.74^{*,\#5}$	$0.73^{*,\#6}$, $0.81^{**,\#7}$, $0.84^{**,\#8}$, $0.83^{**,\#9}$	$0.86^{***,\#10}$, $0.82^{**,\#11}$, $0.84^{**,\#12}$	$0.76^{**,\#13}$

* —$p \leq 0.05$, ** —$p \leq 0.01$; *** —$p \leq 0.001$; # *n*—multivariable regression model number; GRF—ground reaction force; SI—symmetry index, JI—Jaccard index; [a] determined by pressure insoles; [b] approximated on the basis of the movements of the center of mass.

4. Discussion

The major novel finding here was confirmation of the hypothesis that asymmetries in technique and ground reaction forces are associated with asymmetries in the performance of elite, competitive slalom skiers. More specifically, (i) asymmetries in instantaneous and sectional performance were associated with the largest predictor coefficients for asymmetry in the angle of the shank and hip flexion on the outside leg; and (ii) asymmetry in turning radius demonstrated the largest predictor coefficients for asymmetry in the angle of the shank and GRF on the entire foot of the outside leg.

Our descriptive statistics showed that, on average, these elite alpine skiers performed left and right turns quite symmetrically (Tables 1 and 2), with the only statistically significant difference between these turns being the GRF on the entire foot of the inside leg. In particular, the average mean values for performance were almost identical for the left and right turns (Table 2). Furthermore, the symmetrical indices (SI) were all above 84% (sectional performance), except for instantaneous performance (70%).

This symmetry, which in light of the very small differences in performance of elite alpine skiers [9,29,30] was not unexpected, confirmed that our experimental setup was well suited for observing differences between left and right turns. Previously, the differences in the GRF and temporal parameters associated with left and right slalom turns by highly skilled ski instructors were also reported to be non-significant [23]. Similarly, the mean difference in strength between the dominant and non-dominant legs of elite Austrian alpine skiers was also small [31].

In the present case, the only SI that was markedly lower concerned instantaneous performance (70.6%). Overall, sectional and instantaneous performance demonstrated the most pronounced asymmetries, which was the initial rationale for employing these as measures of alpine skiing performance [5,7,30]. In giant slalom as well, utilization of energy-based performance over an entire section was found to be a valuable measure of performance [9].

However, the Jaccard indices (JI) revealed much more pronounced asymmetry between left and right turns, with the lowest value being only 28.6% (for flexion of the outside knee) and the highest 71.3% (for the overall GRF) (Table 1). The lowest individual JI value for the angle of the outside shank was only 14% (Skier I, Figure 4) and during the steering phase, a difference between left and right turns by this skier was clearly visible. This same skier exhibited the lowest JI for instantaneous performance (Figure 6) and the second lowest for turning radius (Figure 5). At the same time for Skier G, the largest JI for the angle of the outside shank (Figure 4) was associated with the largest JI values for both turning radius (Figure 5) and instantaneous performance (Figure 6). The dependence of sectional and instantaneous performance on the SI for the angles of both the inside and outside shank received further support from the multivariable regression analysis (Models #10–13, Table 3). Similarly, the JI for turning radius proved to be dependent on the corresponding value for the angle of the outside shank (Model #4, Table 3), an observation which in itself clearly demonstrates that asymmetry in technique is associated with asymmetry in performance. Such a relationship is not entirely unexpected, since according to the theory of carving skiing, the inclination of the ski is related to turning radius [32] and, moreover, in the case of slalom skiing, turning radius is related to instantaneous performance [5].

The SI for turning radius was not dependent on the SI for the angle of the outside shank. This independence demonstrates that the mean turn values taken into consideration when calculating SI did not take the profound turn cycle information into account as was the case with JI values in Model #4 (Table 3). The SI for turning radius was negatively correlated with the JI for flexion of the outside hip (predictor coefficient −0.10, Model #5, Table 3). This negative association means that less pronounced asymmetry in flexion of the outside hip should correspond to more asymmetry in the turning radius, an observation that we were unable to explain at present.

The predictor coefficients for JI and SI for the GRF acting on the entire foot of the outside leg were also relatively large in connection with the JI and SI for the turning radius (Models #4 and 5, Table 3). This finding can be explained by the action of radial forces, whose basic biomechanical modeling has shown to be dependent on the turning radius [32,33]. In this context, it is important to emphasize that only the GRF acting on the outside leg, not the overall GRF, was a predictor in the multivariable models. Indeed, in a previous study [5], this overall GRF did not differ between better and poorer slalom skiers. However, in the present investigation, the SI for average velocity was dependent on the corresponding value for the overall GRF in combination with several other "less important" variables with small predictor coefficients (Models #6–9, Table 3). This particularly interesting finding reveals that despite the virtually identical average velocity and overall GRF associated with left and right turns by our elite skiers, the asymmetries in these variables were actually large enough to demonstrate related dependency in the multivariable models (Tables 1 and 2).

The largest predictor coefficients observed in our multivariable models concerned the dependence of the SI for instantaneous performance on the combination of the SI values for the angle of the inside shank and flexion of the outside hip (Model #12, Table 3). The only apparent explanation for this dependency is the speculation that skiing technique influenced how smoothly the skis glide, (e.g., the attack angle defined as the angle between the longitudinal axis of the ski and the ski's center point's velocity vector projected onto a plane parallel to the surface of the snow) [14]) and/or the distribution of pressure under the ski and thereby the ski–snow interaction [34]. Either or both of these influences could exert an impact on energy dissipation.

Finally, some of the symmetry indices (SI) observed here, such as those for turning time, turn length and sectional performance, were dependent on various parameters related to the asymmetry of the inside leg (Models #1–3 and 13). This indicates that asymmetries in performance were also associated with the behavior of the inside leg, which has earlier been suggested to only play a role in maintaining stability while skiing [35]. Ski coaches already pay special attention to the inside leg in connection with training to optimize performance, but our findings provide the first experimental evidence that this is a valid concern.

Although the current investigation was extensive, assessing the full-body three-dimensional kinematics and GRF in connection with 720 slalom turns, like all studies, has certain limitations. Although some researchers question the reliability of inertial measurement systems and GNSS and/or pressure insoles, their reliability for in-field measurements on alpine skiers has already been demonstrated [23–25,35–39] and, moreover, we utilized state-of-the-art technology in this respect, i.e., one of the most up-to-date and accurate Leica Geosystems RTK GNSS systems and the latest version of the Xsens inertial motion capture hardware. However, since it was not possible to install an inertial sensor on a foot in a ski boot, we were unable to monitor flexion of the ankle joint. It would have been possible to measure bending of the ski boot, but this does not entirely reflect the more complicated three-dimensional behavior of the ankle joint (i.e., technique).

In addition, although GRF can certainly be measured most accurately with dynamometers/force-plates [40], the size and weight of these devices disturb the skiing equipment and, thereby, the performance of the skier. To avoid this, we used pressure insoles here, which do not always indicate the magnitude of GRF accurately [41]. On the other hand, direct measurement of the pressure on the soles, an important parameter when skiing [23,35], is especially useful for dealing with asymmetries in pressure on different parts of the foot. To assess a more precise magnitude of the GRF, we performed biomechanical modeling of this parameter based on the acceleration of the center of mass monitored by three-dimensional kinematics, as in our previous studies [11,42].

As is true of virtually all studies on alpine skiing, generalization of our present results, despite the relatively large size of our study population, is not straightforward. The snow, terrain and weather were nearly ideal during our testing and similar studies under varying conditions are now required.

5. Conclusions

In conclusion, the application of descriptive statistical analysis to left and right turns by elite slalom skiers revealed that with respect to technique, ground reaction forces and performance, these turns were quite symmetrical, with the only significant difference being related to the mean GRF on the entire inside foot. Furthermore, all symmetry indices for skiing technique and performance were >92%, with the exception of those for instantaneous (70.6%) and sectional performance (84.2%), demonstrating the relevance of these latter two parameters in connection with the analysis of skiing asymmetry. The Jaccard index, which takes into account behavior within the turn cycle, was found to be more sensitive to asymmetries than the symmetry index, which is based solely on the mean values of the parameters. Although the movements of elite slalom skiers were found to be quite symmetrical, this is the first demonstration that asymmetry in their skiing technique and ground reaction forces influences asymmetry in their performance. These findings constitute experimental support for the efforts of coaches to achieve symmetrical skiing technique, not only in order to decrease the risk of injury [31], but also to optimize overall performance.

Author Contributions: Conceptualization, M.S. and H.-C.H.; methodology, M.S. and J.O.; formal analysis, J.O. and M.S.; data collection and handling, M.S. and J.O.; writing—preparation of the first draft, M.S.; writing—review and editing, all authors; visualization, J.O. and M.S.; supervision, M.S.; project administration, M.S.; funding acquisition, H.-C.H. and N.Š. All authors have read and agreed to the published version of the manuscript.

Acknowledgments: The authors would like to sincerely thank all the skiers and their coaches for their helpful cooperation. Many thanks also to Alessandro Galloppini and Mads Kjær Madsen Mads for their help with the data collection and to Uwe Kersting for performing inertial motion capture.

References

1. Supej, M.; Cernigoj, M. Relations between different technical and tactical approaches and overall time at men's world cup giant slalom races. *Kinesiol. Slov.* **2006**, *12*, 63–69.
2. Supej, M.; Holmberg, H.C. A new time measurement method using a high-end global navigation satellite system to analyze alpine skiing. *Res. Q. Exerc. Sport* **2011**, *82*, 400–411. [CrossRef] [PubMed]
3. Fasel, B.; Spörri, J.; Kröll, J.; Müller, E.; Aminian, K. A Magnet-Based Timing Tystem to Detect Gate Crossings in Alpine Ski Racing. *Sensors* **2019**, *19*, 940. [CrossRef]
4. Supej, M. Gate-to-Gate Synchronized Comparison of Velocity Retrieved from a High-End Global Navigation Satellite System in Alpine Skiing. In Proceedings of the 28th International Conference on Biomechanics in Sports, Melbourne, Australia, 2–6 July 2012.
5. Supej, M.; Kipp, R.; Holmberg, H.C. Mechanical parameters as predictors of performance in alpine World Cup slalom racing. *Scand. J. Med. Sci. Sports* **2011**, *21*, e72–e81. [CrossRef] [PubMed]
6. Hébert-Losier, K.; Supej, M.; Holmberg, H.C. Biomechanical factors influencing the performance of elite alpine ski racers. *Sports Med.* **2014**, *44*, 519–533. [CrossRef] [PubMed]
7. Supej, M. Differential specific mechanical energy as a quality parameter in racing alpine skiing. *J. Appl. Biomech.* **2008**, *24*, 121–129. [CrossRef]
8. Federolf, P.A. Quantifying instantaneous performance in alpine ski racing. *J. Sports Sci.* **2012**, *30*, 1063–1068. [CrossRef] [PubMed]
9. Spörri, J.; Kröll, J.; Schwameder, H.; Müller, E. The role of path length- and speed-related factors for the enhancement of section performance in alpine giant slalom. *Eur. J. Sport Sci.* **2018**, *18*, 911–919. [CrossRef]
10. Supej, M.; Nedergaard, N.J.; Nord, J.; Holmberg, H.C. The impact of start strategy on start performance in alpine skiing exists on flat, but not on steep inclines. *J. Sports Sci.* **2019**, *37*, 647–655. [CrossRef]
11. Supej, M.; Holmberg, H.C. How gate setup and turn radii influence energy dissipation in slalom ski racing. *J. Appl. Biomech.* **2010**, *26*, 454–464. [CrossRef]
12. Supej, M.; Kugovnik, O.; Nemec, B. New advances in racing slalom technique. *Kinesiol. Slov.* **2002**, *8*, 25–29.
13. Supej, M.; Kugovnik, O.; Nemec, B. Modelling and simulation of two competition slalom techniques. *Kinesiology* **2004**, *36*, 206–212.
14. Reid, R.C.; Haugen, P.; Gilgien, M.; Kipp, R.W.; Smith, G.A. Alpine Ski Motion Characteristics in Slalom. *Front. Sports Act. Living* **2020**, *2*. [CrossRef]
15. Meyer, F.; Le Pelley, D.; Borrani, F. Aerodynamic drag modeling of alpine skiers performing giant slalom turns. *Med. Sci. Sports Exerc.* **2012**, *44*, 1109–1115. [CrossRef]

16. Supej, M.; Sætran, L.; Oggiano, L.; Ettema, G.; Šarabon, N.; Nemec, B.; Holmberg, H.C. Aerodynamic drag is not the major determinant of performance during giant slalom skiing at the elite level. *Scand. J. Med. Sci. Sports* **2013**, *23*, e38–e47. [CrossRef]
17. Gilgien, M.; Kröll, J.; Spörri, J.; Crivelli, P.; Müller, E. Application of dGNSS in alpine ski racing: Basis for evaluating physical demands and safety. *Front. Physiol.* **2018**, *9*, 145. [CrossRef]
18. Federolf, P.; Scheiber, P.; Rauscher, E.; Schwameder, H.; Lüthi, A.; Rhyner, H.U.; Müller, E. Impact of skier actions on the gliding times in alpine skiing. *Scand. J. Med. Sci. Sports* **2008**, *18*, 790–797. [CrossRef] [PubMed]
19. Maloney, S.J. The Relationship Between Asymmetry and Athletic Performance: A Critical Review. *J. Strength Cond. Res.* **2019**, *33*, 2579–2593. [CrossRef]
20. Bell, D.R.; Sanfilippo, J.L.; Binkley, N.; Heiderscheit, B.C. Lean mass asymmetry influences force and power asymmetry during jumping in collegiate athletes. *J. Strength Cond. Res.* **2014**, *28*, 884–891. [CrossRef]
21. Hoffman, J.R.; Ratamess, N.A.; Klatt, M.; Faigenbaum, A.D.; Kang, J. Do bilateral power deficits influence direction-specific movement patterns? *Res. Sports Med.* **2007**, *15*, 125–132. [CrossRef]
22. Beck, O.N.; Azua, E.N.; Grabowski, A.M. Step time asymmetry increases metabolic energy expenditure during running. *Eur. J. Appl. Physiol.* **2018**, *118*, 2147–2154. [CrossRef]
23. Vaverka, F.; Vodickova, S. Laterality of the lower limbs and carving turn. *Biol.Sport* **2010**, *27*, 129–134. [CrossRef]
24. Supej, M. 3D measurements of alpine skiing with an inertial sensor motion capture suit and GNSS RTK system. *J. Sports Sci.* **2010**, *28*, 759–769. [CrossRef]
25. Krüger, A.; Edelmann-Nusser, J. Application of a full body inertial measurement system in alpine skiing: A comparison with an optical video based system. *J. Appl. Biomech.* **2010**, *26*, 516–521. [CrossRef]
26. Rauch, H.E.; Tung, F.; Striebel, C.T. Maximum likelihood estimates of linear dynamic systems. *AIAA J.* **1965**, *3*, 1445–1450. [CrossRef]
27. Dempster, W.T. *Space Requirements of the Seated Operator: Geometrical, Kinematic, and Mechanical Aspects of the Body with Special Reference to the Limbs*; Wright Air Development Center: Wright-Patterson Air Force Base, OH, USA, 1955.
28. Jaccard, P. Distribution florale dans une portio des Alpes du Jura. *Bull. Soc. Vaud. Sc. Nat.* **1901**, *37*, 547–579. [CrossRef]
29. Gilgien, M.; Reid, R.; Raschner, C.; Supej, M.; Holmberg, H.C. The Training of Olympic Alpine Ski Racers. *Front. Physiol.* **2018**, *9*, 1772. [CrossRef]
30. Supej, M.; Holmberg, H.C. Recent Kinematic and Kinetic Advances in Olympic Alpine Skiing: Pyeongchang and Beyond. *Front. Physiol.* **2019**, *10*, 111. [CrossRef]
31. Steidl-Muller, L.; Hildebrandt, C.; Muller, E.; Fink, C.; Raschner, C. Limb symmetry index in competitive alpine ski racers: Reference values and injury risk identification according to age-related performance levels. *J. Sport Health Sci.* **2018**, *7*, 405–415. [CrossRef] [PubMed]
32. Howe, J. *The New Skiing Mechanics: Including the Technology of Short Radius Carved Turn Skiing and the Claw Ski*; McIntire: Waterford, Ireland, 2001.
33. Lind, D.A.; Sanders, S.P. *The Physics of Skiing: Skiing at the Triple Point*; Springer: New York, NY, USA, 2013.
34. Federolf, P.; Roos, M.; Lüthi, A.; Dual, J. Finite element simulation of the ski–snow interaction of an alpine ski in a carved turn. *Sports Eng.* **2010**, *12*, 123–133. [CrossRef]
35. Falda-Buscaiot, T.; Hintzy, F.; Rougier, P.; Lacouture, P.; Coulmy, N. Influence of slope steepness, foot position and turn phase on plantar pressure distribution during giant slalom alpine ski racing. *PLoS ONE* **2017**, *12*, e0176975. [CrossRef]
36. Zorko, M.; Nemec, B.; Babic, J.; Lesnik, B.; Supej, M. The waist width of skis influences the kinematics of the knee joint in alpine skiing. *J. Sports Sci. Med.* **2015**, *14*, 606–619. [PubMed]
37. Spörri, J.; Kröll, J.; Fasel, B.; Aminian, K.; Müller, E. Course setting as a prevention measure for overuse injuries of the back in alpine ski racing: A kinematic and kinetic study of giant slalom and slalom. *Orthop. J. Sports Med.* **2016**, *4*, 2325967116630719. [CrossRef] [PubMed]
38. Spörri, J.; Kröll, J.; Fasel, B.; Aminian, K.; Müller, E. Standing Height as a Prevention Measure for Overuse Injuries of the Back in Alpine Ski Racing: A Kinematic and Kinetic Study of Giant Slalom. *Orthop. J. Sports Med.* **2018**, *6*, 2325967117747843. [CrossRef]
39. Spörri, J.; Kröll, J.; Haid, C.; Fasel, B.; Müller, E. Potential mechanisms leading to overuse injuries of the back in alpine ski racing: A descriptive biomechanical study. *Am. J. Sports Med.* **2015**, *43*, 2042–2048. [CrossRef]

40. Lüthi, A.; Federolf, M.; Fauve, M.; Oberhofer, K.; Rhyner, H.; Ammann, W.; Stricker, G.; Shiefermüller, C.; Eitzlmair, E.; Schwameder, H.; et al. Determination of forces in carving using three independent methods. In *Science and Skiing III*; Müller, E., Bacharach, D., Klika, R., Lindinger, S., Schwameder, H., Eds.; Meyer & Meyer Sport: Oxford, UK, 2005; pp. 96–106.
41. Stricker, G.; Scheiber, P.; Lindenhofer, E.; Müller, E. Determination of forces in alpine skiing and snowboarding: Validation of a mobile data acquisition system. *Eur. J. Sport Sci.* **2010**, *10*, 31–41. [CrossRef]
42. Supej, M.; Hébert-Losier, K.; Holmberg, H.C. Impact of the steepness of the slope on the biomechanics of World Cup slalom skiers. *Int. J. Sports Physiol. Perform.* **2015**, *10*, 361–368. [CrossRef]

5

Does Beef Protein Supplementation Improve Body Composition and Exercise Performance?

Pedro L. Valenzuela [1], Fernando Mata [2], Javier S. Morales [3], Adrián Castillo-García [4] and Alejandro Lucia [3,*]

[1] Department of Systems Biology, University of Alcalá, 28805 Madrid, Spain; pedrol.valenzuela@edu.uah.es
[2] NutriScience, Nutrition & Health Sciences, 14002 Córdoba, Spain; fernando.mata@nutriscience.pt
[3] Faculty of Sport Sciences, Universidad Europea de Madrid and Research Institute 'i+12' (Hospital 12 de Octubre), 28670 Madrid, Spain; javiersalvador.morales@universidadeuropea.es
[4] Fissac-Physiology, health and physical activity, 28015 Madrid, Spain; castillogarcia.adrian@gmail.com
* Correspondence: alejandro.lucia@universidadeuropea.es

Abstract: Protein supplementation might improve body composition and exercise performance. Supplements containing whey protein (WP) have received the most attention, but other protein sources such as beef protein (BP) are gaining popularity. We conducted a systematic review and meta-analysis of randomized controlled trials that compared the effects of exercise training combined with BP, WP or no protein supplementation (NP), on body composition or exercise performance. Secondary endpoints included intervention effects on total protein intake and hematological parameters. Seven studies (n = 270 participants) were included. No differences were found between BP and WP for total protein intake (standardized mean difference (SMD) = 0.04, p = 0.892), lean body mass (LBM) (SMD = −0.01, p = 0.970) or fat mass (SMD = 0.07, p = 0.760). BP significantly increased total daily protein intake (SMD = 0.68, p < 0.001), LBM (SMD = 0.34, p = 0.049) and lower-limb muscle strength (SMD = 0.40, p = 0.014) compared to NP, but no significant differences were found between both conditions for fat mass (SMD = 0.15, p = 0.256), upper-limb muscle strength (SMD = 0.16, p = 0.536) or total iron intake (SMD = 0.29, p = 0.089). In summary, BP provides similar effects to WP on protein intake and body composition and, compared to NP, might be an effective intervention to increase total daily protein intake, LBM and lower-limb muscle strength.

Keywords: resistance training; exercise; nutrition; muscle mass; hypertrophy

---

1. Introduction

Protein supplementation might increase muscle anabolism and, if combined with exercise training, could also improve physical performance [1–3]. The anabolic response to protein intake can be affected not only by factors such as individual nutritional state, digestive/absorption capacity, or sensitivity of muscle anabolic pathways, but also by the source of protein [4]. In this regard, numerous protein sources have been investigated for their effect on muscle anabolism, including milk [5], eggs [6], soy [7], rice [8] or bovine colostrum [9]. Although supplements containing whey protein (WP) have received the most attention due to their high content in leucine and potential anabolic effect [10,11], beef protein (BP) has gained popularity in recent years [12].

Acute ingestion of BP can increase muscle protein synthesis in both young and older individuals [13–15], and these benefits seem to be maximized when combined with exercise training (particularly resistance training) [16]. There is thus biological rationale to support BP supplementation as a potentially effective strategy for improving lean body mass (LBM) and physical performance (notably, muscle strength). However, the evidence on the effectiveness of BP supplementation for increasing muscle mass or performance is mixed, with some studies reporting benefits compared to no protein supplementation [17,18] but others finding no such benefits [19,20]. Moreover, the effectiveness of BP for improving body composition or performance compared to WP remains unclear [18,19,21,22].

On the other hand, owing to its high content in heme iron, BP supplementation could also increase total iron intake and thus theoretically benefit hematological parameters, and indeed some benefits have been reported [20,22]. However, to our knowledge, there is not yet meta-analytical evidence on the potential benefits of BP supplementation.

Given the purported benefits of BP supplementation on body composition and performance, and the lack of consensus on its actual effectiveness, the main aim of this systematic review and meta-analysis was to compare the effects of BP, WP or no protein supplementation (NP) combined with exercise training on body composition and exercise performance. Changes in nutritional intake and hematological parameters were also analyzed as secondary endpoints.

2. Materials and Methods

The conduct and reporting of the current systematic review and meta-analysis conform to the Preferred Reporting Items for Systematic Reviews and Meta-Analyses (PRISMA) [23].

2.1. Systematic Search

Relevant articles were identified by title and abstract in the electronic databases MEDLINE, Web of Science and SportDiscus (since inception to 5 May 2019) using the following search strategy: (beef OR meat) AND (supplement*) AND (athlet* OR train* OR "physical activity" OR exercise). The electronic search was supplemented by a manual review of reference lists from relevant publications and reviews to find additional publications on the subject. Gray literature (abstracts, conference proceedings or editorials) and reviews were excluded.

2.2. Study Selection and Data Extraction

Studies were eligible for inclusion if they met each of the following criteria: (a) analyzed the effect of BP supplementation on at least one endpoint related to body composition or exercise performance; (b) duration of the exercise training + supplementation intervention ≥4 weeks; (c) used a randomized controlled trial design that included one group performing exercise training in combination with BP supplementation and 1+ groups performing the same exercise program as those receiving BP, but with WP or NP. Case studies were excluded, as well as those in which BP was combined with WP or other protein/'anabolic' supplements (e.g., creatine).

Two reviewers (P.L.V. and F.M.) independently extracted the following data from each study: number of participants within each group, participants' characteristics, exercise and nutritional intervention's characteristics, endpoints, measurement methods and results. Disagreements were resolved through discussion with a third reviewer (J.S.M.).

Endpoints data were registered as mean and standard deviation (SD). When the standard error of the mean (SEM) but not the SD was available, the latter was calculated from the square root of the sample size multiplied by the SEM. If data were provided as a figure, we used a specific software (WebPlotDigitalizer 4.2, San Francisco, CA, USA) for data extraction. We contacted the authors when necessary to request additional information. In this regard, the authors of two studies [17,19] provided us with the required specific data upon request. Fat-free mass was taken as a surrogate of LBM if the latter was not reported.

2.3. Quality Assessment

Study quality was evaluated using the 'risk-of-bias' assessment tool following the recommendations by the Cochrane Handbook for Systematic Reviews of Interventions [24]. Two authors (A.C.G. and

J.S.M.) analyzed the following criteria: random sequence generation and allocation concealment (selection bias), blinding of participants and research staff to group allocation (performance bias), blinding of outcome assessor (detection bias), incomplete outcome data (attrition bias), and selective reporting (reporting bias). Quality assessment by both reviewers was compared and disagreements in scores were resolved through discussion with a third reviewer (P.L.V.).

2.4. Statistical Analysis

We performed a meta-analysis when a minimum of three studies compared the effects (pre- and post-intervention data) of BP vs. WP or NP for a given endpoint. The pooled standardized mean difference (SMD) between interventions (post- *minus* pre-intervention data) and 95% confidence interval (CI) were computed using a random effects model. A conservative Pearson' r value of 0.7 was used for the computation of the within-group SD [25], and a sensitivity analysis (r = 0.2, 0.5 or 0.9) was then performed when a significant result was found. Begg's test was used to determine the presence of publication bias. We considered that the analysis of an outcome was at risk of bias when Begg's test was significant (i.e., $p < 0.05$). The Q and I^2 statistics were used to assess heterogeneity between studies. I^2 values of 25, 50, and 75% were considered reflective of low, moderate, and large heterogeneity, respectively.

All statistical analyses were performed using the statistical software package Comprehensive Meta-analyis 2.0 (Biostat; Englewood, NJ, USA) setting the level of significance at 0.05.

3. Results

3.1. Included Studies

From the retrieved articles, seven (including 270 participants in total) [17–22,26] met all inclusion criteria and were included in the systematic review (Figure 1, Table 1).

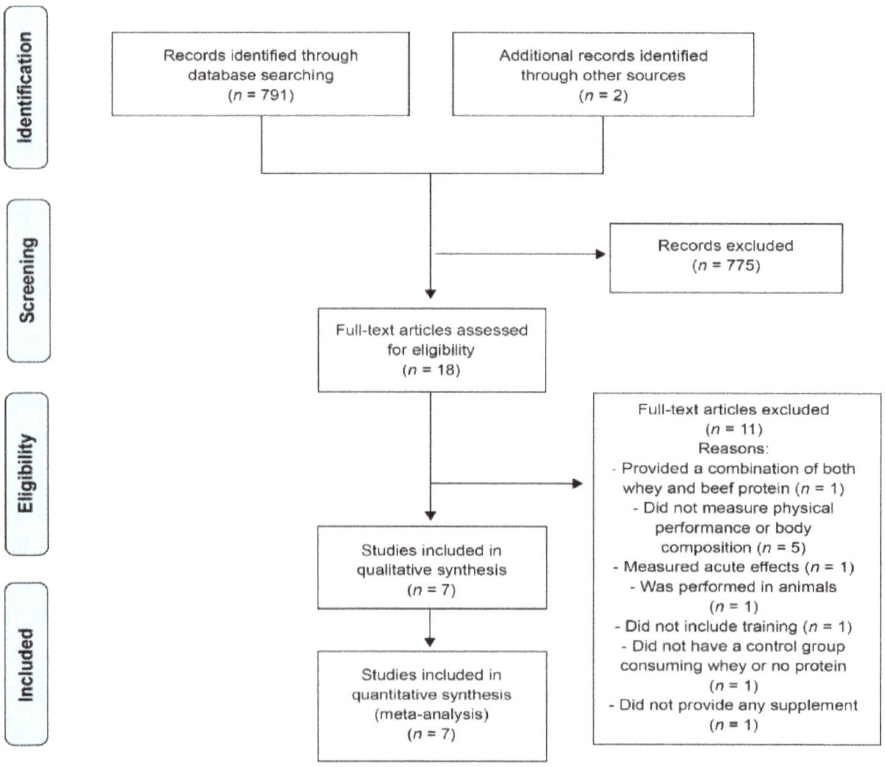

Figure 1. Flow chart of literature search.

Table 1. Main characteristics of the included studies.

Study	Participants and Group Assignment	Duration	Exercise Training Protocol (Common to all Study Groups)	Baseline Protein Intake	BP Group	WP Group	NP Group	Additional Group	Measurements	Main Outcomes
Burke et al. [20]	28 runners (18–24 years, 14 female) stratified by iron status, use of iron supplements, and gender, and randomized into a BP (*n* = 14) or NP group (*n* = 14)	8 weeks	Maintained their typical exercise regime	~1.7 g/kg/day	255 g of lean beef supplement per week + multivitamin daily	–	Multivitamin daily	–	-Dietary intake -Blood analysis -Body composition (plethysmography) -VO_{2max}	-No differences in body composition -↑heme iron intake in females -↑hematocrit in females -No differences in VO_{2max}
Daly et al. [17]	100 females (60–90 years) randomized into a BP (*n* = 53) or NP group (*n* = 47)	4 months	RT 2 times per week	~1.1–1.3 g/kg/day	220 g lean red meat (45 g protein) 6 days per week + 1 vitamin D3 capsule (1000-IU) daily	–	1 serving pasta or rice daily (25–35 g CHO) + 1 vitamin D3 capsule (1000-IU) daily	–	-Dietary intake -Physical activity -Body composition (DXA) -Muscle and fat CSA and muscle density (peripheral quantitative computed tomography) -Muscle function (TUG, FSST, and 30-s STS) -Strength (1RM estimated from 3 RM) -Blood analysis	-↑Protein intake -↑LBM -↑Leg LBM -No differences in BMD -↑Muscle strength -No differences in muscle function. -↑IGF-I -↓IL-6 -No differences in blood lipids or blood pressure.
Naclerio et al. [21]	24 active males (~26–29 years) randomized into a BP, WP or NP group (*n*=8 each)	8 weeks	RT 3 times per week	~1.5 g/kg/day	20 g of beef supplement (16.4 g protein) + 250 mL of orange juice per day	20 g of WP + 250 mL of orange juice per day	20 g of CHO + 250 mL of orange juice per day	–	-Body composition (plethysmography) -Limb circumference -Strength (1 RM) -Muscle thickness (ultrasound)	-↑*biceps brachialis* thickness -No differences in limb circumference or body composition. -No differences in strength.
Naclerio et al. [22]	24 male master triathletes (35–60 years) randomized into a BP, WP or NP group (*n* = 8 each)	10 weeks	ET 4–6 times per week	~1.3–1.5 g/kg/day	20 g of beef supplement (16.4 g protein) per day	20 g of WP per day	20 g of CHO per day	–	-Body composition (plethysmography) -VO_{2max} -Muscle thickness (ultrasound) -Blood analysis	-No differences in body composition. -↓BM -↑heme iron intake. -↑ferritin concentrations -↑muscle thickness -No differences in VO_{2max}

Table 1. *Cont.*

Study	Participants and Group Assignment	Duration	Exercise Training Protocol (Common to all Study Groups)	Baseline Protein Intake	BP Group	WP Group	NP Group	Additional Group	Measurements	Main Outcomes
Naclerio et al. [19]	27 active males and females (~24–28 years) randomized into a BP, WP or NP group (*n* = 8 each)	8 weeks	RT 3 times per week	~1.1–1.5 g/kg/day	20 g of beef supplement (16.4 g protein) + 250 mL of orange juice per day	20 g of WP + 250 mL of orange juice per day	20 g of CHO + 250 mL of orange juice per day	-	-Body composition (plethysmography) -Strength (total weight lifted) -Muscle thickness (ultrasound) -Blood analysis -Saliva analysis	-No differences in body composition nor muscle thickness. -↓HNP1-3 and saliva flow rate. -No differences in strength.
Negro et al. [26]	26 male and female healthy subjects (~24 years) randomized into a BP (*n* = 12) or NP group (*n* = 14)	8 weeks	RT 3 times per week	~1.0 g/kg/day	135 g (20 g protein) of tinned beef per day	-	No supplement provided	-	-Strength (1 RM) -Body composition (bioimpedance)	-↑FFM and ↓FM -No differences in LBM -No differences in strength.
Sharp et al. [18]	41 male and female trained subjects (18–30 years) randomized into a WP (*n* = 10, 5 male), BP (*n* = 10, 5 male), chicken protein (*n* = 11, 5 male) or NP group (*n* = 10, 4 male)	8 weeks	RT 3 times per week and HIIT 2 times per week.	~2.0–2.2 g/kg/day	46 g of isolated BP per day	46 g of WP per day	46 g of CHO per day	46 g of chicken protein per day	-Dietary intake -Body composition (DXA). -Anaerobic peak power (10-second sprint) -Strength (1RM) -Gastrointestinal symptoms	-↑LBM and ↓FM compared to CHO. -No differences in body composition compared to other protein sources. -No differences in strength. -↓improvement in peak power compared to WP. -No differences in gastrointestinal symptoms.

Abbreviations: BM, body mass; BMD, bone mineral density; BP, beef protein; CHO, carbohydrates; CSA, cross-sectional area; DXA, dual-energy X-ray absorptiometry; ET, endurance training; FFM, fat-free mass; FM, fat mass; FSST, 4-square step test; HIIT, high intensity interval training; HNP1-3, human neutrophil peptides; IGF-1, insulin-like growth factor 1; IL-6, interleukin-6; LBM, lean body mass; NP, no protein supplementation; RM, repetition maximum; RT, resistance training; STS, sit-to-stand test; TUG, timed-up-and-go test; VO_{2max}, maximal oxygen uptake; WP, whey protein. ↑, increase; ↓, reduce.

3.2. *Quality Assessment and Publication Bias*

The risk of bias in the included studies was overall low (Figure 2). Three of seven studies [18,20,26] failed to perform/report an appropriate random sequence generation or allocation concealment. Three studies (where BP was provided as lean beef) were at a high risk of performance bias because participants were not blinded to group allocation [17,20,26].

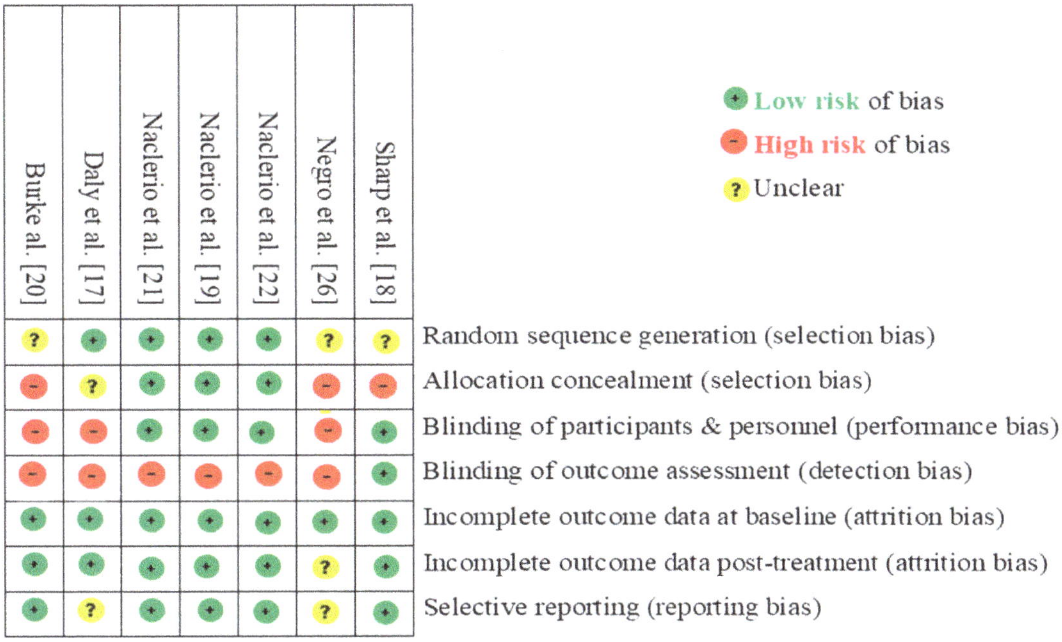

Figure 2. Quality assessment of the included studies.

3.3. *Participants and Intervention Characteristics*

Five studies [18–21,26] analyzed young male and female active/trained subjects whose age ranged between ~18 and 30 years, one [22] analyzed master male athletes (35 to 60 years), and another one [17] assessed women aged 60 to 90 years.

The duration of the interventions ranged from 8 to 16 weeks. BP was supplied as isolated BP (powder form) in four studies [18,19,21,22] or as a lean beef supplement in a remainder of studies [17,20,26]. The amount of protein was specified in all but one study [20], and ranged from 16.4 to 46 g/day. BP was compared with NP in all studies, and with WP in four of them [18,19,21,22]. The nutritional intervention was combined with a resistance ('strength') exercise training program (2 to 3 sessions/ week) in five studies [17–19,21,26] or with aerobic exercise training (four to six sessions/week) in one study [22]. One study [20] only reported that participants were cross-country runners who maintained their typical usual exercise regime during the intervention.

3.4. *Body Composition*

Four studies [18,19,21,22] compared the effects of BP and WP on body composition, with none reporting significant differences. Thus, the meta-analysis showed no differences between both conditions for LBM (SMD = −0.01, p = 0.970, Figure 3A), with no signs of heterogeneity (I^2 = 0%, Q = 0.152) or publication bias (p = 0.202). Similarly, no differences were found between BP and WP for fat mass (SMD = 0.07, p = 0.760, Figure 3B), with no signs of heterogeneity (I^2=0%, Q = 0.012) or publication bias (p = 0.054).

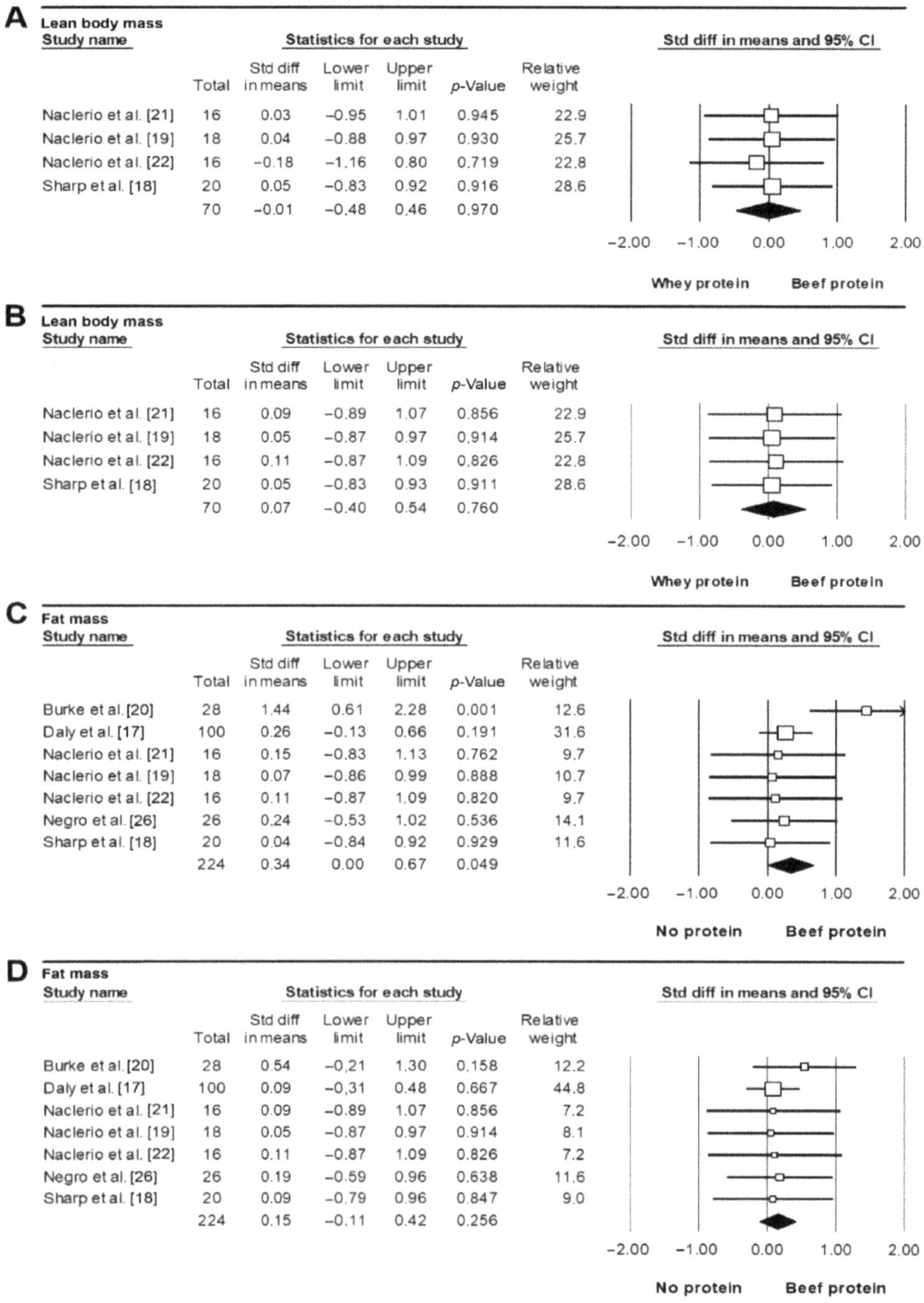

Figure 3. Effects on lean body (**A**) and fat mass (**B**) of beef vs. whey protein supplementation and effects on lean body (panel **C**) and fat mass (panel **D**) of beef vs. no protein supplementation. Each forest plot displays the pooled standardized difference in means and 95% confidence interval.

All included studies compared the effects of BP vs. NP on body composition. The meta-analysis showed a beneficial effect of BP over NP for LBM (SMD = 0.34, $p = 0.049$, Figure 3C), with no signs of heterogeneity ($I^2 = 4.326\%$, $Q = 6.271$) or publication bias ($p = 0.500$). This effect remained significant for $r = 0.9$ (SMD = 0.52, $p = 0.032$) or almost significant for 0.5 (SMD = 0.26, $p = 0.051$), but differences did not reach statistical significance for $r=0.2$ (SMD = 0.21, $p = 0.112$). No differences were found between BP and NP for fat mass (SMD = 0.15, $p = 0.256$, Figure 3D), with no signs of heterogeneity ($I^2 = 0\%$, $Q = 1.238$) or publication bias ($p = 0.500$).

Three studies [19,21,22] analyzed changes in muscle thickness using ultrasonography, but we could not meta-analyze their results because these studies analyzed different muscles. One study [19] found no benefits on muscle thickness with BP vs. WP or NP. However, the other two reported an improvement in the thickness of the *biceps brachialis* [21] or *vastus medialis* muscle [22] with BP compared to WP or NP. One study [22] also analyzed changes in thigh and arm circumference and found larger benefits with BP vs. WP or NP. Finally, one study [17] that analyzed thigh muscle cross-sectional area as well bone mineral density (femoral neck, total hip and lumbar spine) using dual-energy X-ray absorptiometry found no differences between BP and NP.

3.5. Exercise Performance

All retrieved studies analyzed the effects of BP on 1+ markers of exercise performance. Four studies [17,18,21,26] analyzed the effects of BP vs. NP on lower-limb maximal strength (deadlift, leg press, knee extension). Of these, three [18,21,26] found similar increases in strength with both conditions, and one study [17] found an 18% greater increase in leg extension strength with BP than with NP. The meta-analysis showed a beneficial effect of BP over NP (SMD = 0.40, $p = 0.014$, Figure 4A), with no signs of heterogeneity ($I^2 = 0\%$, $Q = 2.954$) or publication bias ($p = 0.367$). This effect remained significant for r=0.5 (SMD = 0.33, $p = 0.040$), but not for $r = 0.2$ (SMD = 0.26, $p = 0.098$) or 0.9 (SMD = 0.42, $p = 0.150$). Three studies [18,21,26] that assessed changes in upper-limb maximal muscle strength (bench press, 1-repetition maximum [1RM]) found no differences between BP and NP, and the meta-analysis showed no differences between both conditions for this outcome (SMD = 0.16, $p = 0.536$, $I^2 = 0\%$, $Q = 0.058$, Begg's p-value = 0.148, Figure 4B).

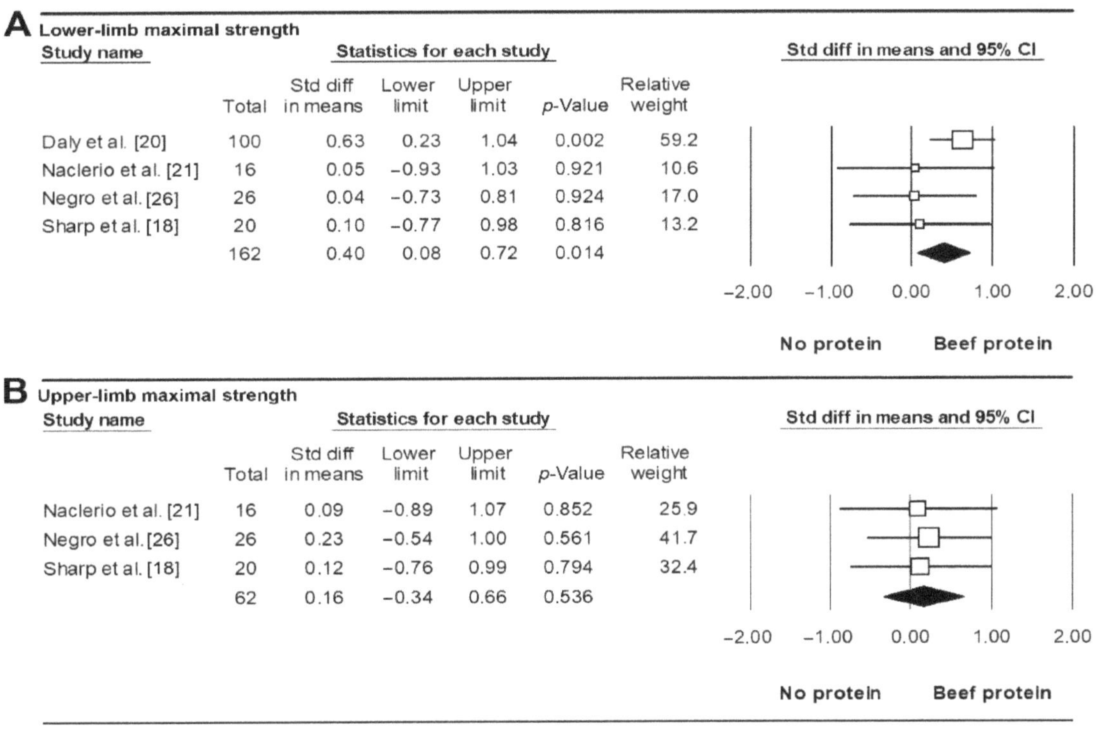

Figure 4. Effects on lower- (**A**) and upper-limb maximal strength (**B**) of beef vs. no protein supplementation. Each forest plot displays the pooled standardized difference in means and 95% confidence interval.

Two studies [18,21] also compared the gains in 1RM with BP over WP and neither found additional benefits. Finally, no benefits were reported with BP vs. NP for maximal oxygen uptake [20,22], anaerobic peak power [18] or total weight lifted during a resistance training session [19].

3.6. Nutritional Intake

Except for one study [26], where the baseline protein intake of the participants was described as ~1.0 g/kg/day, the mean total protein intake (in g/kg/day) during the intervention was consistently reported and ranged from 1.3 to 2.2 g/kg/day (BP), 1.7 to 2.2 g/kg/day (WP), and 1.1 to 2.0 g/kg/day (NP). The total protein intake was higher in BP than NP (SMD = 0.68, $p < 0.001$, Figure 5A; $I^2 = 0\%$, $Q = 1.226$, Begg's $p = 0.403$). This effect remained for $r = 0.2$ (SMD = 0.42, $p = 0.006$), 0.5 (SMD = 0.53, $p = 0.001$) or 0.9 (SMD = 1.17, $p < 0.001$). By contrast, no differences in protein intake were found for BP vs. WP (SMD = 0.04, $p = 0.892$, Figure 5B), with no heterogeneity between studies ($I^2 = 0\%$, $Q = 0.016$) and no signs of publication bias ($p = 0.500$).

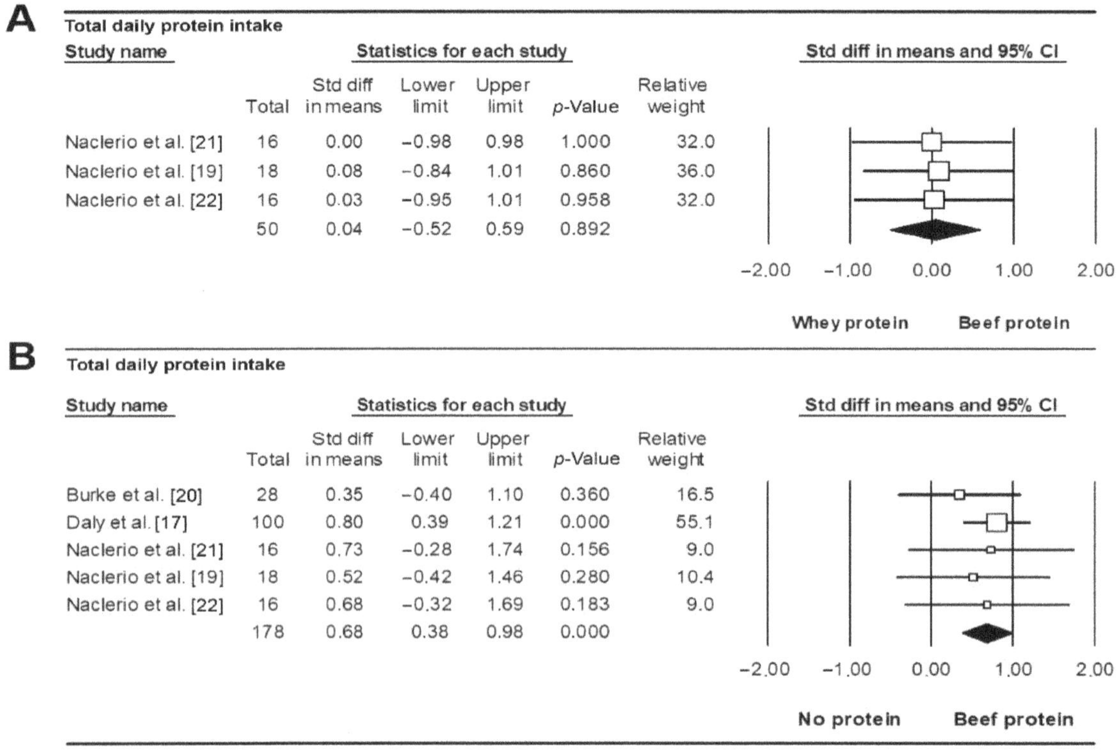

Figure 5. Effects on total daily protein intake of beef vs. whey (**A**) or no protein supplementation (**B**). Each forest plot displays the pooled standardized difference in means and 95% confidence interval.

Five studies [17,19–22] analyzed changes in fat intake with BP vs. NP, with no significant differences between conditions (SMD = −0.11, $p = 0.587$) and with no heterogeneity between studies ($I^2 = 3.8\%$, $Q = 4.158$) and no publication bias ($p = 0.110$). Three of these studies [19,21,22] also analyzed the changes in fat intake with BP vs. WP, and the meta-analysis showed a higher fat intake with the former (SMD = 0.71, $p = 0.015$), with no heterogeneity ($I^2 = 0\%$, $Q = 0.195$) or bias between studies ($p = 0.148$). This effect remained significant for $r = 0.9$ (SMD = 1.22, $p < 0.001$), but not for 0.5 (SMD = 0.55, $p = 0.056$) or 0.2 (SMD = 0.44, $p = 0.128$).

Three studies [17,20,22] analyzed changes in iron intake with BP vs. NP. The meta-analysis showed a non-significant trend towards a higher iron intake with BP (SMD = 0.29, $p = 0.089$), which was significant for $r = 0.9$ (SMD = 0.46, $p = 0.006$), but not for $r = 0.5$ (SMD = 0.22, $p = 0.180$) or 0.2 (SMD = 0.18, $p = 0.285$).

3.7. Hematological Parameters

Two studies [20,22] analyzed the effects of BP vs. NP on hematological parameters, with one study reporting an increased ferritin concentration [22] and the other study finding an increased hematocrit (although significance was only reached for the female participants) [20].

Three studies [17–19] analyzed the effects of BP vs. NP on lipid profile, and two of them [18,19] also compared BP and WP. None of them found differences between interventions for any of the analyzed variables (i.e., total cholesterol, LDL and HDL-cholesterol, or triglycerides). However, no meta-analysis could be performed because the mean and SD values for baseline and post-intervention were not available for all the studies.

4. Discussion

Protein supplementation might be a potentially beneficial strategy for maximizing exercise training-related gains in body composition and performance [2], with WP receiving the most attention to date. This systematic review and meta-analysis showed that, when combined with exercise training, BP supplementation provides benefits on protein intake and LBM that are similar to those elicited by WP. Our results also show that BP supplementation might be an effective means of increasing total daily protein intake compared to NP, and suggest it might be also useful for improving LBM and lower-limb muscle strength, although these results should be corroborated in further studies.

The popularity of WP compared to other protein sources is mainly based on a higher digestibility of the former together with a greater content of essential amino acids such as leucine [27]. Indeed, WP has proven to stimulate muscle protein synthesis to a greater extent than other popular protein sources such as casein or soy [28,29]. The ingestion of BP has also demonstrated promising anabolic effects, with the ingestion of 30 g (equivalent to 113 g of lean beef) increasing muscle protein synthesis by ~50% compared with fasting conditions [13–15]. Moreover, the combination of BP and exercise training might provide additional benefits, as the increase in muscle protein synthesis observed after BP intake followed by a resistance training session is higher than that observed with the former alone [15,16]. However, WP has been reported to have a higher digestibility (as reflected by a higher Protein Digestibility Corrected Amino Acid Score, 1.00 vs. 0.92) as well as a greater content of essential amino acids than BP (52% vs. 44% of total protein, respectively), including more leucine (13.6% vs. 8.8%) and lysine (10.6% vs. 8.9%) and a similar methionine content (2.5% vs. 2.3%) [27]. Of note, in human muscle, essential amino acids make up to 45% of the total protein content, and 9.4%, 8.7% and 2.2% of the protein comes from leucine, lysine and methionine, respectively [27]. Burd et al. [30] compared the mean muscle protein synthesis response to the ingestion of 30 g of protein coming from skimmed milk or beef after a resistance training session. Skimmed milk (from which WP is obtained) was more rapidly digested and absorbed than beef, thereby resulting in a greater leucine availability, and a higher stimulation of muscle protein synthesis in the early phase after exercise (0–2 h), but not for the whole recovery period (0–5 h post-exercise) [30]. Thus, these results suggest that milk/WP might be more effective than BP for the stimulation of muscle anabolism during the early postprandial stage, but that no overall differences are found between these protein sources. In line with these findings, our results support similar mid/long-term (≥4 weeks) benefits of WP or BP supplementation on LBM.

On the other hand, the present study shows that BP might be effective compared to NP for increasing LBM and lower-limb muscle strength, although the magnitude of the benefit was small (SMD <0.50 in both cases) and this result should be confirmed in further studies as sensitivity analyses raised concern about statistical significance. Furthermore, no consistent benefits were observed on physical performance, as reflected by the lack of differences for upper-limb muscle strength. Given the abovementioned anabolic potential of BP, which also resulted in a higher total daily protein intake than NP, we expected greater benefits of BP on LBM and physical performance compared to NP. One of the factors that might explain the small benefits obtained in these endpoints is that participants already consumed an 'optimal' quantity of protein in their diet (1.1 to 2.0 g/kg/day for the NP group, above the current international recommendations for the general adult population of 0.8 g/kg/day [31]). Of note, a protein intake higher than 0.8 g/kg/day is recommended to promote skeletal muscle anabolism in physically active individuals (i.e., 1.0, 1.3, and 1.6 g/kg/day for individuals with minimal, moderate, and intense physical activity levels, respectively; [32]) as well as in older people (>1.2 g/kg/day, [33]) such as those included in the study of Daly et al. [17]. However, a recent meta-analysis found no additional benefits on LBM when protein intake was greater than 1.6 g/kg/day [2]. Thus, the daily protein intake of the participants in the studies analyzed here could be considered within the 'optimal' range even without protein supplementation. Greater benefits might perhaps have been observed in individuals with a baseline protein intake below the recommended levels.

Another purported benefit of supplementation with BP is the potential increase in iron intake, which might theoretically improve hematological parameters. In this regard, our results show a non-significant trend towards an increased iron intake with BP compared to NP. Two studies [20,22] analyzed the specific changes in heme iron intake and both found increased values with BP—although only in the female participants in one study [20]—compared to WP or NP. In line with these results, although we could not perform a meta-analysis of hematological parameters, preliminary evidence suggests that BP could provide benefits at hematological level, such as increased hematocrit levels in collegiate distance runners [20] or enhanced iron (ferritin) deposits in master-age triathletes [22]. Future research should confirm if BP might serve as an effective intervention to counteract hematological conditions such as anemia in individuals with deficient iron intake.

An interesting finding was that, when compared to WP, BP supplementation seemed to increase the total daily intake of fat. However, in sensitivity analysis, this effect did not reach statistical significance and no differences in total daily fat intake were observed between BP and NP. Thus, there is not yet clear evidence to support that BP *per se* significantly increases fat intake. Moreover, no differences have been reported in lipid profile (e.g., cholesterol levels) or in fat mass with BP compared to WP or NP. However, more research is needed in the field.

Some limitations must be noted, notably the small number of studies included, the small sample size of most studies or the lack of participants' blinding to group allocation in some of them. The included studies provided BP in different forms (powder or lean beef), which might have affected digestibility/absorption rates and potentially, anabolic responses [34]. However, although minced beef is more rapidly digested/absorbed than beef steak resulting in a greater amino acid availability, no differences have been reported in post-prandial muscle protein synthesis [35]. Future research should confirm if providing BP in isolate form (powder) results in a greater anabolic response than lean beef. The type of exercise training intervention did also differ between studies, with some including resistance training and others using endurance training. In this regard, resistance training is more effective for promoting muscle protein synthesis and muscle mass accretion than endurance exercise [36], and this might have acted as a confounding variable in our findings. However, protein supplementation can also provide benefits in individuals performing endurance exercise training, notably by avoiding muscle catabolism—especially during periods of negative energy intake—and through the enhancement of recovery and the promotion of exercise-induced adaptations [37]. On the other hand, we combined studies with participants of wide age ranges, including individuals aged 60 to 90 years. In this regard, aging is associated with an impaired anabolic response to both aminoacidemia and acute physical exercise [38], which might have acted as a confounding factor in our results. Interestingly, the study that included older adults was the one reporting the greatest increases in muscle strength [17]. Thus, BP supplementation might be particularly useful for this population segment. However, statistical analyses showed no heterogeneity between studies for the outcomes that we analyzed.

On the other hand, the benefits of supplementing with BP—and of every diet in general—should be viewed under the context of its sustainability, that is, it should have a low environmental impact that contributes to food and nutrition security and to a healthy lifestyle for present and future generations [39]. Diets that primarily contain animal-derived food sources are associated with higher greenhouse gas emissions, and indeed beef production/consumption is the food source that results in greater gas emissions (>70 kg CO_2/kg) [40]. By contrast, the production of dairy products (such as milk or WP), and especially of plant-based protein foods, is associated with lower moderate greenhouse gas emissions [41]. Thus, a balance between environmental sustainability and optimal dietary intake (particularly regarding protein consumption) should be sought, and WP might be a more recommendable option in this regard.

5. Conclusions

This systematic review and meta-analysis of randomized controlled trials showed no mid/long-term (≥4 weeks) differences between BP and WP on total daily protein intake or body composition (LBM, fat mass), and thus both protein sources might be similarly effective to promote increases in LBM. However, BP resulted in a greater total daily protein intake than NP, and our results suggest that BP might represent an effective strategy for increasing LBM and lower-limb muscle strength. However, these and other potential benefits (including preliminary data on heme iron intake and ferritin levels) should be confirmed in future studies.

Author Contributions: Conceptualization, P.L.V. and F.M.; Data curation, P.L.V. and F.M.; Formal analysis, P.L.V.; Funding acquisition, A.L.; Investigation, P.L.V.; Methodology, P.L.V., J.S.M. and A.C.-G.; Project administration, P.L.V.; Resources, P.L.V.; Software, P.L.V.; Supervision, P.L.V. and A.L.; Validation, A.L.; Visualization, A.C.-G.; Writing—original draft, P.L.V. and A.L.; Writing—review and editing, P.L.V., F.M., J.S.M., A.C.-G. and A.L.

References

1. Cermak, N.M.; Res, P.T.; de Groot, L.C.; Saris, W.H.M.; Loon, L.J.C. Van Protein supplementation augments the adaptive response of skeletal muscle to resistance-type exercise training: A meta-analysis. *Am. J. Clin. Nutr.* **2012**, *96*, 1454–1464. [CrossRef]
2. Morton, R.W.; Murphy, K.T.; McKellar, S.R.; Schoenfeld, B.J.; Henselmans, M.; Helms, E.; Aragon, A.A.; Devries, M.C.; Banfield, L.; Krieger, J.W.; et al. A systematic review, meta-analysis and meta-regression of the effect of protein supplementation on resistance training-induced gains in muscle mass and strength in healthy adults. *Br. J. Sports Med.* **2018**, *52*, 376–384. [CrossRef]
3. Pasiakos, S.M.; McLellan, T.M.; Lieberman, H.R. The Effects of Protein Supplements on Muscle Mass, Strength, and Aerobic and Anaerobic Power in Healthy Adults: A Systematic Review. *Sports Med.* **2014**, *45*, 111–131. [CrossRef]
4. Stokes, T.; Hector, A.J.; Morton, R.W.; McGlory, C.; Phillips, S.M. Recent perspectives regarding the role of dietary protein for the promotion of muscle hypertrophy with resistance exercise training. *Nutrients* **2018**, *10*, 180. [CrossRef]
5. Elliot, T.A.; Cree, M.G.; Sanford, A.P.; Wolfe, R.R.; Tipton, K.D. Milk ingestion stimulates net muscle protein synthesis following resistance exercise. *Med. Sci. Sports Exerc.* **2006**, *38*, 667–674. [CrossRef]
6. Moore, D.; Robinson, M.; Fry, J.; Tang, J.; Glover, E.; Wilkinson, S.; Prior, T.; Tarnopolsky, M.; Philips, S. Ingested protein dose response of muscle and albumin protein synthesis after resistance exercise in young men. *Am. J. Clin. Nutr.* **2009**, *89*, 161–168. [CrossRef]
7. Yang, Y.; Churchward-Venne, T.A.; Burd, N.A.; Breen, L.; Tarnopolsky, M.A.; Phillips, S.M. Myofibrillar protein synthesis following ingestion of soy protein isolate at rest and after resistance exercise in elderly men. *Nutr. Metab.* **2012**, *9*, 1. [CrossRef]
8. Joy, J.M.; Lowery, R.P.; Wilson, J.M.; Purpura, M.; De Souza, E.O.; Wilson, S.M.; Kalman, D.S.; Dudeck, J.E.; Jäger, R. The effects of 8 weeks of whey or rice protein supplementation on body composition and exercise performance. *Nutr. J.* **2013**, *12*, 1–7. [CrossRef]
9. Duff, W.; Chilibeck, P.; Rooke, J.; Kaviani, M.; Krentz, J.; Haines, D. The Effect of Bovine Colostrum Supplementation in Older Adults during Resistance Training. *Int. J. Sport Nutr. Exerc. Metab.* **2014**, *24*, 276–285. [CrossRef]

10. Cribb, P.J.; Williams, A.D.; Hayes, A.; Carey, M.F. The Effect of Whey Isolate and Resistance Training on Strength, Body Composition and Plasma Glutamine. *Int. J. Sport Nutr. Exerc. Metab.* **2006**, *16*, 494–509. [CrossRef]
11. Volek, J.S.; Volk, B.M.; Gómez, A.L.; Kunces, L.J.; Kupchak, B.R.; Freidenreich, D.J.; Aristizabal, J.C.; Saenz, C.; Dunn-Lewis, C.; Ballard, K.D.; et al. Whey Protein Supplementation During Resistance Training Augments Lean Body Mass. *J. Am. Coll. Nutr.* **2013**, *32*, 122–135. [CrossRef]
12. Gorissen, S.H.M.; Rémond, D.; van Loon, L.J.C. The muscle protein synthetic response to food ingestion. *Meat Sci.* **2015**, *109*, 96–100. [CrossRef]
13. Symons, T.; Schutzler, S.E.; Cocke, T.L.; Chinkes, D.L.; Wolfe, R.R.; Paddon-Jones, D. Aging does not impair the anabolic response to a protein-rich meal. *Am. J. Clin. Nutr.* **2007**, *86*, 451–456. [CrossRef]
14. Symons, T.; Sheffield-Moore, M.; Wolfe, R.R.; Paddon-Jones, D. A Moderate Serving of High-Quality Protein Maximally Stimulates Skeletal Muscle Protein Synthesis in Young and Elderly Subjects. *J. Am. Diet. Assoc.* **2009**, *109*, 1582–1586. [CrossRef]
15. Robinson, M.J.; Burd, N.A.; Breen, L.; Rerecich, T.; Yang, Y.; Hector, A.J.; Baker, S.K.; Phillips, S.M. Dose-dependent responses of myofibrillar protein synthesis with beef ingestion are enhanced with resistance exercise in middle-aged men. *Appl. Physiol. Nutr. Metab.* **2013**, *38*, 120–125. [CrossRef]
16. Symons, T.; Sheffield-Moore, M.; Mamerow, M.M.; Wolfe, R.R.; Paddon-Jones, D. The anabolic response to resistance exercise and a protein-rich meal is not diminished by age. *J. Nutr. Health Aging* **2011**, *15*, 376–381. [CrossRef]
17. Daly, R.M.; O'Connell, S.L.; Mundell, N.L.; Grimes, C.A.; Dunstan, D.W.; Nowson, C.A. Protein-enriched diet, with the use of lean red meat, combined with progressive resistance training enhances lean tissue mass and muscle strength and reduces circulating IL-6 concentrations in elderly women: A cluster randomized controlled trial. *Am. J. Clin. Nutr.* **2014**, *99*, 899–910. [CrossRef]
18. Sharp, M.H.; Lowery, R.P.; Shields, K.A.; Lane, J.R.; Gray, J.L.; Partl, J.M.; Hayes, D.W.; Wilson, G.J.; Hollmer, C.A.; Minivich, J.R.; et al. The Effects of Beef, Chicken, or Whey Protein Post-Workout on Body Composition and Muscle Performance. *J. Strength Cond. Res.* **2018**, *32*, 2233–2242. [CrossRef]
19. Naclerio, F.; Larumbe-Zabala, E.; Ashrafi, N.; Seijo, M.; Nielsen, B.; Allgrove, J.; Earnest, C.P. Effects of protein–carbohydrate supplementation on immunity and resistance training outcomes: A double-blind, randomized, controlled clinical trial. *Eur. J. Appl. Physiol.* **2017**, *117*, 267–277. [CrossRef]
20. Burke, D.E.; Johnson, J.V.; Vukovich, M.D.; Kattelmann, K.K. Effects of Lean Beef Supplementation on Iron Status, Body Composition and Performance of Collegiate Distance Runners. *Food Nutr. Sci.* **2012**, *03*, 810–821. [CrossRef]
21. Naclerio, F.; Seijo-Bujia, M.; Larumbe-Zabala, E.; Earnes, C. Carbohydrates Alone or Mixing With Beef or Whey Protein Promote Similar Training Outcomes in Resistance Training Males: A Double Blind, Randomized Controlled Clinical Trial. *Int. J. Sport Nutr. Exerc. Metab.* **2017**, *27*, 408–420. [CrossRef] [PubMed]
22. Naclerio, F.; Seijo, M.; Larumbe-Zabala, E.; Ashrafi, N.; Christides, T.; Karsten, B.; Nielsen, B.V. Effects of Supplementation with Beef or Whey Protein Versus Carbohydrate in Master Triathletes. *J. Am. Coll. Nutr.* **2017**, *36*, 593–601. [CrossRef] [PubMed]
23. Moher, D.; Liberati, A.; Tetzlaff, J.; Altman, D.G.; Altman, D.; Antes, G.; Atkins, D.; Barbour, V.; Barrowman, N.; Berlin, J.A.; et al. Preferred reporting items for systematic reviews and meta-analyses: The PRISMA statement. *PLoS Med.* **2009**, *6*, e1000097. [CrossRef] [PubMed]
24. Higgins, J.P.T.; Altman, D.G.; Gøtzsche, P.C.; Jüni, P.; Moher, D.; Oxman, A.D.; Savović, J.; Schulz, K.F.; Weeks, L.; Sterne, J.A.C. The Cochrane Collaboration's tool for assessing risk of bias in randomised trials. *BMJ* **2011**, *343*, 1–9. [CrossRef] [PubMed]
25. Rosenthal, R. *Meta-Analytic Procedures for Social Research*; Sage: Newbury Park, CA, USA, 1991.
26. Negro, M.; Vandoni, M.; Ottobrini, S.; Codrons, E.; Correale, L.; Buonocore, D.; Marzatico, F. Protein supplementation with low fat meat after resistance training: Effects on body composition and strength. *Nutrients* **2014**, *6*, 3040–3049. [CrossRef] [PubMed]
27. Van Vliet, S.; Burd, N.A.; van Loon, L.J.C. The Skeletal Muscle Anabolic Response to Plant- versus Animal-Based Protein Consumption. *J. Nutr.* **2015**, *145*, 1981–1991. [CrossRef] [PubMed]
28. Tang, J.E.; Moore, D.R.; Kujbida, G.W.; Tarnopolsky, M.A.; Phillips, S.M. Ingestion of whey hydrolysate, casein, or soy protein isolate: Effects on mixed muscle protein synthesis at rest and following resistance exercise in young men. *J. Appl. Physiol.* **2009**, *107*, 987–992. [CrossRef] [PubMed]

29. Burd, N.A.; Yang, Y.; Moore, D.R.; Tang, J.E.; Tarnopolsky, M.A.; Phillips, S.M. Greater stimulation of myofibrillar protein synthesis with ingestion of whey protein isolate v. micellar casein at rest and after resistance exercise in elderly men. *Br. J. Nutr.* **2012**, *108*, 958–962. [CrossRef]
30. Burd, N.A.; Gorissen, S.H.; Van Vliet, S.; Snijders, T.; Van Loon, L.J.C. Differences in postprandial protein handling after beef compared with milk ingestion during postexercise recovery: A randomized controlled trial. *Am. J. Clin. Nutr.* **2015**, *102*, 828–836. [CrossRef]
31. Trumbo, P.; Schlicker, S.; Yates, A.; Poos, M. Dietary reference intakes for energy, carbohydrate, fiber, fat, fatty acids, cholesterol, protein and amino acids. *J. Am. Diet. Assoc.* **2002**, *102*, 1621–1630. [CrossRef]
32. Wu, G. Dietary protein intake and human health. *Food Funct.* **2016**, *7*, 1251–1265. [CrossRef] [PubMed]
33. Traylor, D.A.; Gorissen, S.H.M.; Phillips, S.M. Perspective: Protein requirements and optimal intakes in aging: Arewe ready to recommend more than the recommended daily allowance? *Adv. Nutr.* **2018**, *9*, 171–182. [CrossRef] [PubMed]
34. Trommelen, J.; Betz, M.W.; van Loon, L.J.C. The Muscle Protein Synthetic Response to Meal Ingestion Following Resistance-Type Exercise. *Sports Med.* **2019**, *49*, 185–197. [CrossRef] [PubMed]
35. Pennings, B.; Groen, B.B.L.; Van Dijk, J.W.; De Lange, A.; Kiskini, A.; Kuklinski, M.; Senden, J.M.G.; Van Loon, L.J.C. Minced beef is more rapidly digested and absorbed than beef steak, resulting in greater postprandial protein retention in older men. *Am. J. Clin. Nutr.* **2013**, *98*, 121–128. [CrossRef] [PubMed]
36. Egan, B.; Zierath, J.R. Exercise metabolism and the molecular regulation of skeletal muscle adaptation. *Cell Metab.* **2013**, *17*, 162–184. [CrossRef] [PubMed]
37. Moore, D.R.; Camera, D.M.; Areta, J.L.; Hawley, J. A Beyond muscle hypertrophy: Why dietary protein is important for endurance athletes. *Appl. Physiol. Nutr. Metab.* **2014**, *11*, 1–11. [CrossRef] [PubMed]
38. Breen, L.; Phillips, S.M. Skeletal muscle protein metabolism in the elderly: Interventions to counteract the "anabolic resistance" of ageing. *Nutr. Metab.* **2011**, *8*, 68. [CrossRef] [PubMed]
39. MacDiarmid, J.I. Is a healthy diet an environmentally sustainable diet? *Proc. Nutr. Soc.* **2013**, *72*, 13–20. [CrossRef]
40. Scarborough, P.; Appleby, P.N.; Mizdrak, A.; Briggs, A.D.M.; Travis, R.C.; Bradbury, K.E.; Key, T.J. Dietary greenhouse gas emissions of meat-eaters, fish-eaters, vegetarians and vegans in the UK. *Clim. Chang.* **2014**, *125*, 179–192. [CrossRef]
41. Gorissen, S.H.M.; Witard, O.C. Characterising the muscle anabolic potential of dairy, meat and plant-based protein sources in older adults. *Proc. Nutr. Soc.* **2018**, *77*, 20–31. [CrossRef]

6

Anthropometric Characteristics, Maximal Isokinetic Strength and Selected Handball Power Indicators are Specific to Playing Positions in Elite Kosovan Handball Players

Jeton Havolli [1,2], Abedin Bahtiri [1], Tim Kambič [3,4], Kemal Idrizović [2], Duško Bjelica [2] and Primož Pori [4,*]

[1] Department of Physical Culture, Sport and Recreation, Kolegji Universi (Universi College) Prishtina, 10000 Prishtina, Kosovo; jeton.havolli@kolegjiuniversi-edu.net (J.H.); abedinbahtiri@gmail.com (A.B.)
[2] Faculty of Sport and Physical Education, 81400 Nikšić, Montenegro; kemali@ucg.ac.me (K.I.); dbjelica@ucg.ac.me (D.B.)
[3] Department of Research and Education, General Hospital Murska Sobota, 9000 Murska Sobota, Slovenia; tim.kambic@gmail.com
[4] Department of Sports Medicine, Faculty of Sport, University of Ljubljana, 1000 Ljubljana, Slovenia
* Correspondence: primoz.pori@fsp.uni-lj.si

Abstract: Anthropometric characteristics and physical performance are closely related to the game demands of each playing position. This study aimed to first examine the differences between playing positions in anthropometric characteristics and physical performance with special emphasis on the isokinetic strength of elite male handball players, and secondly to examine the correlations of the latter variables with ball velocity. Anthropometric characteristics, maximal isokinetic strength, sprinting and vertical jumping performance, and ball velocity in the set shot and jump shot were obtained from 93 elite handball players (age 22 ± 5 years, height 184 ± 8 cm, and weight 84 ± 14 kg) pre-season. Wing players were shorter compared to other players, and pivots were the heaviest. Wings had the fastest 20 m sprints, and, along with backcourt players, jumped higher, had better maximal knee isometric strength, and achieved the highest ball velocity compared to pivots and goalkeepers, respectively. There were no significant differences between playing positions in unilateral and bilateral maximal leg strength imbalances. Ball velocity was significantly correlated with height, weight, squat jump and maximal torque of extensors and flexors. Our study suggest that shooting success is largely determined by the player's height, weight, muscle strength and power, while it seems that anthropometric characteristics and physical performance are closely related to the game demands of each playing position.

Keywords: morphology; isokinetic; sprints; vertical jump performance; handball shooting

---

1. Introduction

Handball is an Olympic team sport [1,2], split into two periods (each 30 min long) and consisting of a high degree of body contact and predominantly aerobic activities separated by anaerobic bouts of sprints, jumps, throws, changes of directions in the offense (counterattack and attack buildup) and defense [2,3]. Therefore, competition success in elite handball is not only closely related to the technical and tactical skills of each individual or team, but also to the players' anthropometric characteristics, physical performance (e.g., maximal strength and power as measured using strength, sprinting, and jumping tests), and handball shooting performance [3–5].

To date, only a few studies evaluating the physical and physiological demands in handball matches have shown significant differences between playing positions [6–8]. Results obtained during gameplay have shown that backcourt players cover larger distances and spend less time standing and walking, and, together with pivots, have higher in-game heart rates and spend longer durations at higher intensities (>80% maximal heart rate) [7]. In contrast, wing players are faster than other playing positions, and pivots endure more body impact than other players [6]. Furthermore, similar differences between playing positions were also obtained in anthropometric characteristics [9,10] and physical performance [11–16]. Wings are the shortest, have significantly lower body mass and body mass index (BMI) than other players; pivots are the heaviest, whereas other playing positions do not differ in height [9–16]. Research comparing playing positions in sprinting (e.g., sprints on 20–30 m) and jumping performance (squat jump (SJ) and/or countermovement jumps (CMJs)) is relatively scarce, and there are some discrepancies in sprinting times and jump heights among studies [11,14–16]. Nevertheless, backcourt players and wings demonstrated the fastest sprinting times [14,15], while CMJ height was the highest in wings [14], compared to pivots and goalkeepers [15].

Isokinetic dynamometry has long been the gold standard for assessing changes to an athlete's maximal muscle strength/torque during the season [17,18] and risk of injury (measured as imbalances between agonist and antagonist muscles or bilateral differences) in different types of a team sport [19]. In the past, only a few studies have evaluated isokinetic maximal knee strength and strength imbalances in male handball players [19–21], with the majority of studies having been performed on female handball players, focusing on shoulder muscle strength, and several on knee muscle strength in relation to shoulder and knee injuries [18,22–25]. Evidence from two studies evaluating isokinetic maximal strength in male handball players has suggested no differences between dominant and nondominant lower limb knee extensor and flexor strength, as well as normal hamstring-to-quadriceps ratio on both limbs at 60°/s and 180°/s [19,20]. However, no studies in handball have investigated isokinetic maximal strength of the knee joint according to playing position. Furthermore, it also remains to be elucidated the potential role of playing position on development of muscle strength imbalances between and within legs as a product of specific game demands. Such findings would serve as excellent feedback to practitioners to focus on preventing potential injuries and to improve player performance.

Ball velocity has been recognized as one of the most important determinants of game performance [14]. Maximal ball velocity is achieved through a proximal-to-distal manner; this movement allows momentum of force to transfer from the lower limb and/or pelvis through the trunk to the throwing arm, thereby enabling higher velocities of the shot [26]. During the game, the majority of shots are performed using two shooting techniques: a three-step jump shot and a standing set shot from the ground. Both techniques use two different kinetic strategies (braking the body with lead leg in the standing set shot vs. opposed leg movement during the flight phase of the three-step jump shot) [27,28], while ball velocity in both is influenced by an optimal proximal–distal principle, trunk movement, and maximal arm rotation [26,28]. It is well established that elite players are able to maintain an optimal proximal-to-distal principle and arm movement while performing different shooting techniques [27]. Lower ball velocity has been associated with lower strength in the lower and upper limbs, leading to inefficient transfer of power from the proximal (pelvis, trunk) to distal (shooting arm) parts of the body [29]. Backcourt players and wings shoot the ball faster compared to pivots or goalkeepers [14,15,30]. For overhead throws, only inconsistent correlations have been reported between ball velocity and anthropometric characteristics or physical performance, and this is likely due to the complex nature of this movement [10,11,13,31,32]. Body height and weight were the only anthropometric characteristics significantly correlated with ball velocity of the standing shot [11] and/or three-step running shot [10,13,31], whereas two additional studies reported significant correlations with lower limb strength (1-RM half back squat) [31], standing long jump, 30 m sprint, and maximal oxygen uptake (estimated from 20 m shuttle run) [31]. Other studies have failed to detect such correlations [11,13]; therefore, additional studies are warranted to transfer these findings into training settings.

Based on the identified gaps in the knowledge of the anthropometric characteristics, maximal strength and power performance, and handball shooting performance of elite handball players, our study consisted of three aims. The first aim of the study was to provide further evidence on the isokinetic maximal strength and potential limb imbalances between playing positions in elite male handball players. The second aim was to examine the differences in anthropometric characteristics, sprinting and vertical jump performance between playing positions, and the last aim was to investigate the correlations between handball-specific performance (e.g., ball velocity) and selected anthropometric characteristics and physical performance indicators.

2. Materials and Methods

2.1. Study Design

The study was designed as a cross-sectional study of a sample of elite Kosovo handball players. Measurements were conducted two weeks before the start of a competitive season, at the end of August 2019. Testing procedures were split into three days. On the first day anthropometric characteristics (height, weight, wingspan, and thigh circumference) and body composition (skeletal muscle mass and fat mass) were measured, and familiarization with all testing procedures was conducted. On the second day, following a standardized warm-up procedure, sprinting performance (20 m sprints), vertical jump performance (CMJ and SJ), and shooting performance (shooting velocity of three-step set shot and jump shot) were assessed. Finally, during the last day measurements of unilateral isokinetic knee flexor and extensor torque at 60°/s and 180°/s were conducted after the standardized warm-up. Forty-eight hours of rest were given between the second and third testing day to minimize any potential effects of fatigue. Testing procedures were performed by experienced strength and conditioning specialists.

2.2. Subjects

A total of 93 elite male handball players from Kosovo's first handball league were enrolled into the study, age (mean (SD)) 22 (1) years, height 184.0 (7.83) cm, weight 84.10 (13.74) kg, and with 8 (4) years of professional playing experience. The sample consisted of 35 (37.63%) backcourt players, 26 (27.96%) wing players, 15 (16.13%) pivots, and 17 (18.28%) goalkeepers. Playing positions were determined according to registration data obtained from the Handball Federation of Kosovo. Players' adherence was consistent throughout the study, and no injuries or other health issues were reported.

Prior to enrolment into the study, we informed all participants about the aims of our study, methods and procedures, and potential testing risks. Measurements were performed at the end of the last week of the specific preparation phase for the upcoming season, with at least 48 h of rest after the last training session, and 10–14 days prior to beginning of the season. The exclusion criteria were: fewer than two years of professional playing experience, age younger than 18 years, and any recent musculoskeletal injuries (<6 months). All participants signed a written consent prior to inclusion in the study. The study design was approved by the Ethics Committee of Universi College Prishtina (document number: 488/18), while the study was conducted according to the Declaration of Helsinki guidelines for the use of human participants.

2.3. Procedures

2.3.1. Anthropometric and Body Composition Measurement

Prior to physical performance measurements on the first testing day, anthropometric and bioimpedance measurements were obtained according to the international guidelines [33]. Body height and weight were measured while standing barefoot using a SECA 763 stadiometer with electronic scale (Seca Instruments Ltd., Hamburg, Germany) to the nearest cm and kg, respectively. The wingspan was measured using a horizontal wall-mounted scale to the nearest cm, with arms abducted at 90° from a neutral position and back facing towards the wall, and thigh circumference was measured using a tape measure while standing at 2/3 of the distance between the lateral epicondyle of the knee and the greater trochanter on the dominant leg. Skeletal muscle mass and fat mass measurements were obtained using a Biospace Inbody 720 bioimpedance device (Inbody Co., Leicester, United Kingdom). Participants were asked to place toes and heels on the anterior and posterior electrodes of the weighting platform, and to firmly grasp the hand grip with both hands. Measurements were taken early in the morning, and participants were advised to avoid any moderate to vigorous physical activity a day before the measurement [34].

2.3.2. Sprint Performance Measurement

After the general 15-min warm-up (10 min running, and 5 min of whole-body dynamic mobility exercises) and an additional three repetitions of progressive acceleration from faster to sprint running, participants performed two 20 m sprints, with 3 min of rest between each exertion. Prior to testing, four photocell gates (Polifemo Radio Light, Microgate, Bolzano, Italy) were placed at the start, at 5 m, at 10 m, and at 20 m. The dominant foot (lead-off foot) [35] was placed one meter behind the first photocell. The time recording was automatically initialized when a participant crossed the first photocell gate and stopped when the participant crossed the last photocell gate at 20 m distance. Participants were instructed to sprint at least 25 m in order to reach the highest maximum sprinting speed. The fastest of the two split times on 5 m, 10 m, and 20 m distances was used in the final analysis [4]. All measurements were performed indoors.

2.3.3. Vertical Jump Performance Measurement

Vertical jump performance, measured as jump height (cm), was evaluated from the CMJ and SJ using an OptoJump infrared timing system (Microgate, Bolzano, Italy). The participants first performed three trials of CMJs followed by three trials of SJs [15]. One minute of rest was given between two trials. Prior to performing both jumps, participants were instructed about the jumping technique and later performed at least two submaximal familiarization repetitions of CMJs and SJs to learn proper jumping techniques [4]. The CMJ was performed by flexing the knee to a squat position (approximately 90° of knee flexion) from an upright position and then immediately extending the hips and the knee into a vertical jump, whereas the SJ was performed by jumping to vertical from squat position (90° of knee flexion) [20]. When approaching the landing position, participants were advised to land with extended knees to avoid any measurement error resulting from prolonged flight time. Both jumps were performed with hands placed on hips and with legs straightened during the flight. The jump height was calculated from the recorded flight time (height = [gravitational acceleration (9.81 m/s^2) × flight time2] × 8 – 1) [4], and the highest jump was used in the final analysis.

2.3.4. Handball Shooting Performance Measurement

Handball shooting performance was evaluated by measuring the ball velocity of a three-step set shot from the ground and the ball velocity of a three-step jump shot from the 9-m line, using the Bushnell Radar (Bushnell, Overland Park, KS, USA) with a measurement error of ±1.60 km/h (www.bushnellspeedster.com). The investigator measured ball velocity while standing at the 9-m line within 1 m of the participant performing the throw. After the warm-up, each participant performed one familiarization shot and two test shots of each shot type, with one minute of rest between shots [14,15].

2.3.5. Maximal Isokinetic Strength Measurement

Isokinetic concentric torque of knee extensors and flexors was measured using an isokinetic dynamometer Biodex Pro 4 (Biodex Medical Systems, Shirley, New York, NY, USA) at 60°/s and 180°/s according to previous guidelines and studies [18,36]. Prior to testing day, the machine was calibrated according to manufacturer guidelines, using a long shoulder attached to the axis of the apparatus, generating a standard torque of 67.8 Nm.

Prior to testing, each participant completed a standardized warm-up protocol consisting of 10 min of light jogging, followed by short dynamic stretching exercises for lower limbs, and ending with a single 8-repetition set of squat and hip thrust exercises. After the general warm-up, the participants were seated upright in the dynamometer chair with restraining belts fastened across the chest, pelvis, and leg thigh to minimize body movement or any potential compensation of synergist muscles. Later, we aligned the dynamometer axis of rotation to the participant's knee joint axis of rotation using the lateral epicondyle as the anatomic mark. Additionally, gravitation torque error was measured prior to each trial, and the starting leg was randomly selected for each participant. The range of motion was set at 80°, from 90° to 10° of knee flexion.

Prior to measuring maximal effort, each participant first performed a specific warm-up on the dynamometer consisting of 10 submaximal concentric contractions of knee flexion and extension at 60°/s. The maximal test was conducted after 2 min of rest, with participants performing five maximal concentric knee extensions and flexions. Verbal encouragement was given by the investigator during the test to ensure participants performed at their maximal effort. The maximal value out of five measurements was normalized to body weight (N/kg) and used in the final statistical analysis. In addition, bilateral differences between left and right maximal isometric torque (left leg/right leg maximal isometric torque × 100%) and unilateral hamstring-to-quadriceps maximal isometric torque (hamstring/quadriceps maximal isometric torque × 100%) [37] was calculated prior to further statistical analysis.

2.4. Statistical Analysis

Categorical variables are presented as frequencies and percentages, and numeric variables are presented as means and standard deviations, unless otherwise stated. All numeric variables were firstly screened for assumptions of normality of distribution and homogeneity of variances using the Shapiro–Wilk test and the Levene's test, respectively. This was screened for the whole sample and according to each playing position. The difference between playing positions was calculated using one-way analysis of variance (ANOVA) for normally distributed variables and homogeneous variances, otherwise, the Kruskal–Wallis test was applied. When one-way ANOVA detected significant differences between playing positions, an additional post hoc analysis was performed using the Tukey's honest significance test or pairwise comparisons, depending on the dispersion of variances between playing positions. Correlations between anthropometric, physical, and handball performance were assessed using Spearman's rank correlation coefficient. All statistical analyses were performed using IBM SPSS version 21 (SPSS Inc., Armonk, New York, NY, USA), and the level of significance was set at p-value < 0.05.

3. Results

There were statistically significant differences for playing positions in all measured anthropometric characteristics and skeletal muscle mass and fat mass (all p-values < 0.01; Table 1). The wings were significantly shorter compared to backcourt players ($p < 0.001$), pivots ($p = 0.035$), and goalkeepers ($p = 0.018$). Similar significant differences were obtained in weight (pivots vs. wing, $p < 0.001$; wings vs. backcourt players, $p < 0.001$), wingspan (wings vs. pivots, $p < 0.001$; wings vs. backcourt players, $p < 0.001$; wings vs. goalkeepers, $p = 0.038$), and thigh circumference (wings vs. pivots, $p < 0.001$; wings vs. backcourt players, $p = 0.041$). Additionally, pivots were heavier than goalkeepers ($p < 0.001$) and backcourt players ($p = 0.003$) and had larger thigh circumference compared to goalkeepers ($p < 0.001$) and backcourt players ($p < 0.001$), whereas backcourt players were heavier than goalkeepers ($p = 0.015$).

Table 1. Differences between playing positions in anthropometric characteristics and body composition.

	Backcourt Player (N = 34)	Wing (N = 26)	Pivot (N = 15)	Goalkeeper (N = 17)	p
Height (cm)	187 (8)[1]	179 (7)	185 (7) [1]	185 (6) [1]	<0.001
Weight (kg)	87 (11) [1,2]	75 (9)	102 (11) [1,2]	78 (10)	<0.001
Wingspan (cm)	190 (9) [1]	180 (8)	191 (9) [1]	186 (8) [1]	<0.001
Thigh circ. (cm)	60 (5) [1]	57 (5)	68 (5) [1,2,3]	58 (5)	<0.001
Skeletal muscle mass (kg)	44 (5) [1,2]	38 (4)	47 (5) [1,2]	37 (4)	<0.001
Body fat mass (kg)	12 (5)	10 (4)	23 (8) [1,2,3]	15 (7) [1]	<0.001

Cir.–circumference, [1]—significantly different from the wing, [2]—significantly different from the goalkeeper, [3]—significantly different from backcourt players.

Body composition measurements revealed that goalkeepers had significantly less skeletal muscle mass than backcourt players ($p < 0.001$) and pivots ($p < 0.001$), while wings had less skeletal muscle mass than backcourt players ($p < 0.001$) and pivots ($p < 0.001$). Pivots, on the other hand, had significantly more fat mass than wings ($p < 0.001$), backcourt players ($p < 0.001$) and goalkeepers ($p = 0.005$). Lastly, goalkeepers also had significantly more muscle mass than wings ($p = 0.010$).

Similar to the anthropometric characteristics, the playing positions differed in maximal isokinetic concentric extensor strength at 60°/s and 180°/s ($p < 0.001$), concentric knee flexion of the left knee at 60°/s ($p = 0.007$), and borderline significance of the right knee ($p = 0.070$) (Table 2). Pivot players displayed lower isokinetic concentric torque of knee extensors and flexors compared with wings and backcourt players at 60°/s and 180°/s, respectively, whereas backcourt players were superior compared to goalkeepers at 60°/s and 180°/s of knee flexion and extension. Additionally, wings performed better than goalkeepers at 60°/s and 180°/s of knee extension and flexion. Otherwise, no differences between playing positions were obtained in hamstring-to-quadriceps ratio (HQR) and in bilateral differences in maximal concentric torque of extensors and flexors at 60°/s and 180°/s.

Table 2. Differences among playing positions in isokinetic concentric torque.

	Backcourt Player (N = 34)	Wing (N = 26)	Pivot (N = 15)	Goalkeeper (N = 17)	p
Extension left knee at 60°/s (Nm/kg)	2.80 (0.58)	2.88 (0.55)	2.23 (0.45) [1,2]	2.53 (0.32) [1,2]	<0.001
Extension right knee at 60°/s (Nm/kg)	2.86 (0.45)	2.83 (0.56)	2.30 (0.43) [1,2]	2.50 (0.35) [2]	<0.001
Extension left knee at 180°/s (Nm/kg)	1.80 (0.32)	1.85 (0.28)	1.42 (0.28)[1,2]	1.49 (0.29) [1,2]	<0.001
Extension right knee at 180°/s (Nm/kg)	1.79 (0.27)	1.73 (0.36)	1.45 (0.27) [1,2]	1.51 (0.24) [2]	<0.001
Flexion left knee at 60°/s (Nm/kg)	1.74 (0.38)	1.74 (0.38)	1,50 (0.63) [1,2]	1.52 (0.24) [1,2]	0.007
Flexion right knee at 60°/s (Nm/kg)	1.78 (0.25)	1.70 (0.39)	1.57 (0.59)	1.53 (0.39)	0.070
Flexion left knee at 180°/s (Nm/kg)	1.33 (0.29)	1.33 (0.30)	1.07 (0.34) [1,2]	1.11 (0.26) [1,2]	0.002
Flexion right knee at 180°/s (Nm/kg)	1.32 (0.25)	1.21 (0.28)	1.08 (0.34) [2]	1.12 (0.22) [2]	0.012
Bilateral ratio left–right knee extension at 60°/s (%)	98.23 (15.08)	102.36 (9.97)	95.95 (7.04)	96.95 (7.04)	0.251
Bilateral ratio left–right knee flexion at 60°/s (%)	98.50 (21.14)	103.16 (11.35)	95.17 (10.47)	102.86 (20.42)	0.059
Bilateral ratio left–right knee extension at 180°/s (%)	101.89 (19.47)	110.65 (16.02)	100.71 (13.56)	98.58 (11.86)	0.112
Bilateral ratio left–right knee flexion at 180°/s (%)	101.43 (17.55)	109.70 (19.37)	97.76 (9.74)	98.59 (13.11)	0.068
HQR left knee at 60°/s (%)	63.23 (17.97)	60.84 (11.78)	70.29 (36.66)	59.93 (6.39)	0.725
HQR right knee at 60°/s (%)	63.56 (12.52)	60.54 (11.69)	69.40 (28.23)	61.06 (12.21)	0.958
HQR left knee at 180°/s (%)	74.18 (15.22)	71.55 (11.83)	77.35 (27.68)	74.67 (13.42)	0.596
HQR right knee at 180°/s (%)	74.32 (14.73)	70.90 (12.91)	74.58 (21.80)	74.17 (10.87)	0.704

HQR–hamstring-to-quadriceps torque ratio, [1]—significantly different from the wing, [2]—significantly different from backcourt players.

Measurements of sprinting and vertical jump performance showed significant differences between playing positions (all p-values < 0.01; Table 3). Wing players were significantly faster than backcourt players (5 m, $p = 0.042$; 10 m, $p = 0.001$; and 20 m, $p = 0.027$), goalkeepers (5 m, $p = 0.013$; 10 m, $p = 0.001$; and 20 m, $p = 0.001$), and pivots (5 m, $p = 0.001$ and 20 m, $p < 0.001$). At the 10-m time gate, backcourt players were significantly faster than goalkeepers ($p < 0.001$). Moreover, backcourt players and wings jumped significantly higher compared to pivots (backcourt players vs. pivots: CMJ, $p = 0.007$, SJ, $p = 0.027$; wings vs. pivots: CMJ, $p < 0.001$, SJ, $p < 0.001$) and goalkeepers (backcourt players vs. pivots: CMJ, $p = 0.006$; wings vs. goalkeepers: CMJ, $p < 0.001$, SJ, $p = 0.004$), respectively.

Table 3. Differences between playing positions in sprinting, vertical jump performance, and handball shooting performance.

	Backcourt Player (N = 34)	Wing (N = 26)	Pivot (N = 15)	Goalkeeper (N = 17)	*p*
Sprint 5 m (s)	1.05 (0.08) [1]	1.01 (0.08)	1.11 (0.09) [1]	1.10 (0.12) [1]	0.006
Sprint 10 m (s)	1.83 (0.20) [1]	1.75 (0.24)	1.93 (0.30)	1.97 (0.13) [1,3]	0.003
Sprint 20 m (s)	3.31 (0.24) [1]	3.15 (0.19)	3.44 (0.22) [1]	3.42 (0.17) [1]	<0.001
SJ (cm)	30 (5)	32 (6)	25 (6) [1,3]	26 (4) [1,3]	<0.001
CMJ (cm)	34 (4)	37 (6)	29 (6) [1,3]	31 (5) [1]	<0.001
Set shot (km/h)	89 (7) [1,2]	84 (9) [2]	89 (5) [2]	79 (6)	<0.001
Jump shot (km/h)	88 (7) [1,2]	83 (9) [2]	87 (9) [2]	77 (6)	<0.001

SJ–squat jump, CMJ–countermovement jump, [1]—significantly different from the wing, [2]—significantly different from the goalkeeper, [3]—significantly different from backcourt players.

There were also significant differences in ball velocity among playing positions (both *p*-values <0.001). Post hoc analysis showed that goalkeepers shoot the ball at significantly lower velocity while shooting from ground position (all *p*-values < 0.01) or while performing a three-step jump shot (all *p*-values < 0.01).

Correlations between handball shooting performance and sprinting, jumping, and maximal strength performance are shown in Table 4. With the exception of body fat mass and thigh circumference, all other anthropometric characteristics were significantly correlated with the ball velocity of a three-step set shot and jump shot. A higher SJ was significantly correlated with the ball velocity of the set shot, and borderline significant with the ball velocity of the jump shot. Maximal isokinetic torque of knee flexors and extensors was significantly correlated with ball velocity of both shot types. Lastly, HQR at 60°/s was significantly correlated with the ball velocity of the set shot.

Table 4. Correlations between playing positions in sprinting, vertical jump performance, and handball shooting performance.

	Set Shot (m/s)		Jump Shot (m/s)	
	Spearman Rho	*p*	Spearman Rho	*p*
Height (cm)	0.330	0.001	0.263	0.011
Weight (kg)	0.303	0.003	0.282	0.006
Skeletal muscle mass (kg)	0.522	<0.001	0.473	<0.001
Body fat mass (kg)	−0.116	0.267	−0.083	0.428
Wingspan (cm)	0.387	<0.001	0.349	0.001
Thigh circumference (cm)	0.183	0.080	0.166	0.112
Sprint 20 (s)	0.061	0.566	−0.018	0.862
SJ (cm)	0.210	0.043	0.185	0.076
CMJ (cm)	0.128	0.221	0.057	0.585
Knee extension torque at 60°/s (Nm)	0.219	0.035	0.340	0.001
Knee extension torque at 180°/s (Nm)	0.352	0.001	0.419	<0.001
Knee flexion torque at 60°/s (Nm)	0.493	<0.001	0.465	<0.001
Knee flexion torque at 180°/s (Nm)	0.477	<0.001	0.460	<0.001
HQR at 60°/s (%)	0.317	0.002	0.171	0.101
HQR at 180°/s (%)	0.139	0.185	0.061	0.564

SJ–squat jump, CMJ–countermovement jump, HQR–hamstring-to-quadriceps torque ratio.

4. Discussion

In the present study, we identified differences between playing positions in anthropometric characteristics, isometric maximal leg strength, sprinting and vertical jumping performance, and established new evidence on the relationship between anthropometry, physical performance, and ball velocity as an indicator of game performance. The most novel findings of this study were related to isokinetic performance, adding to the few reports of the isokinetic maximal strength and strength imbalances in elite male handball players that have been published to our knowledge [19–21]. Our results suggest that maximal knee flexor and extensor strength is related to playing position, whereas no differences between playing positions were observed in bilateral muscle imbalances or the ratios between knee joint agonists and antagonists.

In the previous studies of sports performance in elite handball, the investigators applied different methods to assess maximal leg strength. Most of those studies on elite male handball players used different variations of maximal squat tests to determine maximal leg strength [4,11,15,32], while (only) a small body of evidence used isokinetic testing [19,20], despite it being considered the gold standard for assessing quadriceps and hamstring maximal strength and muscle imbalances [17,18]. Most studies measuring maximal isokinetic knee strength were performed with females [18,24,38,39], likely due to higher rates of anterior cruciate ligament injuries, compared with males [40], while only two isokinetic studies included male handball players [19,20]. In the latter studies, male handball players were recognized as functionally balanced athletes, where maximal unilateral (50–69%) and bilateral (10–15%) muscle strength differences were in the normal range [19,20]. This was similarly demonstrated in our study, although there were no bilateral differences in maximal strength of flexors and extensors, or muscle imbalances between hamstrings and quadriceps on each leg at 60°/s and 180°/s. Our relative values of maximal flexion and extension torque at 60°/s and 180°/s (N/kg) were also similar to a report by Gonzalez-Rave et al. [20]. Additionally, our study also evaluated the difference between playing positions in relative maximal strength and muscle imbalances. Backcourt and wing players were the strongest in extension and flexion, independent of muscle mass at both angular velocities. These results may potentially be associated with game demands, as wings and backcourt players perform the most jumps and throws [7]. In contrast, all playing positions showed symmetrical strength (unilateral and bilateral ratios in the normal range) between legs and within each leg analysis.

Studies have suggested that anthropometric characteristics are related to playing position. In our study, wing players were the shortest, had the lowest body weight, shortest wingspan and smallest thigh circumference, while pivots had the highest body weight, skeletal muscle mass, and body fat mass content. These results were in line with previous studies [7,10,13–16] from elite and sub-elite male handball players. Despite the similar ages of players and the differences between playing positions in body weight and height, our subsample of backcourt players, pivots, and goalkeepers was generally shorter and lighter than players competing on elite German [10,14], Norwegian [15], and national teams playing in the World Championship [9]. Thus, these differences can be explained by the level of play and age. Players competing in lower leagues were generally shorter [10], independent of playing position, whereas pivots in higher leagues were heavier and had the highest body mass index [14]. Also, younger elite handball players were shorter, lighter, had lower free fat mass and body mass index values compared to elite adult players [16].

The fastest sprint times were recorded in wing players compared to other playing positions on each of three time gates (5 m, 10 m, and 20 m). Similar variations in sprinting performance at 20 m were observed in the other two studies consisting of handball players performing in elite European leagues [14,15]. In addition to the fastest times recorded by wings, backcourt players were also faster than goalkeepers on 10-m sprints, similar to data obtained by Haugen et al. [15] (wings, 2.78 (0.08) s; backcourt players, 2.83 (0.11) s; goalkeepers, 2.94 (0.10) s). Partly contrary to our findings, one study reported significant differences between playing positions only on longer sprint distances (30 m), postulating equal starting acceleration of all playing positions, which likely contributed to the longer competitive career and a higher level of competition [14]. Moreover, sprinting performance is closely related to the in-game demands of each playing position. Data derived from game movement analysis has shown that wing players have a higher frequency of performed sprints, with the longest duration, time, and fraction of distance covered compared to pivots and backcourt players [7].

Vertical jumping is an important movement performed during the course of the game [7]. In previous studies, the best vertical jumps were performed by the wings (39–50 cm) and backcourt players (38–47 cm), compared to pivots (35–43 cm) and goalkeepers (35–47 cm) [14,15]. Similar differences between playing positions were also obtained in our study. Nevertheless, jump performance was lower compared to data from two samples of elite European Championship players [14,15], but comparable to a similar level of play [16], thus, our results were likely influenced by the level of play and quality of the training regime.

Handball scoring efficiency is largely dependent on ball velocity. In our study, ball velocity was highest in backcourt players and lowest in wings and goalkeepers. A similar superiority was also obtained in other samples of elite players [13–15], although the maximal shooting velocities of our participants (88.94 km/h) were only comparable to one study (90.72 km/h) [14], while others performed better (94.32–96.84 km/h) [13,15]. The best shooting performance from three-step shots was reported in a sample of Tunisian national team players (99.67 km/h), although it showed no significant difference between playing positions, likely due to its small sample size (N = 21) [11].

The kinematics of overhead shoots is a highly complex whole-body movement [26], with many studies undertaken to identify the possible determinants of shooting success [10,11,13,31,32]. Our results supported previous findings that suggest body height and mass may influence shooting velocities from a standing [11] and/or jumping position [10,13,31]. In contrast, several studies investigating the correlations between physical performance and ball velocity have been inconclusive [11,13,31,32]. Others, including our study, reported significant correlations between ball velocity and sprinting time, lower limb maximal strength, and endurance [31,32], while others failed to reach such conclusions [11,13]. Furthermore, our results also highlighted the importance of lower limb muscle mass and strength as an initiator of proximal-to-distal principal during the shot [41]. When an optimal sequence of force translation from proximal muscles of legs, pelvis, and trunk to throwing arm is achieved, the highest force production in the leg muscles can substantially contribute to higher ball velocities [27,29,32], as confirmed in our study. Similarly, recent study has suggested that jump height in the CMJ is significantly correlated with jump height while performing a jump shot in a game-based performance test [42]. During the handball game, this may present an advantage over the opponent, as the three-step jump shot is the most frequently executed shot [26]. In addition to faster ball-shooting velocity, the importance of jump height may also explain the higher frequency of jumps and shots performed during the game by backcourt players compared to pivots and goalkeepers [7]. However, as a handball shot is a complex, multi-joint movement, more research is needed to determine new potential physical performance determinants of shooting success (e.g., ball velocity).

In summary, the results of this study may further clarify several important aspects of the anthropometric and physical aspects of handball performance with special reference to playing position. Firstly, we confirmed previously reported variations between playing positions in anthropometric characteristics, sprinting, jumping, and handball shooting performance. Secondly, and most importantly, our study was one of the first to establish new evidence on the isokinetic maximal strength of lower limbs. We provided novel data for maximal torque of extensors and flexors in elite handball as well as demonstrated that male handball players are symmetrical with no significant maximal strength deficits between, and within, knee extensors and flexors. Lastly, our study also established further evidence on the potential role of various physical performance aspects in handball success as measured by ball velocity. Despite presenting novel findings on one of the largest samples in male handball performance research, some limitations must be acknowledged. Most of our sample were members of Kosovo's national handball team, but none of them played abroad in higher-ranking leagues or the European Championship league. As Kosovo is a young country with very few professional handball opportunities, our results may be affected by the playing level, training process, and relative lack of experience of the players. Nevertheless, our data showed results comparable to other elite playing countries, e.g., Germany and Norway, therefore, we believe that strong professional handball foundations have been built in Kosovo.

5. Conclusions

In conclusion, our study clearly demonstrated the importance of anthropometry, jumping performance, and maximal isometric strength to handball performance. In future sports practice, more emphasis should be given to handball-specific resistance training for players to gain more muscle mass of lower (legs and pelvis) and upper limbs (shoulders and arms), which will afterwards manifest in better jumping, sprinting, and shooting performance. Special consideration must be given to resistance training of pivots and goalkeepers to improve their muscle strength and shooting performance [2], as they were outperformed by wings and backcourt players. Furthermore, we also propose the routine inclusion of isometric measurement of shoulder and knee joint maximal torques to monitor changes of maximal muscle strength during the course of the handball season and to detect potential muscle imbalances, which may contribute to higher injury incidence. In line with this, more studies on elite and sub-elite handball players should be conducted to provide new practical evidence of the importance of isokinetic testing and to further determine several important aspects of physical performance in relation to handball shooting performance.

Author Contributions: Conceptualization, J.H., T.K., K.I., D.B. and P.P.; methodology, J.H., T.K., K.I., D.B. and P.P.; software, J.H., A.B.; validation, J.H., A.B. and P.P.; formal analysis, J.H., T.K. and P.P.; investigation, J.H., A.B. and P.P; resources, J.H. and A.B.; data curation, T.K.; writing—original draft preparation, J.H., T.K. and P.P.; writing—review and editing, J.H., A.B.,T.K., K.I., D.B. and P.P.; visualization, J.H., T.K. and P.P.; supervision, K.I., D.B.,P.P.; project administration, J.H., A.B. and P.P. All authors have read and approved the final version of the manuscript.

Acknowledgments: The authors would like to thank all participants for their efforts during the study, and Jožef Šimenko, for his valuable feedback during the preparation of the manuscript. No external funds were used in the present study.

References

1. Saavedra, J.M. Handball Research: State of the Art. *J. Hum. Kinet.* **2018**, *63*, 5–8. [CrossRef] [PubMed]
2. Ziv, G.A.L.; Lidor, R. Physical characteristics, physiological attributes, and on-court performances of handball players: A review. *Eur. J. Sport Sci.* **2009**, *9*, 375–386. [CrossRef]
3. Karcher, C.; Buchheit, M. On-court demands of elite handball, with special reference to playing positions. *Sport Med.* **2014**, *44*, 797–814. [CrossRef] [PubMed]
4. Ortega-Becerra, M.; Pareja-Blanco, F.; Jiménez-Reyes, P.; Cuadrado-Peñafiel, V.; González-Badillo, J.J. Determinant Factors of Physical Performance and Specific Throwing in Handball Players of Different Ages. *J. Strength Cond. Res.* **2018**, *32*, 1778–1786. [CrossRef]
5. Gorostiaga, E.M.; Granados, C.; Ibanez, J.; Izquierdo, M. Differences in physical fitness and throwing velocity among elite and amateur male handball players. *Int. J. Sports Med.* **2005**, *26*, 225–232. [CrossRef]
6. Barbero, J.C.; Granda-Vera, J.; Calleja-González, J.; Del Coso, J. Physical and physiological demands of elite team handball players. *Int. J. Perform. Anal. Sport* **2014**, *14*, 921–933. [CrossRef]
7. Póvoas, S.C.A.; Ascensão, A.A.M.R.; Magalhães, J.; Seabra, A.F.; Krustrup, P.; Soares, J.M.C.; Rebelo, A.N. Physiological demands of elite team handball with special reference to playing position. *J. Strength Cond. Res.* **2014**, *28*, 430–442. [CrossRef]
8. Michalsik, L.; Aagaard, P. Physical demands in elite team handball: Comparisons between male and female players. *J. Sport Med. Phys. Fit.* **2015**, *55*, 878–891.
9. Ghobadi, H.; Rajabi, H.; Farzad, B.; Bayati, M.; Jeffreys, I. Anthropometry of world-class elite handball players according to the playing position: Reports from men's handball world championship 2013. *J. Hum. Kinet.* **2013**, *39*, 213–220. [CrossRef]

10. Fieseler, G.; Hermassi, S.; Hoffmeyer, B.; Schulze, S.; Irlenbusch, L.; Bartels, T.; Delank, K.S.; Laudner, K.G.; Schwesig, R. Differences in anthropometric characteristics in relation to throwing velocity and competitive level in professional male team handball: A tool for talent profiling. *J. Sports Med. Phys. Fit.* **2017**, *57*, 985–992.
11. Chaouachi, A.; Brughelli, M.; Levin, G.; Boudhina, N.B.B.; Cronin, J.; Chamari, K. Anthropometric, physiological and performance characteristics of elite team-handball players. *J. Sports Sci.* **2009**, *27*, 151–157. [CrossRef] [PubMed]
12. Hermassi, S.; Laudner, K.G.; Schwesig, R. Playing level and position differences in body characteristics and physical fitness performance among male team handball players. *Front. Bioeng. Biotechnol.* **2019**, *7*, 149. [CrossRef] [PubMed]
13. Schwesig, R.; Hermassi, S.; Fieseler, G.; Irlenbusch, L.; Noack, F.; Delank, K.-S.; Shephard, R.J.; Chelly, M.S. Anthropometric and physical performance characteristics of professional handball players: Influence of playing position. *J. Sports Med. Phys. Fit.* **2017**, *57*, 1471–1478.
14. Krüger, K.; Pilat, C.; Ückert, K.; Frech, T.; Mooren, F.C. Physical Performance Profile of Handball Players Is Related to Playing Position and Playing Class. *J. Strength Cond. Res.* **2014**, *28*, 117–125. [CrossRef] [PubMed]
15. Haugen, T.A.; Tønnessen, E.; Seiler, S. Physical and physiological characteristics of male handball players: Influence of playing position and competitive level. *J. Sports Med. Phys. Fit.* **2016**, *56*, 19–26.
16. Nikolaidis, P.T.; Ingebrigtsen, J.; Póvoas, S.C.; Moss, S.; Torres-Luque, G.; Pantelis, N. Physical and physiological characteristics in male team handball players by playing position-Does age matter. *J. Sports Med. Phys. Fit.* **2015**, *55*, 297–304.
17. Maurelli, O.; Bernard, P.L.; Dubois, R.; Ahmaidi, S.; Prioux, J. Effects of the Competitive Season on the Isokinetic Muscle Parameters Changes in World-Class Handball Players. *J. Strength Cond. Res.* **2019**, *33*, 2778–2787. [CrossRef]
18. Xaverova, Z.; Dirnberger, J.; Lehnert, M.; Belka, J.; Wagner, H.; Orechovska, K. Isokinetic strength profile of elite female handball players. *J. Hum. Kinet.* **2015**, *49*, 257–266. [CrossRef]
19. Teixeira, J.; Carvalho, P.; Moreira, C.; Santos, R. Isokinetic assessment of muscle imbalances and bilateral differences between knee extensores and flexores' strength in basketball, footbal, handball and volleyball athletes. *Int. J. Sport Sci.* **2014**, *4*, 1–6.
20. Gonzalez-Rave, J.M.; Juarez, D.; Rubio-Arias, J.A.; Suarez, V.J.; Martinez-Valencia, M.A.; Abian-Vicen, J. Isokinetic leg strength and power in elite handball players. *J. Hum. Kinet.* **2014**, *41*, 227–233. [CrossRef]
21. Carvalho, A.; Mourão, P.; Abade, E. Effects of Strength Training Combined with Specific Plyometric exercises on body composition, vertical jump height and lower limb strength development in elite male handball players: A case study. *J. Hum. Kinet.* **2014**, *41*, 125–132. [CrossRef] [PubMed]
22. Andrade, M.D.S.; Fleury, A.M.; de Lira, C.A.B.; Dubas, J.P.; da Silva, A.C. Profile of isokinetic eccentric-to-concentric strength ratios of shoulder rotator muscles in elite female team handball players. *J. Sports Sci.* **2010**, *28*, 743–749. [CrossRef] [PubMed]
23. Dos Santos Andrade, M.; de Lira, C.A.B.; Vancini, R.L.; de Almeida, A.A.; Benedito-Silva, A.A.; da Silva, A.C. Profiling the isokinetic shoulder rotator muscle strength in 13-to 36-year-old male and female handball players. *Phys. Ther. Sport* **2013**, *14*, 246–252. [CrossRef] [PubMed]
24. Risberg, M.A.; Steffen, K.; Nilstad, A.; Myklebust, G.; Kristianslund, E.; Moltubakk, M.M.; Krosshaug, T. Normative quadriceps and hamstring muscle strength values for female, healthy, elite handball and football players. *J. Strength Cond. Res.* **2018**, *32*, 2314. [CrossRef]
25. Steffen, K.; Nilstad, A.; Kristianslund, E.K.; Myklebust, G.; Bahr, R.; Krosshaug, T. Association between lower extremity muscle strength and noncontact ACL injuries. *Med. Sci. Sport Exerc.* **2016**, *48*, 2082–2089. [CrossRef]
26. Bencke, J.; van den Tillaar, R.; Møller, M.; Wagner, H. Throwing Biomechanics: Aspects of Throwing Performance and Shoulder Injury Risk. In *Handball Sports Medicine*; Laver, L., Landreau, P., Seil, R., Popović, N., Eds.; Springer: Berlin/Heidelberg, Germany, 2018; pp. 69–79.
27. Wagner, H.; Pfusterschmied, J.; Klous, M.; von Duvillard, S.P.; Müller, E. Movement variability and skill level of various throwing techniques. *Hum. Mov. Sci.* **2012**, *31*, 78–90. [CrossRef]
28. Wagner, H.; Pfusterschmied, J.; von Duvillard, S.P.; Müller, E. Performance and kinematics of various throwing techniques in team-handball. *J. Sports Sci. Med.* **2011**, *10*, 73.
29. Wagner, H.; Buchecker, M.; Von Duvillard, S.P.; Müller, E. Kinematic description of elite vs. low level players in team-handball jump throw. *J. Sports Sci. Med.* **2010**, *9*, 15.

30. Michalsik, L.; Madsen, K.; Aagaard, P. Physiological capacity and physical testing in male elite team handball. *J. Sport Med. Phys. Fit.* **2015**, *55*, 415–429.
31. Zapartidis, I.; Kororos, P.; Christodoulidis, T.; Skoufas, D.; Bayios, I. Profile of young handball players by playing position and determinants of ball throwing velocity. *J. Hum. Kinet.* **2011**, *27*, 17–30. [CrossRef]
32. Hermassi, S.; Chelly, M.S.; Wagner, H.; Fieseler, G.; Schulze, S.; Delank, K.-S.; Shephard, R.J.; Schwesig, R. Relationships between maximal strength of lower limb, anthropometric characteristics and fundamental explosive performance in handball players. *Sport. Sport.* **2019**, *33*, 96–103. [CrossRef] [PubMed]
33. Stewart, A.D.; Marfell-Jones, M.; Olds, T.; De Ridder, J.H. *International Standards for Anthropometric Assessment*; International Society for the Advancement of Kinanthropometry: Wellington, New Zealand, 2012.
34. Lee, L.-W.; Liao, Y.-S.; Lu, H.-K.; Hsiao, P.-L.; Chen, Y.-Y.; Chi, C.-C.; Hsieh, K.C. Validation of two portable bioelectrical impedance analyses for the assessment of body composition in school age children. *PLoS ONE* **2017**, *12*, e0171568. [CrossRef] [PubMed]
35. Van Melick, N.; Meddeler, B.M.; Hoogeboom, T.J.; Nijhuis-van der Sanden, M.W.G.; van Cingel, R.E.H. How to determine leg dominance: The agreement between self-reported and observed performance in healthy adults. *PLoS ONE* **2017**, *12*, e0189876. [CrossRef] [PubMed]
36. Kovaleski, J.E.; Heitman, R.J. Testing and training the lower extremity. In *Isokinetics in Human Performance*; Brown, L.E., Ed.; Human Kinetics: Champagne, IL, USA, 2000; pp. 171–195.
37. Croisier, J.-L.; Ganteaume, S.; Binet, J.; Genty, M.; Ferret, J.-M. Strength Imbalances and Prevention of Hamstring Injury in Professional Soccer Players: A Prospective Study. *Am. J. Sports Med.* **2008**, *36*, 1469–1475. [CrossRef] [PubMed]
38. Andrade, M.D.S.; De Lira, C.A.B.; Koffes, F.D.C.; Mascarin, N.C.; Benedito-Silva, A.A.; Da Silva, A.C. Isokinetic hamstrings-to-quadriceps peak torque ratio: The influence of sport modality, gender, and angular velocity. *J. Sports Sci.* **2012**, *30*, 547–553. [CrossRef] [PubMed]
39. Lund-Hanssen, H.; Gannon, J.; Engebretsen, L.; Holen, K.; Hammer, S. Isokinetic muscle performance in healthy female handball players and players with a unilateral anterior cruciate ligament reconstruction. *Scand. J. Med. Sci. Sports* **1996**, *6*, 172–175. [CrossRef] [PubMed]
40. Myklebust, G.; Maehlum, S.; Holm, I.; Bahr, R. A prospective cohort study of anterior cruciate ligament injuries in elite Norwegian team handball. *Scand. J. Med. Sci. Sports* **1998**, *8*, 149–153. [CrossRef]
41. Herring, R.M.; Chapman, A.E. Effects of changes in segmental values and timing of both torque and torque reversal in simulated throws. *J. Biomech.* **1992**, *25*, 1173–1184. [CrossRef]
42. Wagner, H.; Sperl, B.; Bell, J.W.; Von Duvillard, S.P. Testing specific physical performance in male team handball players and the relationship to general tests in team sports. *J. Strength Cond. Res.* **2019**, *33*, 1056–1064. [CrossRef]

7

Satiating Effect of High Protein Diets on Resistance-Trained Individuals in Energy Deficit

Justin Roberts [1,*], Anastasia Zinchenko [2,3], Krishnaa T. Mahbubani [4], James Johnstone [1], Lee Smith [1], Viviane Merzbach [1], Miguel Blacutt [3], Oscar Banderas [3], Luis Villasenor [3], Fredrik T. Vårvik [3] and Menno Henselmans [3]

1 School of Psychology and Sport Science, Cambridge Centre for Sport and Exercise Sciences, Anglia Ruskin University, East Road, Cambridge CB1 1PT, UK; james.johnstone@anglia.ac.uk (J.J.); lee.smith@anglia.ac.uk (L.S.); viviane.merzbach@anglia.ac.uk (V.M.)

2 Department of Biochemistry, Kings College, University of Cambridge, Kings Parade, Cambridge CB2 1ST, UK; a.zinchenko@live.de

3 International Scientific Research Foundation for Fitness and Nutrition, 1073 LC Amsterdam, The Netherlands; miguelblacutt@hotmail.com (M.B.); oscarbanderastk@gmail.com (O.B.); luis@villasenor.net (L.V.); ftvaarvik@gmail.com (F.T.V.); menno.henselmans@gmail.com (M.H.)

4 Department of Surgery, Addenbrookes Hospital, Cambridge CB2 0QQ, UK; ktam2@cam.ac.uk

* Correspondence: Justin.roberts@anglia.ac.uk

Abstract: Short-term energy deficit strategies are practiced by weight class and physique athletes, often involving high protein intakes to maximize satiety and maintain lean mass despite a paucity of research. This study compared the satiating effect of two protein diets on resistance-trained individuals during short-term energy deficit. Following ethical approval, 16 participants (age: 28 $\pm$ 2 years; height: 1.72 $\pm$ 0.03 m; body-mass: 88.83 $\pm$ 5.54 kg; body-fat: 21.85 $\pm$ 1.82%) were randomly assigned to 7-days moderate (PRO_{MOD}: 1.8 $g \cdot kg^{-1} \cdot d^{-1}$) or high protein ($PRO_{HIGH}$: 2.9 $g \cdot kg^{-1} \cdot d^{-1}$) matched calorie-deficit diets in a cross-over design. Daily satiety responses were recorded throughout interventions. Pre-post diet, plasma ghrelin and peptide tyrosine tyrosine (PYY), and satiety ratings were assessed in response to a protein-rich meal. Only perceived satisfaction was significantly greater following PRO_{HIGH} (67.29 $\pm$ 4.28 v 58.96 $\pm$ 4.51 mm, $p = 0.04$). Perceived cravings increased following PRO_{MOD} only (46.25 $\pm$ 4.96 to 57.60 $\pm$ 4.41 mm, $p = 0.01$). Absolute ghrelin concentration significantly reduced post-meal following PRO_{MOD} (972.8 $\pm$ 130.4 to 613.6 $\pm$ 114.3 $pg \cdot mL^{-1}$; $p = 0.003$), remaining lower than PRO_{HIGH} at 2 h (-0.40 ± 0.06 v -0.26 ± 0.06 $pg \cdot mL^{-1}$ normalized relative change; $p = 0.015$). Absolute PYY concentration increased to a similar extent post-meal (PRO_{MOD}: 84.9 $\pm$ 8.9 to 147.1 $\pm$ 11.9 $pg \cdot mL^{-1}$, PRO_{HIGH}: 100.6 $\pm$ 9.5 to 143.3 $\pm$ 12.0 $pg \cdot mL^{-1}$; $p < 0.001$), but expressed as relative change difference was significantly greater for PRO_{MOD} at 2 h (+0.39 $\pm$ 0.20 $pg \cdot mL^{-1}$ v -0.28 ± 0.12 $pg \cdot mL^{-1}$; $p = 0.001$). Perceived hunger, fullness and satisfaction post-meal were comparable between diets ($p > 0.05$). However, desire to eat remained significantly blunted for PRO_{MOD} ($p = 0.048$). PRO_{HIGH} does not confer additional satiating benefits in resistance-trained individuals during short-term energy deficit. Ghrelin and PYY responses to a test-meal support the contention that satiety was maintained following PRO_{MOD}, although athletes experiencing negative symptoms (i.e., cravings) may benefit from protein-rich meals as opposed to over-consumption of protein.

Keywords: dietary protein; satiety; ghrelin; peptide YY; resistance training

---

1. Introduction

Weight loss is an essential component of success for many strength athletes, as well as individuals involved in general strength training. Weight class athletes restrict dietary energy intake typically for 7–21 days prior to a competition [1], or during phases of training, to enhance the strength to body-mass ratio, improve body composition, and increase the competitive advantage in weight class events [2]. For physique/ bodybuilding athletes, similar practices of caloric restriction often occurs for longer time periods i.e., >12 weeks to reach a very low body fat percentage, often going below 5% to improve aesthetical appearance and succeed in bodybuilding competitions [2,3]. During dieting phases many athletes may substantially increase their protein intake, as this practice has been shown to be beneficial to maintain lean mass whilst reducing body-fat [4–13]. Although the recommended daily intake of protein for healthy adults has been indicated at 0.83 $g{\cdot}kg^{-1}{\cdot}d^{-1}$ ([14] with habitual protein intakes being reportedly greater at ~1.2 $g{\cdot}kg^{-1}{\cdot}d^{-1}$ [15]), protein requirements for resistance-trained individuals to achieve maximal fractional synthetic rate and strength performance may exceed these recommendations ranging from 1.3 to 1.8 $g{\cdot}kg^{-1}{\cdot}d^{-1}$ [16,17]. During acute energy deficit, protein requirements may be subtly higher at 1.8–2.0 $g{\cdot}kg^{-1}{\cdot}d^{-1}$ to offset lean muscle losses. There is, however, controversy as to whether substantially higher protein intakes ranging from 2.3 to 3.1 $g{\cdot}kg^{-1}{\cdot}d^{-1}$ may in fact yield optimal results [13] with evidence that resistance-trained athletes consume protein intakes as high as 4.3 $g{\cdot}kg^{-1}{\cdot}d^{-1}$ [18].

Higher protein intakes may also provide an additional benefit of increased satiety. A recent meta-analysis by Dhillon et al. (2016) concluded that higher protein meals (ranging from 97 to 188 g) increased fullness ratings more than lower protein meals [19]. However, this analysis focused on short-term studies (up to 10 h) in untrained individuals and can therefore not necessarily be extrapolated to longer-term satiety over several days/ weeks. There may be a possibility that a person becomes accustomed to a high protein intake and that a further increase in protein intake does not result in additional satiety. This point can be particularly important for strength athletes who generally consume a higher protein diet beyond the recommended levels for maximal performance [16,17].

Very few long-term, randomized, controlled trials have examined satiety and *ad libitum* energy intake in normal weighted individuals following a low-protein vs a high-protein diet [20–22]. Only three studies have been conducted on resistance-trained individuals showing that a higher protein intake may be beneficial for muscle retention and well-being following a weight loss diet [4,6,23]. Walberg et al. have shown that even though a higher protein diet (1.6 $g{\cdot}kg^{-1}{\cdot}d^{-1}$) during an extreme weight loss intervention (18 $kcal{\cdot}kg^{-1}$) led to positive nitrogen balance compared to a lower protein group (0.8 $g{\cdot}kg^{-1}{\cdot}d^{-1}$); it also led to reduced maximal isometric muscular endurance in weight lifters [6]. In a different study, 2.3 $g{\cdot}kg^{-1}{\cdot}d^{-1}$ protein intake was shown to be beneficial for muscle retention in 40% energy deficit compared to the 1.0 $g{\cdot}kg^{-1}{\cdot}d^{-1}$ control group [4]. However, higher protein intake was also associated with increased fatigue for participants in this study, although this has been contested elsewhere [23].

The finding of increased fatigue is particularly important considering that many athletes increase their protein intake during caloric restriction in order to limit muscle loss, reduce hunger and increase the feeling of satiety [13]. An increase in fatigue can result in decreased motivation to train [4], reduced training efficiency and thus have a negative effect on athletic performance [6] particularly during the competition preparation phase, in which many weight-class strength athletes undergo weight loss interventions. It is important to note that the control condition examined in this study [4] represented an unusually low protein intake (1.0 $g{\cdot}kg^{-1}{\cdot}d^{-1}$) for strength athletes that is below the established recommendations [16]. Equally so, very high protein intakes, exceeding these recommendations, may not only negatively impact on an athletes' well-being and reduce the effort given to training, but also carries the risk of displacement of other nutrients.

Therefore, the aim of this study was to compare the satiating effect of two diets with a different protein content in resistance-trained subjects in energy deficit, participant well-being and training motivation. A moderately high protein diet (PRO_{MOD}) with an intake corresponding to the recommendation for maximal performance (1.8 $g{\cdot}kg^{-1}{\cdot}d^{-1}$) [16,17] and a very high protein diet (PRO_{HIGH}) with a protein intake of 2.9 $g{\cdot}kg^{-1}{\cdot}d^{-1}$ were used as main interventions. It was hypothesised that a protein intake of 2.9 $g \cdot kg^{-1} \cdot d^{-1}$ would not impact on satiety levels more so than an intake of 1.8 $g \cdot kg^{-1} \cdot d^{-1}$ but may reduce the motivation to train.

2. Materials and Methods

2.1. Participants

This study was conducted in accordance with the Declaration of Helsinki, and the protocol was approved by the Faculty of Science and Technology Ethics Committee, Anglia Ruskin University (approval number: FST/FREP/15/595). A priori sample size based on G*power software ($\alpha = 0.05$ and $1\text{-}\beta = 0.80$) using satiety data from Mettler et al. (2010) [4] based on resistance training individuals consuming 2.3 $g \cdot kg^{-1} \cdot d^{-1}$ vs. 1 $g \cdot kg^{-1} \cdot d^{-1}$, estimated 14 in each group. Participants were required to have a resistance training background of >6 months, while actively training >3 h per week, in a similar manner to previous research [4]. This was to ensure participants were undergoing habitual training at the point of study inclusion, and beyond the time-frame typically employed during acute training studies [24–29].

Informed consent was obtained from all individual participants prior to study inclusion. All participants satisfactorily completed a health screen questionnaire, and had no known history of cardiovascular or metabolic abnormalities (e.g., diabetes); or recent viral infections or injuries which would prevent them from maintaining habitual training sessions. As part of the inclusion criteria, participants were required to not have any blood related disorders, no known eating disorders and no known adverse reactions to whey protein supplementation, gluten or coconut oil. Additionally, all participants were required to not be taking any medication/supplementation which could influence satiety levels. Lacto-vegetarians were eligible for the study.

Twenty-two individuals (13 men, 9 women) volunteered for study inclusion. However, five participants withdrew prior to first dietary intervention (due to personal factors conflicting with the study requirements) and one participant did not complete the final assessment, resulting in 16 resistance trained participants in this randomised, controlled trial (9 men, 7 women). None of the participants reported using any anabolic drugs, and were required to refrain from taking additional supplementation (e.g., creatine, beta-alanine) for 4 weeks prior to and during the study. Participant characteristics are shown in Table 1.

Table 1. Participant characteristics and baseline measurements.

Variable	All Participants (n = 16)	Male (n = 9)	Female (n = 7)
Age (years)	28 ± 2	26 ± 2	30 ± 3
Height (m)	1.72 ± 0.03	1.79 ± 0.02	1.63 ± 0.04 *
Body-mass (kg)	88.83 ± 5.54	95.68 ± 5.73	80.01 ± 6.21
Body-fat (%)	21.85 ± 1.82	18.33 ± 1.91	26.37 ± 2.57 *
BIA FM (kg)	25.52 ± 3.37	23.12 ± 3.02	28.60 ± 6.82
BIA FM (%)	27.53 ± 2.46	23.40 ± 1.99	32.84 ± 4.40 *
BIA FFM (kg)	63.31 ± 3.50	72.56 ± 3.05	51.41 ± 3.48 *
BIA FFM (%)	72.47 ± 2.46	76.60 ± 1.99	67.16 ± 4.40 *
PA (°)	8.27 ± 0.16	8.71 ± 0.10	7.70 ± 0.19 *
TBW (%)	52.26 ± 1.77	55.23 ± 1.43	48.43 ± 3.17 *
ICW (%)	58.49 ± 0.81	59.48 ± 0.48	57.23 ± 1.43
ECW (%)	41.48 ± 0.81	40.52 ± 0.84	42.71 ± 1.45

Data presented as mean ± SE. Body-fat (%) refers to estimation via skinfold measures. BIA denotes bioelectrical impedance analysis. FM = fat-mass; FFM = fat-free mass; PA = phase angle; TBW = total body water; ICW = intracellular water; ECW = extracellular water. Hydration markers from BIA. * denotes significantly different to male cohort, $p \leq 0.05$.

2.2. Pre-Intervention Measures

All testing took place within the Cambridge Centre for Sport and Exercise Science, Human Physiology Laboratory, Anglia Ruskin University, Cambridge. Prior to main trial procedures, participants were required to visit the laboratory ~72–96 h prior to start of the first and second trials to ascertain body composition measures required for energy intake calculations. As such, participants were requested to arrive acutely fasted (i.e., no food within 3 h of assessment, and maintain habitual hydration patterns) with last consumption of fluid (~0.5 L water) 1 h prior to assessment to standardise procedures. Body-mass (Seca 799, Hamburg, Germany), height (Seca CE123 stadiometer, Hamburg, Germany) and body composition were assessed under temperature controlled conditions.

Following a standardized 5-min resting period in a supine position, single frequency bioelectrical impedance (Impedimed DF50, Carlsbad, CA, USA) was undertaken for initial assessment of body composition measures, with particular emphasis on hydration indices (to confirm adherence to the pre-testing requirements) and phase angle (a proxy marker of muscle quality to confirm trained status (with >7.0 reported for female athletes, and >8.0 for male athletes from previous research [30]). In addition, estimated body fat was evaluated using an 8 site skinfold calliper assessment (using guidelines outlined by the International Society for the Advancement of Kinanthropometry (ISAK)). All body composition measures were undertaken by the same researcher. Within the same timeframe, participants completed habitual food intake and training diaries.

2.3. Dietary Assessment

As part of pre-intervention measures, and throughout the intervention, participants were requested to maintain habitual food/activity diaries (following individual guidance in diary collation, with emphasis on meal content, portion size and weight, and fluid intake) using the smart phone app/browser program (www.MyFitnessPal.com). This method has been shown to be a reliable food tracking method used in previous studies [31–33]. Diaries were assessed using Nutritics Professional Dietary Analysis software (Nutritics Ltd., Co. Dublin, Ireland). Initial assessment was used to monitor typical food choices and habitual caloric balance (including criterion assessment of training levels). From this, assessment of individual maintenance caloric intake was undertaken using the formula of Katch-McArdle (1996) based on an estimated resting daily energy expenditure (RDEE) of 370 + (21.6 * lean body weight in kg) and adjusted against training requirements and non-exercise adaptive thermogenesis [34], based on previous research [35].

2.4. Experimental Design and Intervention Measures

This study employed an experimental, randomised controlled, counter-balanced, crossover design. Participants were randomly assigned to a 7-day matched calorie-restricted diet (20% from estimated maintenance calories) of either moderate (1.8 $g \cdot kg^{-1} \cdot d^{-1}$) or high (2.9 $g \cdot kg^{-1} \cdot d^{-1}$) total protein intake ($PRO_{MOD}$ and PRO_{HIGH} respectively) with a fixed frequency of 4 meals per day. Guidance on meal intake, food options in line with habitual patterns and portion size was provided to each participant, along with provision of additional whey protein to supplement daily intake where required. Participants visited the laboratory prior to starting the dietary intervention (day 0), and again at on the completion of the 7 days (day 8) for assessment of satiety measures to a test meal (see below). After each diet, participants were required to undertake a 3-day period in which the same meal frequency (4 meals per day) was maintained, and protein intake was fixed (1.8 $g \cdot kg^{-1} \cdot d^{-1}$). However, energy, carbohydrate and fat intake was permitted *ad libitum* at each meal until participants felt full. Perception of satiety was noted by participants across each day during this period. This was included to determine the dieting condition less likely to result in acute post-diet overeating.

Throughout this 10-day period, participants recorded all food and fluid intakes using an individually allocated MyFitnessPal account, and maintained habitual training patterns. Compliance of dietary intake was checked daily by the research team, and further individual support was provided as required to meet expected intakes. At the end of the first dietary period, participants undertook a washout period and returned to habitual intake patterns for 4 weeks before returning to carry out the opposing dietary condition. Mean dietary intakes at baseline and for each intervention are shown in Table 2.

Table 2. Mean dietary intake at baseline and across intervention periods.

Variable	Category	PRO_{MOD}		PRO_{HIGH}	
		PRE	POST	PRE	POST
Energy Intake	($kcal \cdot d^{-1}$)	2359.44 ± 220.84 *	2057.44 ± 104.47	2270.71 ± 150.41 *	2119.44 ± 122.79
	($kcal \cdot kg^{-1} \cdot d^{-1}$)	26.89 ± 1.94	23.83 ± 0.93	25.53 ± 1.17	24.35 ± 0.84
Protein Intake	($g \cdot d^{-1}$)	158.19 ± 13.55	162.94 ± 10.14	166.71 ± 18.33	256.13 ± 16.64 [a,b]
	($g \cdot kg^{-1} \cdot d^{-1}$)	1.80 ± 0.12	1.84 ± 0.02	1.84 ± 0.15	2.89 ± 0.01 [a,b]
	(%EI)	27.79 ± 1.98	31.68 ± 1.33	28.79 ± 2.13	48.44 ± 1.93 [a,b]
Carbohydrate Intake	($g \cdot d^{-1}$)	220.75 ± 25.34	238.75 ± 13.32	221.79 ± 12.07	160.88 ± 13.88 [a,b]
	($g \cdot kg^{-1} \cdot d^{-1}$)	2.57 ± 0.25	2.81 ± 0.18	2.55 ± 0.16	1.90 ± 0.16 [a,b]
	(%EI)	38.08 ± 2.52	46.55 ± 1.32 [a]	40.28 ± 2.45	30.32 ± 1.82 [a,b]
Fat Intake	($g \cdot d^{-1}$)	90.94 ± 11.40	46.88 ± 2.62 [a]	73.79 ± 7.68	47.31 ± 2.80 [a]
	($g \cdot kg^{-1} \cdot d^{-1}$)	1.02 ± 0.11	0.55 ± 0.03 [a]	0.83 ± 0.08 [b]	0.55 ± 0.03 [a]
	(%EI)	14.83 ± 0.77	9.12 ± 0.25 [a]	12.86 ± 0.90 [b]	8.94 ± 0.21 [a]

Data presented as mean ± SE, and for macronutrient categories expressed in grams per day, grams per kg per day, and percentage of energy intake (EI). PRO_{MOD} denotes moderate protein condition (target: 1.80 $g \cdot kg^{-1} \cdot d^{-1}$); PRO_{HIGH} denotes high protein condition (target: 2.90 $g \cdot kg^{-1} \cdot d^{-1}$). * denotes main effect for time ($p = 0.04$), but no significant post-hoc findings. [a] denotes significantly different to PRE within condition ($p \leq 0.005$). [b] denotes significantly different to PRO_{MOD} at same time-point ($p \leq 0.024$).

2.5. Laboratory Measures

Laboratory assessment took place on day 0 and 8 of each main intervention period, in addition to pre-trial body composition measures. Participants were instructed to refrain from strenuous physical activity 24–48 h prior to all laboratory visits, arrive strictly overnight fasted (>12 h) and avoid any undue exertion travelling to the laboratory. Upon arrival, participants were required to rest in a seated position for ~30 min without any undue distractions and complete an online satiety questionnaire (see below). Following this, a venous whole blood sample (T0) was collected from participants by a qualified phlebotomist into duplicate 4 mL K3EDTA vacutainers (Greiner Bio-One GmbH, Kremsmunster, Austria). Once collected, stabilisers were added to each of the samples prior to being centrifuged for 15 min at 3000 g. The plasma layer was pipetted and aliquoted into sterile, non-pyrogenic, polypropylene cryovials (Fisherbrand, Fisher Scientific, Loughborough, UK) and immediately frozen at −20 °C for later assessment of satiety hormones: ghrelin and peptide YY (PYY). Body composition measures (height, weight, bioelectrical impedance) were assessed at the end of each 7-day intervention period as previously described.

2.6. Test Meal and Satiety Measures

At each visit for both intervention conditions, following resting measures, participants consumed a standardised high-protein breakfast meal (Asda Scottish porridge oats (Asda Stores Ltd., Leeds, UK) comprising (per 100g): 367 kcal; 12.0 g protein; 61.0 g carbohydrate; 6.2 g fat), added whey protein (Pure Protein GF-1, USN UK Ltd., Longbridge, Birmingham, UK), coconut oil (Asda 100% raw extra virgin coconut oil, Asda Stores Ltd., Leeds, UK) with 200 mL water under supervision based on individual estimated caloric requirements for the PRO_{HIGH} condition and a protein content of 0.725 $g \cdot kg^{-1}$). On immediate completion of the test meal, a stopwatch was started and participants captured their subjective post-prandial satiety responses using a previously validated satiety/hunger questionnaire based on a standard 100 mm visual analogue scale [36,37] at 15, 30, 60, 90 and 120 min. The questionnaire was based on immediate response to set questions ("How 'hungry' do you feel?"; "How 'full' do you feel?"; "How 'satisfied' do you feel?"; "How 'much' can you eat right now?"). Participants were required to remain in a quiet, seated position during this time with no activity except light reading, and moving to a designated couch (supine position) for collection of blood samples at T60 and T120 (minutes) for assessment of selected satiety hormones. Data was normalised to individual relative change and relative change differences in a similar manner to blood analyses (see Section 2.8 below).

2.7. Post-Laboratory Measures and Support

An online satiety questionnaire was additionally completed at the end of each day across the 7-day intervention, and during the post-diet 3-day *ad libitum* period. The questionnaire captured individual perceived responses to the following questions: (i) how hungry were you today?, (ii) how full were you today?, (iii) how satisfied were you today with your diet?, (iv) how much do you think you can eat right now?, (v) how high have your food cravings been today?, (vi) how often did you feel energetic and active today?, (vii) how often were you in a good mood today?, (viii) how much did you enjoy your training today?, (ix) how much do you feel you can give your best effort at training today?. Mean data was collated for days 1–3 and 5–7 across the intervention period, and for days 1–3 of the *ad libitum* period. To increase dietary compliance during each intervention period, participants were provided with additional whey protein (Pure Protein GF-1, whey protein concentrate/ soya protein isolate, USN UK Ltd., Longbridge, Birmingham, UK) comprising (per 100g): 370 kcal; 71 g protein; 9.8 g carbohydrate; 4.4 g fat.

2.8. Biochemical Analyses

All samples were analysed at the Department of Surgery, Addenbrookes Hospital, Cambridge. Plasma samples with 4-(2-Aminoethyl) benzenesulfonyl fluoride hydrochloride (AEBSF; Sigma, Dorset, UK) to a final concentration of 1 mg·mL^{-1} were frozen to −20 °C within 30 min of centrifuging (15 min at 3000 g). Samples were subsequently thawed aseptically in a 37 °C water bath, centrifuged at 3000 g for 5 min to sediment any cryoprecipitates and then analysed in duplicate using a human total ghrelin ELISA kit or human PYY ELISA kit (EMD Millipore Corporation, Billerica, MA, USA) for ghrelin and PYY measurements according to manufacturers' instructions. ELISA plates were read using a FLUOstar OPTIMA plate reader (BMG Labtech, Aylesbury, UK). In addition to raw concentrations (pg·mL^{-1}), data were individually normalised as relative change (to reflect normalised post-intervention effects) and relative change differences (to reflect normalised intervention effects taking into consideration pre-intervention results) according to the following equations:

Relative change (relative Δ pg·mL^{-1}) = $\frac{y-x}{x}$ where x = the pre-meal resting sample, y = the post-meal at the respective sample time-points (i.e., 60, 120 min);

Relative change difference (relative Δ difference pg·mL^{-1}) = $\left(\frac{y_{post}-x_{post}}{x_{post}}\right) - \left(\frac{y_{pre}-x_{pre}}{x_{pre}}\right)$ where pre is the pre-intervention results, and post is the post-intervention results.

2.9. Statistical Analyses

Statistical analyses were performed using SPSS (v24, IBM, Armonk, NY, USA). Dependent variable distributions were assessed for normality using a Shapiro-Wilk test as well as manual inspections of M-estimators, histograms, stem-and-leaf plots and boxplots. Potential order and treatment effects were assessed prior to main analyses using a paired samples t-test. Baseline participant characteristics (gender) were assessed using an independent samples t-test. A mixed design repeated measures ANOVA (diet, time) was performed for main analyses, with Bonferonni post-hoc comparisons where applicable. Where pertinent, relative change questionnaire scores were assessed using a paired samples t-test. An alpha level of $\leq$0.05 was employed for statistical significance. Data are reported as mean ± S.E.

3. Results

3.1. Nutrition Intake and Body Composition Data

Mean dietary intake across both interventions is shown in Table 2. Prior to starting the first intervention average caloric intake for all participants was significantly greater (2379.81 ± 201.48 kcal·d^{-1}, F = 5.07, $p = 0.013$, $\eta p^2 = 0.25$) in comparison to main intervention intakes, although similar to predicted habitual intakes when taking into consideration rest days (2381.25 ± 131.31 kcal·d^{-1}). Across intervention periods, targeted caloric deficit was achieved in relation to estimated maintenance calories (based on individual requirements for both training and rest days) for both PRO_{MOD} ($-22.9 \pm 1.0\%$) and PRO_{HIGH} ($-21.0 \pm 1.1\%$) conditions.

Whilst protein was generally maintained during PRO_{MOD} compared with pre-intervention intakes, PRO_{HIGH} resulted in an expected increase in relative protein from 1.84 ± 0.15 to 2.89 ± 0.01g·kg^{-1}·d^{-1} ($F = 78.29_{(\text{diet x time})}$, $p < 0.0001$, $\eta p^2 = 0.84$). Post-intervention protein intakes were significantly different between conditions ($p < 0.0001$), with mean intakes demonstrating excellent compliance with target amounts. Relative carbohydrate intake was reduced during PRO_{HIGH} by $25.37 \pm 6.16\%$ from 2.55 ± 0.16 g·kg^{-1}·d^{-1} to 1.90 ± 0.16g·kg^{-1}·d^{-1} ($F = 11.54_{(\text{diet x time})}$, $p = 0.004$, $\eta p^2 = 0.44$), and was significantly lower than $PRO_{MOD\text{-}post}$ ($p < 0.0001$). To meet caloric deficit requirements, during both interventions total fat intake was significantly reduced by $39.42 \pm 5.76\%$ ($p < 0.0001$) and $27.63 \pm 6.35\%$ ($p < 0.0001$) for PRO_{MOD} and PRO_{HIGH} respectively ($F = 4.64_{(\text{diet x time})}$, $p = 0.048$, $\eta p^2 = 0.24$). Following interventions, no differences for fat intake were reported between conditions ($p > 0.05$). However, relative fat intakes pre-intervention were significantly higher for PRO_{MOD} compared to PRO_{HIGH} ($p = 0.008$).

Mean body-mass significantly decreased within both interventions ($F = 24.00_{(\text{time})}$, $p < 0.0001$, $\eta p^2 = 0.62$) by $1.28 \pm 0.30\%$ with PRO_{MOD} (from 88.37 ± 5.42 to 87.18 ± 5.31 kg, $p = 0.001$) and by $1.49 \pm 0.36\%$ with PRO_{HIGH} (from 88.48 ± 5.54 to 87.14 ± 5.42 kg, $p = 0.002$) demonstrating compliance with acute energy deficit based on estimated maintenance calories. This corresponded with a significant within-condition reduction in phase angle ($F = 26.02_{(\text{time})}$, $p < 0.0001$, $\eta p^2 = 0.63$) for both PRO_{MOD} ($-0.41 \pm 0.09°$, $p < 0.0001$) and PRO_{HIGH} ($-0.29 \pm 0.12°$, $p = 0.04$). Short-term energy deficit resulted in a reduction in hydration indices, with both total body water (PRO_{MOD}: 53.14 ± 1.81 to $51.16 \pm 1.59\%$, $p = 0.002$; PRO_{HIGH}: 53.04 ± 1.70 to $51.24 \pm 1.80\%$, $p = 0.018$) and intracellular water (PRO_{MOD}: 59.07 ± 0.75 to $57.88 \pm 0.67\%$, $p = 0.001$; PRO_{HIGH}: 58.89 ± 0.71 to $57.88 \pm 0.81\%$, $p = 0.035$) decreasing within-condition. It was noted that mean training frequency was comparable between dietary conditions (PRO_{MOD}: 6.38 ± 0.63 sessions; PRO_{HIGH}: 7.00 ± 0.50 sessions, $p = 0.44$) across the 10-day intervention period.

3.2. Dietary Intervention Perceived Satiety Responses

Across both dietary interventions, participants maintained a daily satiety questionnaire as previously described. Data, based on absolute values (using a 100 mm visual analogue scale), were averaged for the beginning (days 1–3) and end of each intervention (days 5–7). Mean responses are shown in Table 3. Perception of satisfaction was significantly greater at the end of PRO_{HIGH} ($F = 4.52_{(\text{diet})}$, $p = 0.05$, $\eta p^2 = 0.23$) compared with PRO_{MOD} over days 5–7 (67.29 ± 4.28 mm v 58.96 ± 4.51 mm respectively, $p = 0.04$). Participants also reported a significant mean increase in perception of cravings ($F = 5.93_{(\text{time})}$, $p = 0.028$, $\eta p^2 = 0.28$) within PRO_{MOD} only from days 1–3 (46.25 ± 4.96 mm) to days 5–7 (57.60 ± 4.41 mm, $p = 0.01$). No other differences were reported between conditions, including perceived training enjoyment and motivation to train.

Table 3. Satiety and well-being questionnaire responses during dietary intervention phases.

Question	$PRO_{MOD1–3}$	$PRO_{MOD5–7}$	$PRO_{HIGH1–3}$	$PRO_{HIGH5–7}$
Hunger	48.54 ± 3.48	51.46 ± 4.89	43.33 ± 4.22	41.67 ± 3.68
Fullness	62.29 ± 4.11	58.65 ± 4.64	64.38 ± 3.81	65.52 ± 3.99
Satisfaction	65.42 ± 4.38	58.96 ± 4.51	68.65 ± 2.34	67.29 ± 4.28 [a]
Desire to eat	50.94 ± 5.53	57.92 ± 5.45	45.00 ± 5.13	46.15 ± 5.58
Cravings	46.25 ± 4.96	57.60 ± 4.41 [b]	40.83 ± 4.59	47.19 ± 4.60
Energy	65.00 ± 2.81	67.81 ± 4.54	64.48 ± 3.18	69.06 ± 4.64
Mood	72.92 ± 3.35	67.92 ± 5.33	67.71 ± 3.26	71.88 ± 3.89
Training enjoyment	72.29 ± 4.35	68.23 ± 4.73	71.67 ± 4.48	73.02 ± 4.19
Training motivation	71.67 ± 4.97	66.56 ± 4.68	70.21 ± 3.93	70.83 ± 5.92

Data represent mean scores over days 1–3 and days 5–7 during moderate (PRO_{MOD}) or high (PRO_{HIGH}) diet periods. Data based on arbitrary units (a.u.) from participant responses using a visual analogue scale (VAS, 0–100 mm) and presented as mean ± SE. Question categories paraphrased. [a] denotes significant difference to $PRO_{MOD5–7}$ ($p = 0.04$). [b] denotes significant increase within group compared to days 1–3 ($p = 0.01$).

3.3. Test-Meal Satiety Hormone Responses

Absolute values: Mean plasma ghrelin and PYY concentrations in response to the test-meal are shown in Table 4. No differences were reported for pre- or post-intervention concentrations between conditions ($p > 0.05$) for either analyte prior to consuming the test-meal. However, both ghrelin and PYY were notably lower (albeit non-significant, $p = 0.06$ and $p = 0.11$ respectively) at T0 following PRO_{MOD} compared with pre-intervention data. Plasma ghrelin reduced as expected by T60 in all assessments, but typically increased by T120 ($F = 28.77_{(time)}$, $p < 0.001$, $\eta p^2 = 0.63$), remaining significantly lower than pre-meal concentrations ($p \leq 0.036$). However, following PRO_{MOD}, plasma ghrelin continued to decrease to 613.57 ± 114.26pg·mL^{-1} by T120 ($p = 0.003$ within condition compared to T0) and was significantly different overall compared to pre intervention responses ($p = 0.015$). Across all assessments, plasma PYY significantly increased from T0 to T120 ($F = 33.05_{(time)}$, $p < 0.001$, $\eta p^2 = 0.70$), with no differences reported between pre- or post-intervention concentrations.

Table 4. Mean plasma ghrelin and peptide YY concentrations in response to test meal.

Hormone	Time (mins)	PRO_{MOD}		PRO_{HIGH}	
		PRE	POST	PRE	POST
Ghrelin (pg·mL^{-1})	0	1125.97 ± 125.85	972.81 ± 130.42	920.12 ± 143.43	1088.17 ± 158.77
	60	696.42 ± 96.61 *	659.73 ± 86.39 *	672.27 ± 119.29 *	786.61 ± 117.33 *
	120	758.91 ± 129.38 *	613.57 ± 114.26 *, [a]	714.75 ± 136.56 *	850.60 ± 147.68 *
PYY (pg·mL^{-1})	0	103.62 ± 10.15	84.87 ± 8.94	87.94 ± 11.45	100.65 ± 9.54
	60	130.83 ± 9.09 *	129.38 ± 10.49 *	133.84 ± 15.14 *	141.02 ± 12.23 *
	120	137.60 ± 8.71 *	147.14 ± 11.94 *	142.11 ± 13.29 *	143.34 ± 11.98 *

Data presented as mean ± SE. PRO_{MOD} denotes moderate protein condition; PRO_{HIGH} denotes high protein condition. Time-point 0 refers to resting concentrations pre-feeding; other time-points refer to corresponding time post-breakfast meal. * denotes significant differences to 0 time-point within condition only ($p \leq 0.036$). [a] denotes overall difference to pre intervention responses ($p = 0.015$).

Relative values: Plasma ghrelin and PYY expressed as normalized relative change (individual results and mean data, reflective of intervention diet effect) and normalized relative change difference (mean data, reflective of overall change in comparison to habitual intake) are shown in Figures 1 and 2 respectively. Normalized relative change in ghrelin concentration was significantly lower ($F = 5.90_{(diet \times time)}$, $p = 0.029$, $\eta p^2 = 0.30$) at T120 following PRO_{MOD} (−0.40 ± 0.06 pg·mL^{-1}) compared to PRO_{HIGH} (−0.26 ± 0.06 pg·mL^{-1}, $p = 0.015$), with no prior differences reported at T60 between interventions ($p > 0.05$). Relative change difference in ghrelin concentration was comparable between conditions ($p > 0.05$).

Normalized relative change for PYY increased from 0.59 ± 0.14 pg·mL^{-1} at T60 to 0.79 ± 0.16 pg·mL^{-1} at T120 with PRO$_{MOD}$, but was not deemed significant (p=0.07, main effect for time) in comparison to PRO$_{HIGH}$ (0.46 ± 0.10 pg·mL^{-1} at T60 to 0.51 ± 0.12 pg·mL^{-1} at T120). However, relative change difference for PYY was significantly greater for PRO$_{MOD}$ at both T60 (0.26 ± 0.18 pg·mL^{-1}) and T120 (0.39 ± 0.20 pg·mL^{-1}) compared with negative findings for PRO$_{HIGH}$ at the same time-points (T60: -0.15 ± 0.11 pg·mL^{-1}, T120: -0.28 ± 0.12 pg·mL^{-1}; $p \leq 0.018$).

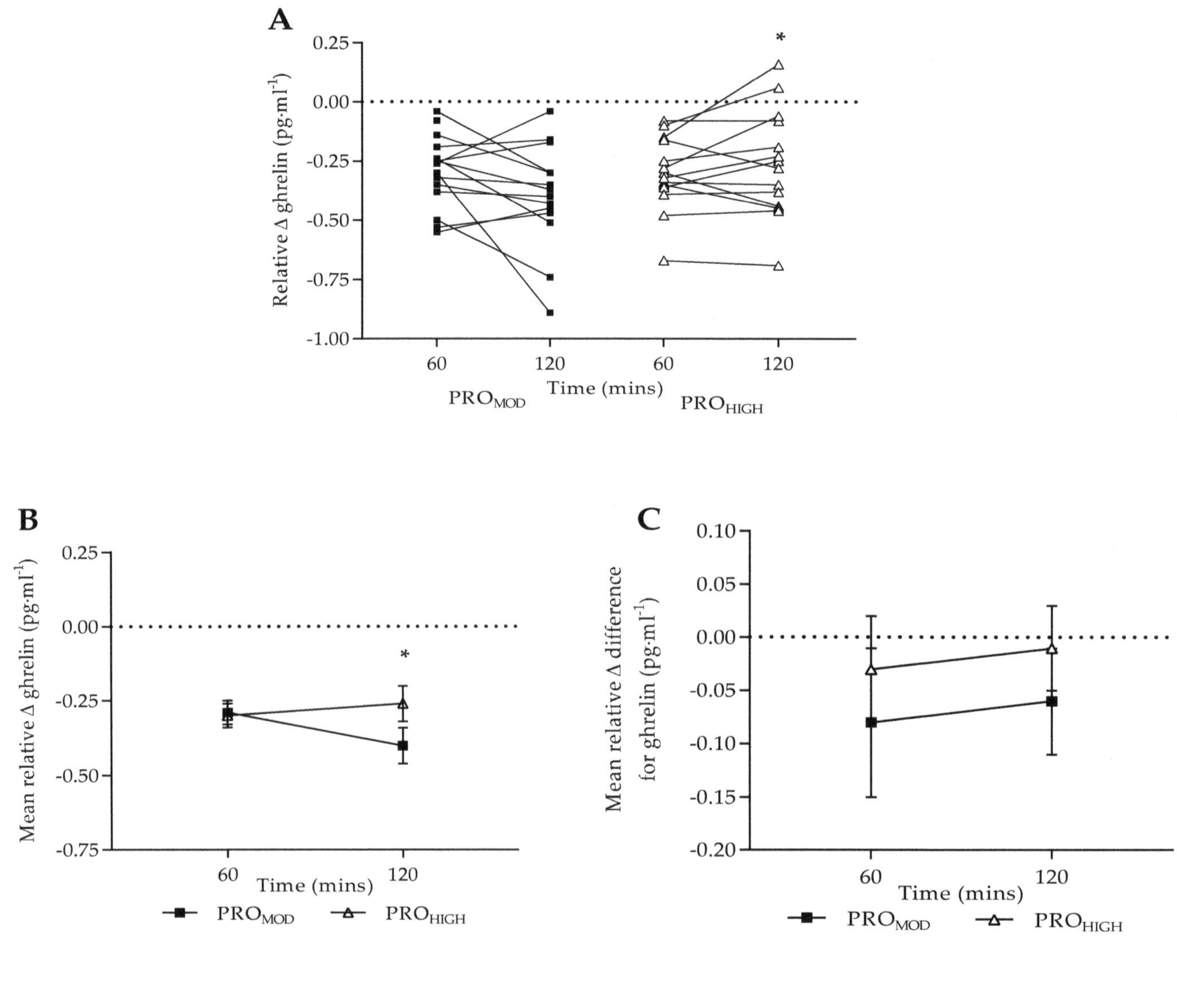

Figure 1. Plasma ghrelin concentrations following test-meal (pg·mL^{-1}; mean $\pm$ SE): (**A**) individual values expressed as normalised relative change to baseline levels; (**B**) mean values expressed as normalised relative change to baseline levels; (**C**) mean relative difference change (taking into consideration pre-intervention results). PRO$_{MOD}$ PRO$_{HIGH}$ denote moderate and high protein conditions. Dashed line provides reference point to pre-meal normalisation. * denotes significant difference overall to PRO$_{MOD}$ at corresponding time-point (p = 0.015).

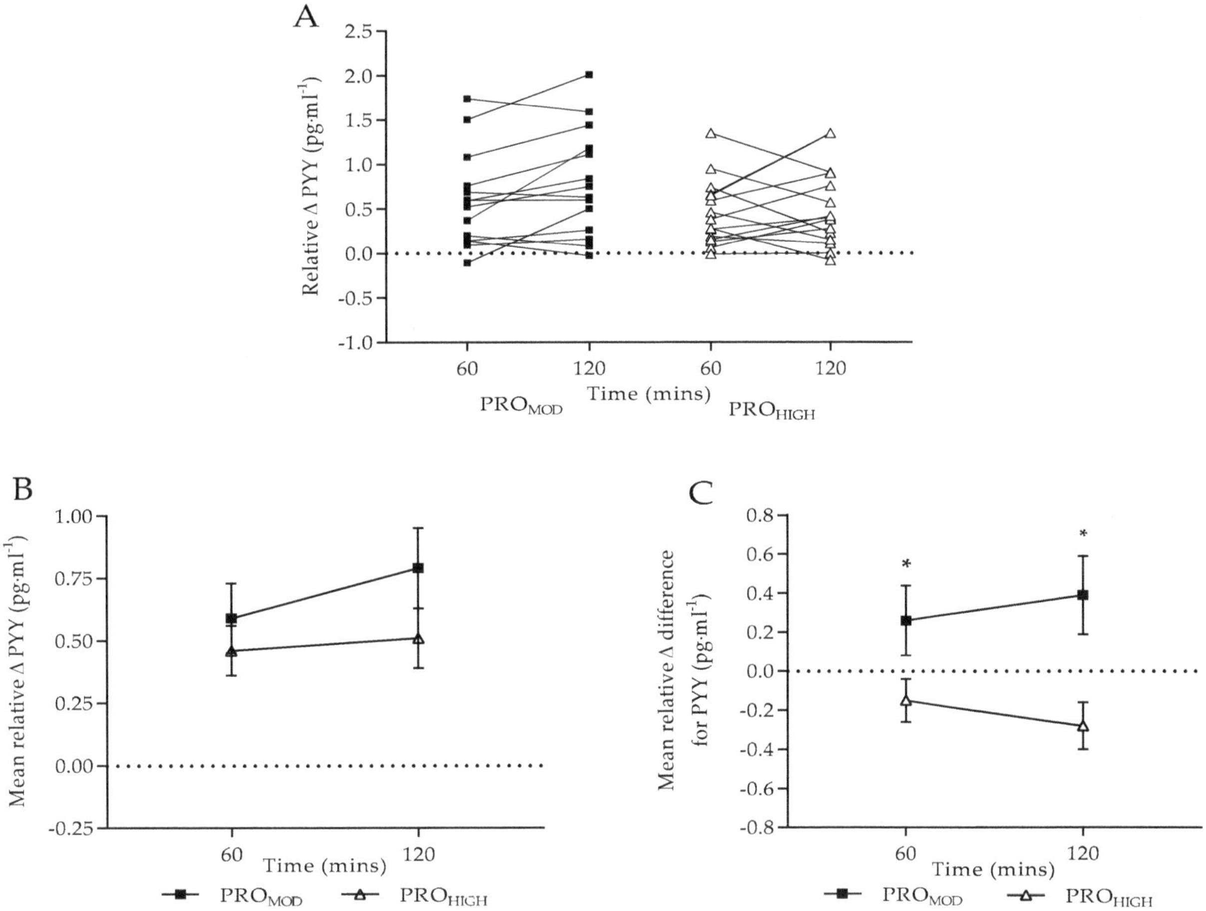

Figure 2. Plasma peptide YY concentrations following test-meal (pg mL^{-1}; mean $\pm$ SE): (**A**) individual values expressed as normalised relative change to baseline levels; (**B**) mean values expressed as normalised relative change to baseline levels; (**C**) mean relative difference change (taking into consideration pre-intervention results). PRO_{MOD} and PRO_{HIGH} denote moderate and high protein conditions. Dashed line provides reference point to pre-meal normalisation. * denotes significant difference between dietary conditions at each time-point ($p \leq 0.018$).

3.4. Test-Meal Satiety Questionnaire Responses

Satiety questionnaire responses to the test-meal following each intervention (normalized relative change) are shown in Figure 3. Perception of hunger was significantly reduced ($F = 15.34_{(time)}$, $p < 0.0001$, $\eta p^2 = 0.51$) for 60 min post test-meal following both interventions ($p \leq 0.024$) with no differences reported between diets ($p > 0.05$). In a similar pattern, perception of fullness significantly increased post-meal ($F = 16.52_{(time)}$, $p < 0.0001$, $\eta p^2 = 0.52$) and remained above pre-meal values at T120 for both interventions ($p \leq 0.05$), with no differences reported between diets ($p > 0.05$). Interestingly, following immediate completion of the test-meal satisfaction was only significantly increased with PRO_{MOD} ($p = 0.006$), beyond which perception of satisfaction remained elevated across all time-points within each dietary condition ($F = 13.65_{(time)}$, $p < 0.0001$, $\eta p^2 = 0.48$). Perception of desire to eat reduced following consumption of the test meal as expected ($F = 16.90_{(time)}$, $p < 0.0001$, $\eta p^2 = 0.53$) and remained lower than pre-meal values for 60 min in both interventions ($p \leq 0.02$). However, perception of desire to eat only remained blunted at T90 and T120 within-PRO_{MOD} only ($p \leq 0.048$).

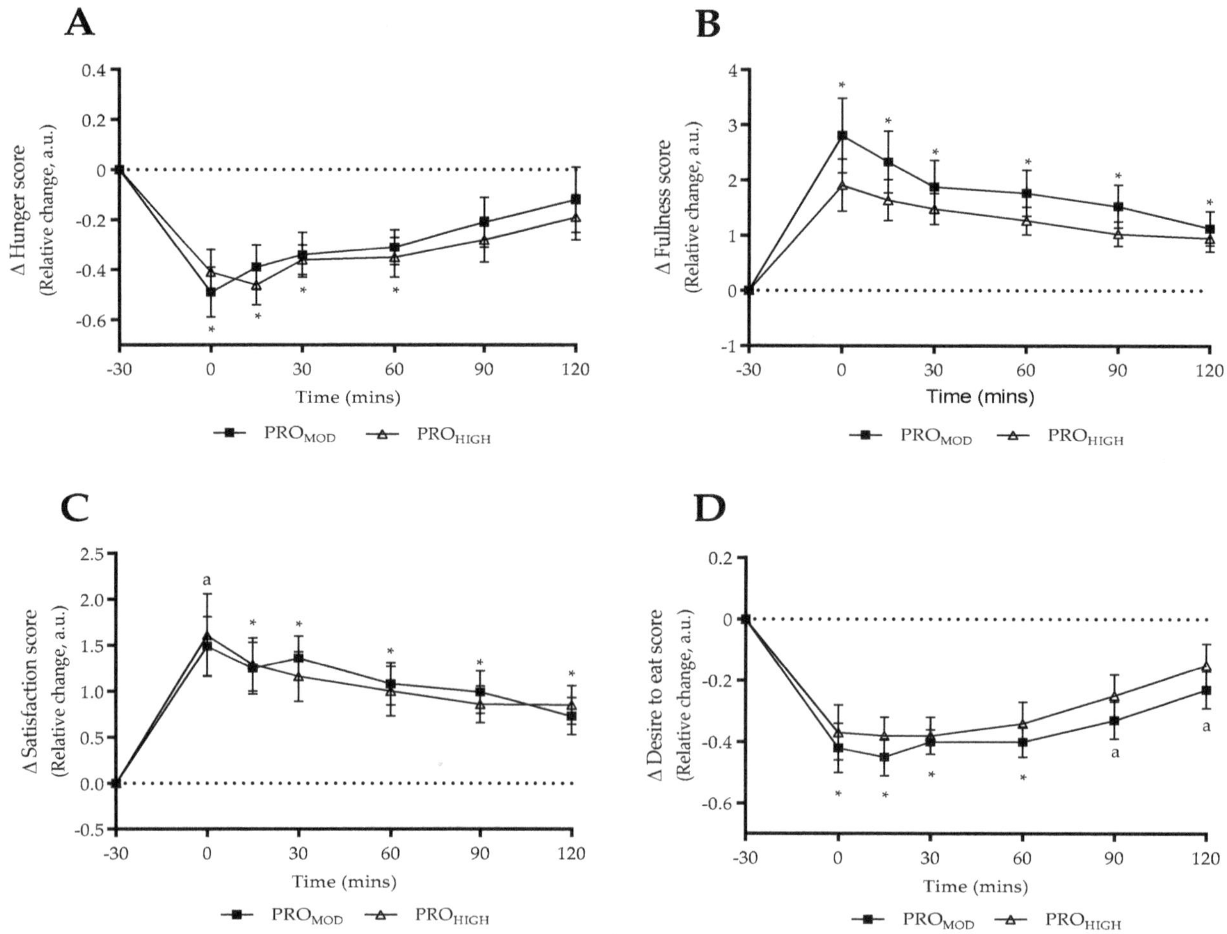

Figure 3. Questionnaire responses in relation to test meal under laboratory conditions. Data expressed as relative change (post diet, normalised) for both moderate (PRO_{MOD}) and high (PRO_{HIGH}) protein conditions (mean ± SE). (**A**) Perception of hunger; (**B**) Perception of fullness; (**C**) Perception of satisfaction; (**D**) Perception of desire to eat. Responses in relation to pre-meal (−30 min) time-point. 0 min denotes immediate completion of test meal. Dashed line provides reference point to pre-meal perceived state. * denotes significant difference compared to pre-meal time-point ($p \leq 0.05$) within both dietary conditions. [a] denotes significant difference compared to pre-meal time-point for PRO_{MOD} only ($p \leq 0.048$). No differences reported between dietary conditions.

Satiety questionnaire responses to the test-meal expressed as normalized relative change difference (taking into consideration pre-intervention responses) are shown in Figure 4. No significant differences were report within or between dietary conditions for perception of hunger, fullness or satisfaction ($p > 0.05$). For perception of desire to eat, a significant main effect for time was reported ($F = 5.43_{(time)}$, $p < 0.0001$, $\eta p^2 = 0.27$), with post-hoc analysis demonstrating a significant increase on immediate completion of the test-meal for PRO_{HIGH} only ($p = 0.028$).

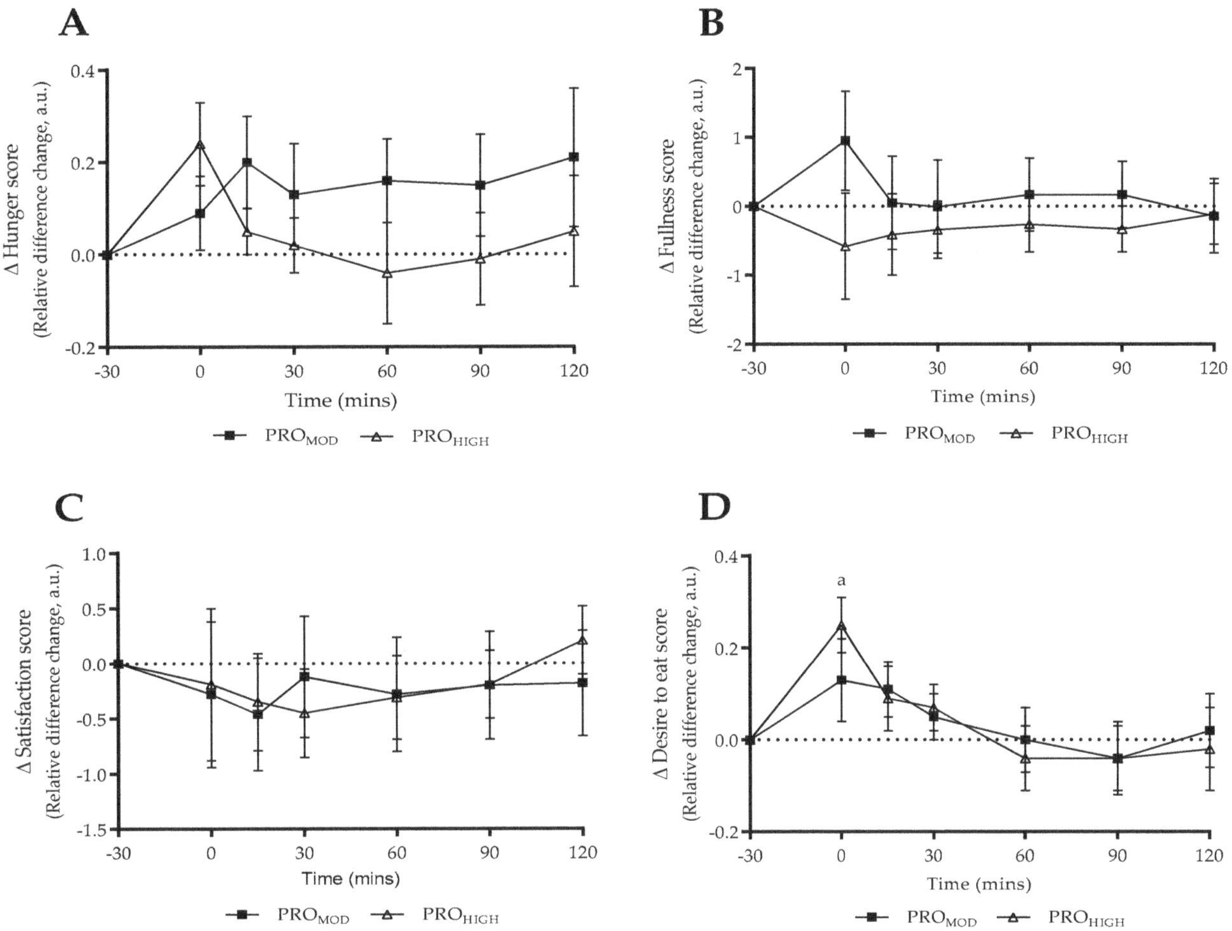

Figure 4. Questionnaire responses in relation to test meal under laboratory conditions. Data expressed as relative difference change (baseline to post diet) for both moderate (PRO_{MOD}) and high (PRO_{HIGH}) protein conditions (mean ± SE). (**A**) Perception of hunger; (**B**) Perception of fullness; (**C**) Perception of satisfaction; (**D**) Perception of desire to eat. Responses in relation to pre-meal (−30 min) time-point. 0 min denotes immediate completion of test meal. Dashed line provides reference point to pre-meal perceived state. [a] denotes difference to pre-meal time-point within PRO_{HIGH} only (p = 0.028). No differences between dietary conditions observed.

3.5. Ad libitum Intake and Satiety Responses

Mean dietary intake during the *ad libitum* phase following each dietary intervention is shown in Table 5. Despite higher absolute energy and fat intakes with PRO_{HIGH}, no significant differences were reported between conditions for any variable ($p > 0.05$). Compliance with target protein intake was met for both conditions. Satiety responses across days 1-3 of the *ad libitum* phase are shown in Table 6, along with delta scores in comparison to days 5-7 of the previous intervention. Perception of hunger was significantly reduced following transition to the *ad libitum* period ($F = 5.18_{(time)}$, $p = 0.038$, $\eta p^2 = 0.26$) within PRO_{MOD} only (−9.67 ± 4.68 mm, $p = 0.046$). Likewise, perception of fullness ($F = 10.33_{(time)}$, $p = 0.006$, $\eta p^2 = 0.41$) and satisfaction ($F = 5.72_{(time)}$, $p = 0.03$, $\eta p^2 = 0.28$) were significantly improved within-condition relative to the end of the PRO_{MOD} diet (fullness: 9.78 ± 3.74 mm, $p = 0.015$; satisfaction: 13.11 ± 4.33 mm, $p = 0.005$). Perceived desire to eat also reduced on transition to an *ad libitum* phase ($F = 14.86_{(time)}$, $p = 0.002$, $\eta p^2 = 0.50$) for PRO_{MOD} only (−16.78 ± 4.54 mm, $p = 0.001$).

A significant interaction effect was reported for perceived cravings ($F = 5.00_{(dietxtime)}$, $p = 0.041$, $\eta p^2 = 0.25$), with post-hoc analysis indicating a significant reduction for PRO_{MOD} (−13.00 ± 4.27 mm, $p = 0.004$). The relative change in perceived cravings for PRO_{MOD} was significantly reduced in comparison to PRO_{HIGH} ($p = 0.04$) following transition to an *ad libitum* phase. Participants reported improvements in general mood within-condition ($p = 0.05$) only. Perceived motivation to train was reportedly improved with PRO_{MOD} ($F = 4.52_{(time)}$, $p = 0.05$, $\eta p^2 = 0.23$) by 8.97 ± 5.08mm ($p = 0.05$). No other differences were reported between dietary conditions during the *ad libitum* phase ($p > 0.05$).

Table 5. Mean dietary intake during *ad libitum* period.

Variable	Category	PRO_{MOD}	PRO_{HIGH}
Energy Intake	($kcal \cdot d^{-1}$)	2197.81 ± 177.58	2348.14 ± 232.46
	($kcal \cdot kg^{-1} \cdot d^{-1}$)	25.64 ± 1.62	26.52 ± 1.81
Protein Intake	($g \cdot d^{-1}$)	162.38 ± 11.18	165.07 ± 12.89
	($g \cdot kg^{-1} \cdot d^{-1}$)	1.85 ± 0.03	1.86 ± 0.07
	(%EI)	30.87 ± 2.13	29.40 ± 1.89
Carbohydrate Intake	($g \cdot d^{-1}$)	214.94 ± 19.61	230.61 ± 24.33
	($g \cdot kg^{-1} \cdot d^{-1}$)	2.57 ± 0.24	2.65 ± 0.23
	(%EI)	39.14 ± 1.98	39.66 ± 1.85
Fat Intake	($g \cdot d^{-1}$)	72.69 ± 9.71	81.29 ± 11.01
	($g \cdot kg^{-1} \cdot d^{-1}$)	0.84 ± 0.09	0.90 ± 0.09
	(%EI)	12.64 ± 0.76	13.29 ± 0.70

Data presented as mean ± SE, and for macronutrient categories expressed in grams per day, grams per kg per day, and percentage of energy intake (EI). PRO_{MOD} denotes post moderate protein condition; PRO_{HIGH} denotes post high protein condition. During *ad libitum* phase, meal frequency set to 4 meals, and target protein intake of 1.80 $g \cdot kg^{-1} \cdot d^{-1}$, otherwise unrestricted. No significant differences reported between conditions.

Table 6. Questionnaire responses during *ad libitum* dietary phase.

Question Category	PRO_{MOD}	PRO_{HIGH}	ΔPRO_{MOD}	ΔPRO_{HIGH}
Hunger	41.67 ± 3.61	40.78 ± 3.48	−9.67 ± 4.68 [a]	−0.89 ± 2.74
Fullness	69.00 ± 4.39	73.39 ± 3.10	9.78 ± 3.74 [a]	7.87 ± 4.61
Satisfaction	73.11 ± 3.80	71.56 ± 3.00	13.11 ± 4.33 [a]	4.26 ± 4.89
Desire to eat	39.67 ± 2.96	38.03 ± 3.62	−16.78 ± 4.54 [a]	−8.12 ± 5.22
Cravings	42.89 ± 4.12	46.15 ± 4.23	−13.00 ± 4.27 [a]	−1.04 ± 5.08 *
Energy	71.33 ± 3.31	71.93 ± 2.91	2.99 ± 4.30	2.87 ± 3.34
Mood	76.11 ± 4.03	77.55 ± 2.09	8.33 ± 3.70 [a]	5.68 ± 2.72 [a]
Training enjoyment	79.35 ± 4.44	74.67 ± 4.51	9.23 ± 6.57	1.67 ± 4.43
Training motivation	78.85 ± 5.39	72.89 ± 4.99	8.97 ± 5.08 [a]	1.33 ± 3.93

Data represent mean scores over days 1–3 during *ad libitum* post diet period. Data based on arbitrary units (a.u.) from participant responses using a visual analogue scale (VAS) and presented as mean ± SE. Δ scores are relative to end of intervention diet. Question categories paraphrased. [a] denotes significant difference within group compared to end of intervention diet ($p \leq 0.05$).* denotes significant difference to ΔPRO_{MOD} ($p = 0.04$).

4. Discussion

The main finding from this study was that the perceived satiating effect of two diets with different protein content was generally comparable in resistance-trained participants undergoing a period of acute energy deficit. Therefore, consuming more protein during acute energy deficit does not appear to improve perceived satiety, as reported elsewhere [38–42]. However, when considering hormonal adaptations to an acute dietary intervention in response to a protein-rich test-meal, a moderate protein, energy deficit diet (1.8 $g \cdot kg^{-1} \cdot d^{-1}$) was deemed more satiating when compared to a high protein (2.9 $g \cdot kg^{-1} \cdot d^{-1}$) diet. These results suggest that whilst in acute energy deficit, a PRO_{MOD} diet may be sufficient to maintain training requirements in accordance with previous recommendations [5,43,44]. It is, however, important to note that a PRO_{HIGH} diet did not appear to disadvantage participants and may offer individual benefits discussed below.

Across the 7-day intervention period, participant responses to the daily satiety questionnaire were largely similar for all categories, with the exception of both cravings and satisfaction (Table 3). By the end of the dietary intervention, whilst consuming a PRO_{MOD} diet, participants reported increased cravings, which was not experienced to the same extent following PRO_{HIGH}. Additionally, perceived satisfaction was not only maintained during PRO_{HIGH}, but was significantly greater than PRO_{MOD} at the end of the intervention period. Similar findings in response to a high protein meal have been observed elsewhere [45]. This implies that during short-term caloric deficit a substantial increase in protein ratio beyond recommended levels for maximal lean muscle gain may be better sustained by resistance trained athletes who are more prone to cravings. Participant well-being, mood, training enjoyment and motivation to train were comparable between dietary conditions. As training frequency was equally maintained across dietary conditions, this inferred that an increase in protein intake beyond 1.8 $g \cdot kg^{-1} \cdot d^{-1}$ did not compromise training responses, and did not result in reduced motivation or perceived energy during training as hypothesized.

In the current study subjects maintained their habitual training routine without any external motivation that was intended to increase their performance. As exercise fatigue has been reported to increase during acute caloric deficit [4], it is possible that participants in the current study subconsciously decreased training effort, despite maintaining session frequency. Interestingly, phase angle (PA) assessed via bioelectrical impedance indicated a significant reduction following both dietary conditions, more notably with PRO_{MOD}. PA has been reported to be a proxy measure of muscle "quality" and is associated with sex, age, body mass index (BMI) and fat mass percentage (FM%) [30,46–48]. A decrease in PA during both dietary conditions may indicate unfavorable changes to muscle integrity as a result of energy restriction. However, the comparable reduction in hydration indices likely infers decreased PA was transient based on acute energy deficit. Our previous findings demonstrated an increase in PA when resistance trainees underwent a period of supervised intensive training to volitional exhaustion during short-term energy deficit when consuming a PRO_{HIGH} diet [30]. It is feasible, therefore, that in order to maintain muscle integrity during periods of acute caloric deficit more intensive training intensity and substantially increased protein intake is required, which is supported elsewhere [13].

Plasma ghrelin responses were comparable with previous research [45,49–52]. However, in response to a laboratory test meal, notable differences were reported between dietary conditions. Following PRO_{MOD}, plasma ghrelin remained significantly reduced at 2 h post-meal indicating a sustained satiating effect. When data was considered as normalized relative change (Figure 1B), this pattern was highlighted further with differences reported between dietary conditions in response to a protein-rich test meal. Furthermore, as no differences were observed between dietary conditions when taking into consideration pre-intervention ghrelin responses (Figure 1C), this would suggest that the satiating effect following PRO_{MOD} was associated with the higher protein content of the test meal.

It should be noted that baseline protein intake for all participants was nearly identical to the protein requirements for the PRO_{MOD} condition. Therefore, the sustained reduction in 2-h ghrelin response observed following PRO_{MOD} may also be related to the energy balance of the individual (both a reduction in caloric and fat intake) across the intervention period [53,54]. It is also noteworthy, that following PRO_{MOD}, plasma ghrelin was reduced at T0 compared with pre-intervention levels which presented an interesting trend ($p = 0.06$, $\eta p^2 = 0.22$) considering the reported increase in cravings within-condition by day 7. As plasma ghrelin followed expected responses pre and post PRO_{HIGH} [55], the findings indicate that satiety may be acutely enhanced by the consumption of a high-protein meal during periods of energy deficit when following a PRO_{MOD} approach. Individuals experiencing periodic cravings when following a PRO_{MOD} diet may therefore benefit by increasing the protein content of individual meals when required [56] without necessarily over-consuming protein.

This may be important considering the potential risks of longer-term consumption of very high protein intakes in some individuals (i.e., those with existing, or predisposition for, kidney disease [57]), and current recognition that high protein diets modulate intestinal microbiota production of tryptophan, leading to elevated metabolites (e.g., indoxyl sulphate) acting as uremic toxins [58,59]. There is also current suggestion that high protein diets may negatively impact intestinal function, potentially via bacterial metabolites produced as a result of undigested proteins [60]. High protein diets, in combination with reduced carbohydrate/fiber intake may reduce short-chain fatty acid concentrations, impacting on colonic environment/mucosa [15] which may influence individual health in the longer term. This supports the contention that a PRO_{MOD} approach may be sufficient for resistance-trained individuals during energy deficit.

On completion of the dietary interventions, absolute plasma PYY did not significantly differ between conditions in response to a standardized test meal, as observed elsewhere [49]. The expected increase in plasma PYY [52] in response to a protein-rich test meal was consistent, with a similar rate of change from T0-T60, following both dietary conditions. It is, however, noteworthy that following PRO_{MOD}, a greater rate of change in plasma PYY from T60-T120 was evident (p = 0.07), which is comparable with the sustained satiating effect observed with plasma ghrelin. When data were compared as normalized relative change (Figure 2B), no differences were reported between dietary conditions (p = 0.06) potentially explained by the mixed individual responses observed. However, when taking into consideration pre-intervention PYY responses (Figure 2C), an overall positive response was observed for PRO_{MOD} at both T60 and T120 in contrast to PRO_{HIGH}. This infers that a PRO_{MOD} intervention improved acute satiety to a greater extent than PRO_{HIGH}. Collectively, these results suggest that individuals may become accustomed to a higher protein intake, and therefore chronic consumption of a PRO_{HIGH} diet may lose its satiating effect over time [61].

Various factors modulate PYY concentrations, including acute/chronic energy balance, as well as nutrient composition of a meal. High protein meal content has been shown to elicit greater PYY secretion leading to short-term sensations of fullness [62,63]. PYY is an agonist at neuropeptide Y2 receptors and increasing levels leads to both reduced hunger perception and food intake [62,64]. In the current study, nutrient composition of the test-meals remained the same across all testing sessions. Therefore, although absolute changes in PYY were not reportedly different between dietary interventions, the relative change difference indicated that both the decrease in caloric intake, along with the higher protein content of the test meal resulted in acute increases in PYY concentrations over the 2-h monitoring period for PRO_{MOD}. Although not significant, the observed increase in absolute PYY concentration for PRO_{HIGH} at T0 may be explained by the increase in dietary protein over the 7-days. However, the hormonal response to a protein-rich meal for PRO_{HIGH} was not considered different to pre-intervention patterns. This further supports the contention that a moderate protein diet favorably improved acute physiological satiety in contrast to very high protein intakes.

Perceived satiety responses to the protein-rich test meal were largely comparable between dietary conditions in contrast to physiological responses. Only "desire to eat" remained significantly reduced until 2 h post-meal with PRO_{MOD} (Figure 3D), which in part supported the satiating effect observed for plasma ghrelin. However, this was not the case for perceived hunger, fullness or satisfaction. Whilst perceived satisfaction was comparable between conditions beyond T15, it was noted that participants reported being more satisfied on completion of the test-meal with PRO_{MOD} (T0, Figure 3C). However, as the mean values at T0 were similar between conditions, it was noted that a trend towards significance was observed for PRO_{HIGH} (p = 0.06) indicating that perceived responses to the test-meal were likely comparable for satisfaction. Overall, our results support previous findings that circulating levels of ghrelin and PYY do not correlate with the subjective perception of appetite [52,65].

Based on the acute energy deficit period undertaken it is feasible that perceived responses may not have changed dramatically compared to habitual intake. Interestingly when test-meal questionnaire responses were normalized in relation to pre-intervention results (Figure 4), no differences were reported between dietary conditions. The only within-condition finding at T0 for "desire to eat" for PRO_{HIGH} (Figure 4D), may be explained by the fact that the protein content of the test-meal was based on the higher protein intervention. Therefore, following a 7-day high protein (2.9 $g \cdot kg^{-1} \cdot d^{-1}$) energy deficit period, it is likely that participants had attained a degree of habituation to the protein intake and hence experienced a greater "desire to eat" on completion of the test-meal. This is, in part, supported by the hunger and fullness scores at T0, albeit non-significant.

On completion of the 7-day dietary intervention, participants then completed a 3-day period in which protein intake was fixed at 1.8 $g \cdot kg^{-1} \cdot d^{-1}$, with *ad libitum* consumption of carbohydrate, fat and energy intake until perceived fullness. This was included to provide insight as whether the preceding intervention increased the likelihood of over-eating on cessation of short-term energy deficit. Although energy and fat intakes were reportedly greater following PRO_{HIGH}, no differences were reported between groups during the *ad libitum* phase, as similarly observed elsewhere [64]. Despite having followed a monitored period of reduced (20%) energy intake, participants tended to only partially increase caloric intake mainly through increased total fat closer to pre-intervention levels. This suggests, at least in the short-term, that resistance-trained athletes are unlikely to over-consume calories on completion of an energy deficit period. This may reflect the tendency to follow habitual dietary intake patterns during periods of training.

In a similar manner, the satiety questionnaire responses during the *ad libitum* period were comparable between dietary conditions. However, when relative responses were compared to the end of the previous intervention period, the change from a PRO_{MOD} approach resulted in significant within-condition improvements in hunger, fullness, satisfaction, desire to eat, as well as general participants' mood and motivation to train. Notably, the reduction in cravings observed following PRO_{MOD} was significantly different to PRO_{HIGH}. Collectively this suggests that whilst a short-term PRO_{MOD} energy deficit period may result in improved hormonal satiety responses, periodic inclusion of higher protein intakes may support sustained periods in which athletes undergo caloric deficit. Alternatively, athletes undergoing periods of energy deficit may physiologically benefit from a PRO_{MOD} approach, but should be mindful of increasing protein content (either based on single meals, or as a dietary approach) when perceived cravings or a reduction in mood and/or training motivation occurs.

On completion of the study, several limitations were noted. Firstly, that in monitoring habitual dietary intake a longer lead in period would have provided clearer insight. All participants were resistance-trained individuals experienced in maintaining individual macronutrient ratios (i.e., $1.8\ g\cdot kg^{-1}\cdot d^{-1}$) and followed regular training routines. Dietary records were kept in the days leading into each testing period prior to each intervention. As such, the observed habitual intake (Table 2) included the requested rest days and therefore did not reflect maintenance intakes expected when taking into consideration training days over a typical week (i.e., $2628 \pm 144\ kcal\cdot d^{-1}$). However, based on the period collected, energy intakes were comparable to expected intakes for less active periods (e.g., $2381 \pm 131\ kcal\cdot d^{-1}$) for this cohort (comprising both male and female athletes). Therefore, although the habitual intakes were comparable prior to each intervention phase, they likely do not reflect accurate mean energy intakes. However, the decrease in body-mass observed across each intervention, along with monitored reduced energy intakes, indicated that participants achieved the 20% energy deficit as expected.

Although training frequency was maintained across both intervention periods, training intensity was not monitored. Therefore, although perceived energy, training motivation and training enjoyment was not different between dietary conditions, it is difficult to know whether participants maintained overall training intensity. It is feasible, as previously mentioned, that fatigue was offset through a subconscious reduction in training intensity during the energy deficit period. Anecdotally, most participants reported that the PRO_{HIGH} diet was challenging (i.e., reduced mental clarity) towards the end of the intervention phase, possibly indicating that such diets may be poorly tolerated in the longer term. Careful attention to monitoring training intensity, along with perceived well-being responses during periods of acute energy deficit may be warranted to ensure performance maintenance.

Another limitation observed was that other gut hormones (i.e., glucagon-like peptide 1 (GLP-1) and cholecystokinin (CCK)) were not assessed in this study. This would have supported our findings in determining that a PRO_{MOD} diet had a greater acute satiating effect after consumption of a high protein meal. GLP-1 for example is secreted in conjunction with PYY, and has been associated with appetite response and decreased food intake [62,66–68]. An increased GLP-1 response to PRO_{MOD} would provide clearer insight that the satiating effect of the test-meal was related to localized stomach/intestinal responses to a protein-rich breakfast meal, and confirmed our reasoning that athletes may become accustomed to chronic consumption of a high protein diet. Likewise, adjunct measurements of CCK released from the duodenum in response to meal consumption influences satiety acutely [62]. Along with reduced ghrelin responses, measures of CCK would have supported the contention that PRO_{MOD} resulted in greater satiety in this cohort.

Whilst the results from this study indicate that a PRO_{MOD} preferentially influences hormonal responses to a test-meal, it is evident that perceived responses were comparable between intervention diets. Further research is therefore warranted to assess whether perceived satiety responses are different when undertaking prolonged energy deficit periods. This is pertinent considering previous research has indicated that fasting ghrelin levels may be increased in response to longer term energy deficit [69,70]. Furthermore, with current recognition that high protein diets (including type of dietary protein) likely modulate gut microbiota, this may have inference to both neurotransmitter and satiety responses (e.g., GLP-1), especially considering inter-individual variance [15].

Although the sample size in the current study was deemed sufficient based on a priori power assessment (comparable to previous research [4]), determination of satiety responses in larger resistance-trained cohorts is also warranted. In addition, with the observation that athletes may benefit from consuming a PRO_{MOD} diet during energy deficit, but periodically include protein-high meals to offset negative symptoms (i.e., cravings), assessment of nutritional periodization during periods of caloric deficit would be beneficial to ascertain sustainability to such diets. Finally, maintenance of training performance and lean gains during periods of acute or chronic energy deficit should be considered to determine whether a PRO_{MOD} diet sustains beneficial responses in resistance-trained athletes.

5. Conclusions

During acute energy deficit in resistance-trained individuals, consuming protein intakes in excess of recommended athlete guidelines did not improve overall perceived satiety in comparison to more habitual, moderate protein intakes. Furthermore, a PRO_{MOD} diet favorably improved hormonal responses to a test-meal compared with a PRO_{HIGH} diet. Therefore, as long as training motivation/ performance is not compromised during short-term energy deficit, moderate protein intakes (1.8 $g \cdot kg^{-1} \cdot d^{-1}$) are likely to be adequate for resistance-trained individuals. The findings also suggest that where individuals experience negative symptoms (i.e., cravings), implementation of periodic high protein meals may be sufficient to maintain satisfaction, and diet sustainability.

Author Contributions: Conceptualization and design of the study was undertaken by M.H., F.T.V., A.Z., J.R. and K.T.M. J.R., A.Z., V.M., K.T.M. were involved with data collection, along with individual participant nutrition tracking support from M.B., O.B., and L.V.; blood collection and assay analyses were undertaken by J.R., V.M. and K.T.M. Formal analysis of data was undertaken by J.R., A.Z. and K.T.M. with support from L.S. and M.H. Original draft preparation was undertaken by J.R. and A.Z., with critical appraisal and editing by all authors. All authors reviewed the paper and approved the final version prior to submission.

Acknowledgments: This study was supported by Ultimate Sports Nutrition (USN) UK Ltd. with provision of whey protein.

References

1. Khodaee, M.; Olewinski, L.; Shadgan, B.; Kiningham, R.R. Rapid weight loss in sports with weight classes. *Curr. Sports Med. Rep.* **2015**, *14*, 435–441. [CrossRef]
2. Rossow, L.M.; Fukuda, D.H.; Fahs, C.A.; Loenneke, J.P.; Stout, J.R. Natural bodybuilding competition preparation and recovery: A 12-month case study. *Int. J. Sports Physiol. Perform.* **2013**, *8*, 582–592. [CrossRef] [PubMed]

3. Robinson, S.L.; Lambeth-Mansell, A.; Gillibrand, G.; Smith-Ryan, A.; Bannock, L. A nutrition and conditioning intervention for natural bodybuilding contest preparation: Case study. *J. Int. Soc. Sports Nutr.* **2015**, *12*, 1–11. [CrossRef] [PubMed]
4. Mettler, S.; Mitchell, N.; Tipton, K.D. Increased protein intake reduces lean body mass loss during weight loss in athletes. *Med. Sci. Sports Exerc.* **2010**, *42*, 326–337. [CrossRef] [PubMed]
5. Tarnopolsky, M.A.; Atkinson, S.A.; MacDougall, J.D.; Chesley, A.; Phillips, S.; Schwarcz, H.P. Evaluation of protein requirements for trained strength athletes. *J. Appl. Physiol.* **1992**, *73*, 1986–1995. [CrossRef] [PubMed]
6. Walberg, J.L.; Leidy, M.K.; Sturgill, D.J.; Hinkle, D.E.; Ritchey, S.J.; Sebolt, D.R. Macronutrient content of a hypoenergy diet affects nitrogen retention and muscle function in weight lifters. *Int. J. Sports Med.* **1988**, *9*, 261–266. [CrossRef] [PubMed]
7. Helms, E.R.; Aragon, A.A.; Fitschen, P.J. Evidence-based recommendations for natural bodybuilding contest preparation: Nutrition and supplementation. *J. Int. Soc. Sports Nutr.* **2014**, *11*, 20. [CrossRef] [PubMed]
8. Lemon, P.W.R. Beyond the zone: Protein needs of active individuals. *J. Am. Coll. Nutr.* **2000**, *19*, 513S–521S. [CrossRef]
9. Phillips, S.M. Dietary protein for athletes: From requirements to metabolic advantage. *Appl. Physiol. Nutr. Metab.* **2006**, *31*, 647–654. [CrossRef]
10. Phillips, S.M.; Moore, D.R.; Tang, J.E. A critical examination of dietary protein requirements, benefits, and excesses in athletes. *Int. J. Sport Nutr. Exerc. Metab.* **2007**, *17*, 58–76. [CrossRef]
11. Layman, D.K.; Boileau, R.A.; Erickson, D.J.; Painter, J.E.; Shiue, H.; Sather, C.; Christou, D.D. A reduced ratio of dietary carbohydrate to protein improves body composition and blood lipid profiles during weight loss in adult women. *J. Nutr.* **2003**, *133*, 411–417. [CrossRef] [PubMed]
12. Stiegler, P.; Cunliffe, A. The role of diet and exercise for the maintenance of fat-free mass and resting metabolic rate during weight loss. *Sports Med.* **2006**, *36*, 239–262. [CrossRef] [PubMed]
13. Helms, E.R.; Zinn, C.; Rowlands, D.S.; Brown, S.R. A systematic review of dietary protein during caloric restriction in resistance trained lean athletes: A case for higher intakes. *Int. J. Sport Nutr. Exerc. Metab.* **2014**, *24*, 127–138. [CrossRef] [PubMed]
14. Rand, W.M.; Pellett, P.L.; Young, V.R. Meta-analysis of nitrogen balance studies for estimating protein requirements in healthy adults. *Am. J. Clin. Nutr.* **2003**, *77*, 109–127. [CrossRef] [PubMed]
15. Blachier, F.; Beaumont, M.; Portune, K.J.; Steuer, N.; Lan, A.; Audebert, M.; Khodorova, N.; Andriamihaja, M.; Airinei, G.; Benamouzig, R.; et al. High-protein diets for weight management: Interactions with the intestinal microbiota and consequences for gut health. A position paper by the my new gut study group. *Clin. Nutr.* **2018**. [CrossRef] [PubMed]
16. Phillips, S.M.; Van Loon, L.J.C. Dietary protein for athletes: From requirements to optimum adaptation. *J. Sports Sci.* **2011**, *29*, S29–S38. [CrossRef] [PubMed]
17. Phillips, S.M. A brief review of higher dietary protein diets in weight loss: A focus on athletes. *Sports Med.* **2014**, *44* (Suppl. 2), S149–S153. [CrossRef]
18. Spendlove, J.; Mitchell, L.; Gifford, J.; Hackett, D.; Slater, G.; Cobley, S.; O'Connor, H. Dietary intake of competitive bodybuilders. *Sport Med.* **2015**, *45*, 1041–1063. [CrossRef]
19. Dhillon, J.; Craig, B.A.; Leidy, H.J.; Amankwaah, A.F.; Osei-Boadi Anguah, K.; Jacobs, A.; Jones, B.L.; Jones, J.B.; Keeler, C.L.; Keller, C.E.; et al. The effects of increased protein intake on fullness: A meta-analysis and its limitations. *J. Acad. Nutr. Diet.* **2016**, *116*, 968–983. [CrossRef]
20. Weigle, D.S.; Breen, P.A.; Matthys, C.C.; Callahan, H.S.; Meeuws, K.E.; Burden, V.R.; Purnell, J.Q. A high-protein diet induces sustained reductions in appetite, ad libitum caloric intake, and body weight despite compensatory changes in diurnal plasma leptin and ghrelin concentrations. *Am. J. Clin. Nutr.* **2005**, *82*, 41–48. [CrossRef]
21. Martens, E.A.; Lemmens, S.G.; Westerterp-Plantenga, M.S. Protein leverage affects energy intake of high-protein diets in humans. *Am. J. Clin. Nutr.* **2013**, *97*, 86–93. [CrossRef] [PubMed]
22. Martens, E.A.; Tan, S.Y.; Dunlop, M.V.; Mattes, R.D.; Westerterp-Plantenga, M.S. Protein leverage effects of beef protein on energy intake in humans. *Am. J. Clin. Nutr.* **2014**, *99*, 1397–1406. [CrossRef] [PubMed]
23. Helms, E.R.; Zinn, C.; Rowlands, D.S.; Naidoo, R.; Cronin, J. High-protein, low-fat, short-term diet results in less stress and fatigue than moderate-protein moderate-fat diet during weight loss in male weightlifters: A pilot study. *Int. J. Sport Nutr. Exerc. Metab.* **2015**, *25*, 163–170. [CrossRef] [PubMed]

24. DeFreitas, J.M.; Beck, T.W.; Stock, M.S.; Dillon, M.A.; Kasishke, P.R. An examination of the time course of training-induced skeletal muscle hypertrophy. *Eur. J. Appl. Physiol.* **2011**, *111*, 2785–2790. [CrossRef] [PubMed]
25. Brown, N.; Bubeck, D.; Haeufle, D.F.B.; Weickenmeier, J.; Kuhl, E.; Alt, W.; Schmitt, S. Weekly time course of neuro-muscular adaptation to intensive strength training. *Front. Physiol.* **2017**, *8*, 329. [CrossRef] [PubMed]
26. Sale, D.G. Neural adaptation to resistance training. *Med. Sci. Sports Exerc.* **1988**, *20* (Suppl. 5), S135–S145. [CrossRef] [PubMed]
27. Trappe, S.; Williamson, D.; Godard, M. Maintenance of whole muscle strength and size following resistance training in older men. *J. Gerontol.* **2002**, *57*, B138–B143. [CrossRef]
28. American College of Sports Medicine. American College of Sports Medicine position stand. Progression models in resistance training for healthy adults. *Med. Sci. Sports Exerc.* **2009**, *41*, 687–708. [CrossRef]
29. Utter, A.C.; Kang, J.; Nieman, D.C.; Brown, V.A.; Dumke, C.L.; McAnulty, S.R.; McAnulty, L.S. Carbohydrate supplementation and perceived exertion during resistance exercise. *J. Strength Cond. Res.* **2005**, *19*, 939–943. [CrossRef]
30. Roberts, J.; Zinchenko, A.; Suckling, C.; Smith, L.; Johnstone, J.; Henselmans, M. The short-term effect of high versus moderate protein intake on recovery after strength training in resistance-trained individuals. *J. Int. Soc. Sports Nutr.* **2017**, *14*, 44. [CrossRef]
31. Antonio, J.; Peacock, C.; Ellerbroek, A.; Fromhoff, B.; Silver, T. The effects of consuming a high protein diet (4.4 g/kg/d) on body composition in resistance-trained individuals. *J. Int. Soc. Sports Nutr.* **2014**, *11*, 19. [CrossRef] [PubMed]
32. Antonio, J.; Ellerbroek, A.; Silver, T.; Orris, S.; Scheiner, M.; Gonzalez, A.; Peacock, C. A high protein diet (3.4 g/kg/d) combined with a heavy resistance training program improves body composition in healthy trained men and women—A follow-up investigation. *J. Int. Soc. Sports Nutr.* **2015**, *12*, 39. [CrossRef] [PubMed]
33. Antonio, J.; Ellerbroek, A.; Silver, T.; Vargas, L.; Peacock, C. The effects of a high protein diet on indices of health and body composition—A crossover trial in resistance-trained men. *J. Int. Soc. Sports Nutr.* **2016**, *13*, 1–7. [CrossRef] [PubMed]
34. McArdle, W.; Katch, F.; Katch, V. *Exercise Physiology: Energy, Nutrition and Human Performance*, 5th ed.; Lippincott Williams and Wilkins: Philadelphia, PA, USA, 2001.
35. Cunningham, J. Body composition and resting metabolic rate: The myth of feminine metabolism. *Am. J. Clin. Nutr.* **1982**, *36*, 721–726. [CrossRef] [PubMed]
36. Stubbs, R.J.; Hughes, D.A.; Johnstone, A.M.; Rowley, E.; Reid, C.; Elia, M.; Stratton, R.; Delargy, H.; King, N.; Blundell, J.E. The use of visual analogue scales to assess motivation to eat in human subjects: A review of their reliability and validity with an evaluation of new hand-held computerized systems for temporal tracking of appetite ratings. *Br. J. Nutr.* **2000**, *84*, 405–415. [CrossRef] [PubMed]
37. Flint, A.; Raben, A.; Blundell, J.E.; Astrup, A. Reproducibility, power and validity of visual analogue scales in assessment of appetite sensations in single test meal studies. *Int. J. Obes. Relat. Metab. Disord.* **2000**, *24*, 38–48. [CrossRef] [PubMed]
38. Raben, A.; Agerholm-Larsen, L.; Flint, A.; Holst, J.J.; Astrup, A. Meals with similar energy densities but rich in protein, fat, carbohydrate, or alcohol have different effects on energy expenditure and substrate metabolism but not on appetite and energy intake. *Am. J. Clin. Nutr.* **2003**, *77*, 91–100. [CrossRef]
39. Bligh, H.F.; Godsland, I.F.; Frost, G.; Hunter, K.J.; Murray, P.; MacAulay, K.; Hyliands, D.; Talbot, D.C.; Casey, J.; Mulder, T.P.; et al. Plant-rich mixed meals based on Palaeolithic diet principles have a dramatic impact on incretin, peptide YY and satiety response, but show little effect on glucose and insulin homeostasis: An acute-effects randomised study. *Br. J. Nutr.* **2015**, *113*, 574–584. [CrossRef]
40. Blatt, A.D.; Roe, L.S.; Rolls, B.J. Increasing the protein content of meals and its effect on daily energy intake. *J. Am. Diet. Assoc.* **2011**, *111*, 290–294. [CrossRef]
41. Wiessing, K.R.; Xin, L.; Budgett, S.C.; Poppitt, S.D. No evidence of enhanced satiety following whey protein- or sucrose-enriched water beverages: A dose response trial in overweight women. *Eur. J. Clin. Nutr.* **2015**, *69*, 1238–1243. [CrossRef]
42. Ravn, A.M.; Gregersen, N.T.; Christensen, R.; Rasmussen, L.G.; Hels, O.; Belza, A.; Raben, A.; Larsen, T.M.; Toubro, S.; Astrup, A. Thermic effect of a meal and appetite in adults: An individual participant data meta-analysis of meal-test trials. *Food Nutr. Res.* **2013**, *57*. [CrossRef] [PubMed]

43. Phillips, S.M.; Chevalier, S.; Leidy, H.J. Protein "requirements" beyond the RDA: Implications for optimizing health. *Appl. Physiol. Nutr. Metab.* **2016**, *41*, 565–572. [CrossRef] [PubMed]
44. Lemon, P.W.; Tarnopolsky, M.A.; MacDougall, J.D.; Atkinson, S.A. Protein requirements and muscle mass/strength changes during intensive training in novice bodybuilders. *J. Appl. Physiol.* **1992**, *73*, 767–775. [CrossRef] [PubMed]
45. Jakubowicz, D.; Froy, O.; Wainstein, J.; Boaz, M. Meal timing and composition influence ghrelin levels, appetite scores and weight loss maintenance in overweight and obese adults. *Steroids* **2012**, *77*, 323–331. [CrossRef] [PubMed]
46. Barbosa-Silva, M.C.G.; Barros, A.J.D.; Wang, J.; Heymsfield, S.B.; Pierson, R.N. Bioelectrical impedance analysis: Population reference values for phase angle by age and sex. *Am. J. Clin. Nutr.* **2005**, *82*, 49–52. [CrossRef] [PubMed]
47. Norman, K.; Stobäus, N.; Pirlich, M.; Bosy-Westphal, A. Bioelectrical phase angle and impedance vector analysis—Clinical relevance and applicability of impedance parameters. *Clin. Nutr.* **2012**, *31*, 854–861. [CrossRef] [PubMed]
48. Souza, M.F.; Tomeleri, C.M.; Ribeiro, A.S.; Schoenfeld, B.J.; Silva, A.M.; Sardinha, L.B.; Cyrino, E.S. Effect of resistance training on phase angle in older women: A randomized controlled trial. *Scand. J. Med. Sci. Sports* **2016**, *8*, 1–9. [CrossRef]
49. Westerterp-Plantenga, M.S.; Lemmens, S.G.; Westerterp, K.R. Dietary protein—Its role in satiety, energetics, weight loss and health. *Br. J. Nutr.* **2012**, *108*, S105–S112. [CrossRef]
50. Gibbons, C.; Caudwell, P.; Finlayson, G.; Webb, D.L.; Hellström, P.M.; Näslund, E.; Blundell, J.E. Comparison of postprandial profiles of ghrelin, active GLP-1, and total PYY to meals varying in fat and carbohydrate and their association with hunger and the phases of satiety. *J. Clin. Endocrinol. Metab.* **2013**, *98*, E847–E855. [CrossRef]
51. Leidy, H.J.; Ortinau, L.C.; Douglas, S.M.; Hoertel, H.A. Beneficial effects of a higher-protein breakfast on the appetitive, hormonal, and neural signals controlling energy intake regulation in overweight/obese, "breakfast-skipping," late-adolescent girls. *Am. J. Clin. Nutr.* **2013**, *97*, 677–688. [CrossRef]
52. Doucet, É.; Laviolette, M.; Imbeault, P.; Strychar, I.; Rabasa-Lhoret, R.; Prud'homme, D. Total peptide YY is a correlate of postprandial energy expenditure but not of appetite or energy intake in healthy women. *Metab. Clin. Exp.* **2008**, *57*, 1458–1464. [CrossRef] [PubMed]
53. OConnor, K.L.; Scisco, J.L.; Smith, T.J.; Young, A.J.; Montain, S.J.; Price, L.L.; Lieberman, H.R.; Karl, J.P. Altered appetite-mediating hormone concentrations precede compensatory overeating after severe, short-term energy deprivation in healthy adults. *J. Nutr.* **2016**, *146*, 209–217. [CrossRef] [PubMed]
54. Moran, L.J.; Luscombe-Marsh, N.D.; Noakes, M.; Wittert, G.A.; Keogh, J.B.; Clifton, P.M. The satiating effect of dietary protein is unrelated to postprandial ghrelin secretion. *J. Clin. Endocrinol. Metab.* **2005**, *90*, 5205–5211. [CrossRef] [PubMed]
55. Leidy, H.J.; Armstrong, C.L.; Tang, M.; Mattes, R.D.; Campbell, W.W. The influence of higher protein intake and greater eating frequency on appetite control in overweight and obese men. *Obesity* **2010**, *18*, 1725–1732. [CrossRef] [PubMed]
56. MacKenzie-Shalders, K.L.; Byrne, N.M.; Slater, G.J.; King, N.A. The effect of a whey protein supplement dose on satiety and food intake in resistance training athletes. *Appetite* **2015**, *92*, 178–184. [CrossRef] [PubMed]
57. Cuenca-Sánchez, M.; Navas-Carrillo, D.; Orenes-Piñero, E. Controversies surrounding high-protein diet intake: Satiating effect and kidney and bone health. *Adv. Nutr.* **2015**, *6*, 260–266. [CrossRef] [PubMed]
58. Tan, X.; Cao, X.; Zou, J.; Shen, B.; Zhang, X.; Liu, Z.; Lv, W.; Teng, J.; Dign, X. Indoxyl sulfate, a valuable biomarker in chronic kidney disease and dialysis. *Hemodial. Int.* **2017**, *21*, 161–167. [CrossRef]
59. Vanholder, R.; Schepers, E.; Pletinck, A.; Nagler, E.V.; Glorieux, G. The uremic toxicity of indoxyl sulfate and p-cresyl sulfate: A systematic review. *J. Am. Soc. Nephrol.* **2014**, *25*, 1897–1907. [CrossRef]
60. Russell, W.R.; Gratz, S.W.; Duncan, S.H.; Holtrop, G.; Ince, J.; Scobbie, L.; Duncan, G.; Johnstone, A.M.; Lobley, G.E.; Wallace, R.J.; et al. High-protein, reduced-carbohydrate weight-loss diets promote metabolite profiles likely to be detrimental to colonic health. *Am. J. Clin. Nutr.* **2011**, *93*, 1062–1072. [CrossRef]
61. Long, S.J.; Jeffcoat, A.R.; Millward, D.J. Effect of habitual dietary-protein intake on appetite and satiety. *Appetite* **2000**, *35*, 79–88. [CrossRef]

62. Batterham, R.L.; Heffron, H.; Kapoor, S.; Chivers, J.E.; Chandarana, K.; Herzog, H.; Le Roux, C.W.; Thomas, E.L.; Bell, J.D.; Withers, D.J. Critical role for peptide YY in protein-mediated satiation and body-weight regulation. *Cell Metab.* **2006**, *4*, 223–233. [CrossRef] [PubMed]
63. Scheid, J.L.; De Souza, M.J. The Role of PYY in Eating Behavior and Diet. In *Handbook of Behavior, Food and Nutrition*; Preedy, V., Watson, R., Martin, C., Eds.; Springer: New York, NY, USA, 2011.
64. Karra, E.; Chandarana, K.; Batterham, R.L. The role of peptide YY in appetite regulation and obesity. *J. Physiol.* **2009**, *587*, 19–25. [CrossRef] [PubMed]
65. Blom, W.A.; Lluch, A.; Stafleu, A.; Vinoy, S.; Holst, J.J.; Schaafsma, G.; Hendriks, H.F. Effect of a high-protein breakfast on the postprandial ghrelin response. *Am. J. Clin. Nutr.* **2006**, *83*, 211–220. [CrossRef] [PubMed]
66. Campbell, M.D.; Gonzalez, J.T.; Rumbold, P.L.; Walker, M.; Shaw, J.A.; Stevenson, E.J.; West, D.J. Comparison of appetite responses to high- and low-glycemic index postexercise meals under matched insulinemia and fiber in type 1 diabetes. *Am. J. Clin. Nutr.* **2015**, *101*, 478–486. [CrossRef] [PubMed]
67. Clayton, D.J.; James, L.J. The effect of breakfast on appetite regulation, energy balance and exercise performance. *Proc. Nutr. Soc.* **2016**, *75*, 319–327. [CrossRef] [PubMed]
68. Clayton, D.J.; Stensel, D.J.; James, L.J. Effect of breakfast omission on subjective appetite, metabolism, acylated ghrelin and GLP-17-36 during rest and exercise. *Nutrition* **2016**, *32*, 179–185. [CrossRef]
69. Iepsen, E.W.; Lundgren, J.; Holst, J.J.; Madsbad, S.; Torekov, S.S. Successful weight loss maintenance includes long-term increased meal responses of GLP-1 and PYY3-36. *Eur. J. Endocrinol.* **2016**, *174*, 775–784. [CrossRef]
70. Sumithran, P.; Prendergast, L.A.; Delbridge, E.; Purcell, K.; Shulkes, A.; Kriketos, A.; Proietto, J. Long-term persistence of hormonal adaptations to weight loss. *N. Engl. J. Med.* **2011**, *365*, 1597–1604. [CrossRef]

8

Effectiveness of Positive and Negative Ions for Elite Japanese Swimmers' Physical Training: Subjective and Biological Emotional Evaluations

Goichi Hagiwara [1,*], Hirotoshi Mankyu [1], Takaaki Tsunokawa [2], Masaru Matsumoto [3] and Hirokazu Funamori [3]

1 National Institute of Fitness and Sports in Kanoya, 1 Shiromizucho, Kanoya-shi, Kagoshima 891-2393, Japan; mankyu@nifs-k.ac.jp
2 Faculty of Health and Sport Science, University of Tsukuba, 1-1-1 Tennodai, Tsukuba-shi, Ibaraki 305-8574, Japan; tsunokawa.takaaki.ke@u.tsukuba.ac.jp
3 Sharp Corporation, 3-1-72 Kitakamei-cho, Yao-shi, Osaka 581-8585, Japan; matsumoto_masaru@sharp.co.jp (M.M.); funamori.hirokazu@sharp.co.jp (H.F.)
* Correspondence: hagiwara-g@nifs-k.ac.jp

Abstract: The purpose of this study is to examine the subjective and objective arousal of elite swimmers during physical training under a positive and negative ion environment. The participants were 10 elite Japanese collegiate swimmers participating in the Fédération Internationale de Natation (FINA) Swimming World Cup (age: 20.80 ± 1.39, five males and five females). Each participant went through two experiments (they were subjected to both the positive and negative ion environment and the control environment) within a four-week interval. The training task was a High-Intensity Interval Training (HIIT) routine for the swimmers. The subjective arousal state was measured using a Two-Dimensional Mood Scale (TDMS). In addition, biological emotional evaluations in the form of an electroencephalogram (EEG) were conducted to assess the arousal state of the elite swimmers. The examination of the change in the arousal level at rest and during training demonstrated that both subjective and objective arousal levels were significantly higher in the positive and negative ion environment than in the control environment. In addition, the average training performance scores were also significantly higher in the positive and negative ion environment than in the control environment. This study posits that the positive and negative ion environment has a positive effect on sports training.

Keywords: training environment; sports; athletes; interval training; biological emotional evaluation; sports sciences

---

1. Introduction

Arousal is a human psychological state and is defined as being "worked up" or energized [1]. In addition, Oxendine [2] proposed that high levels of arousal would benefit, or be essential for, maximal performance; thus, several studies investigated the relationships between arousal and sports performance [1,3,4]. Yamazaki and Sugiyama [4] examined the relationships between subjective arousal level and sports performance and the results indicated that, among Japanese collegiate badminton players, athletes with higher arousal levels had significantly higher shot success rates. In addition, Fronso et al. [5] used an electroencephalogram (EEG) to assess the biological arousal level in Olympic athletes participating in air-pistol shooting, and investigated the relationships between arousal level and sports performance. The results demonstrated that higher levels of arousal were associated with controlled shooting performance. Although subjective evaluations about arousal level have been conducted using questionnaires [1,4,6], few studies about the biological evaluations of psychological arousal level have been attempted.

Air ions are small particles that exist in nature and are positively or negatively charged molecules or atoms in the air [7]; positively charged ions are positive ions and those negatively charged are negative ions [8]. In addition, air ions containing positive and negative ions have certain abilities such as purification of the atmosphere and deodorization [9]. Thus, several studies have been conducted on the relationship between air ions and human emotions.

Previous studies on the relationship between air ions and emotion in humans have been conducted [10]. Flory et al. [11] conducted an experiment where 18 women stayed in a high-density ion environment for over 12 consecutive days and the results indicated that the high-density negative ion environment reduced depression. In addition, other studies that examined the relationship between negative ions and depression [12–15], lower stress [16], and increased well-being [17] have been conducted. Several studies also suggest that relationships exist between positive ion environments and human emotion [10]. For instance, Gianinni et al. [18] examined the correlation between positive air ions and emotion and found that anxiety and excitement significantly increased under this condition. In addition, the relationship between positive ions and feelings of unpleasantness, irritation and anxiety has been verified [18,19].

Although there is some skepticism in the study of ions, the results of the above-mentioned studies confirm that they are connected to emotional changes. In addition, little research has been done on the relationship between positive and negative ions and the emotion and performance of athletes in the field of sports science, and no such research is found in Japan. Thus, the purpose of this study was to examine the subjective and objective arousal of elite Japanese swimmers during physical training in a positive and negative ion environment.

2. Materials and Methods

2.1. Participants and Study Design

Institutional review board approval was obtained from the corresponding author's research institute (National Institute of Fitness and Sports in Kanoya, Institutional Review Board, No.11-6). The participants were informed of the instructions and purpose of this study before the experiment.

The participants were 10 elite Japanese collegiate swimmers participating in the Fédération Internationale de Natation (FINA) Swimming World Cup (age: 20.80 ± 1.39, 5 males and 5 females). Each participant underwent two experiments within a four-week interval. Two types of experimental environment were prepared: a condition in which positive and negative ions were filled up the atmosphere in the experimental room (PNI condition), and a condition in which ions were not generated (control condition). The conditions were blinded by randomly changing the experimental environment to prevent the participants from knowing to which condition they were subjected. The details of randomization are described as follows.

The first experiment was conducted within two days. On the first day, we created a PNI condition and conducted experiments while filling the atmosphere with air ions. The participants were randomly assigned and trained in one of the two environments (in the first experiment, three female and two male athletes performed in the PNI condition). After the experiment in the PNI condition was completed, the experimental laboratory was opened for one day to stop the ionizers and release the PNI from the room. Thereafter, it was confirmed that there were no PNI and the remaining five people (three women, two men) conducted experiments in a control condition. Four weeks after the first experiment, the participants underwent the same procedure and the second experiment was conducted.

The PNI condition was delivered by six Plasmacluster^{TM} ionizers (Sharp Corporation, Sakai-shi, Osaka, Japan) and exposed the participants to positive and negative ions (147,000–164,000 PNI/cm^3). The details of the process for generating positive and negative ions were based on previous research [8]. First, molecules in the air are decomposed by applying positive and negative high voltages to each discharge brush electrode of the ion generation devices, and the devices generate positive ions and negative ions [20].

The ion concentrations were determined by an ion counter (MY1210S, Asahi System Inc., Osaka-shi, Osaka, Japan) by means of the double concentric circle tube method [20]. The room condition was a temperature of 24.0 °C ± 0.5 and humidity was 60% ± 2.0.

The experimental procedure is as follows (Figure 1). First, participants were asked to put on an EEG device for two minutes to investigate their baseline degree of arousal before training. An EEG is an electrical signal generated by the brain and can be used to measure the psychological state of humans in real time. The participants then answered a questionnaire which evaluated their subjective emotional state before the training. A training task was then assigned. The training task was a High-Intensity Interval Training (HIIT) routine for swimmers. Participants conducted eight sets of 20 s of hard exercise and 10 s of rest using a swimming ergometer (Concept2 Inc., Morrisville, VT, USA) (Figure 2). After 8 sets, participants rested for 10 min and then again performed HIIT for 20 s, with one set at maximum power. After the training task, the average load (W) for 8 sets of intervals and the maximum power set of training load (W) after a 10-min rest were evaluated. The training load was set to the load used by the participants in their daily practice. Thus, the training load was set to eight for males and six for females. Thereafter, the EEG of the participants was measured for two minutes to investigate their degree of arousal after training, after which they were required to answer a questionnaire again.

In this study, EEG was also measured during interval training but, since it was accompanied by large movements during training, accurate data could not be acquired due to noise. Therefore, the measurement values were compared for two minutes before and after training. In addition, this study used the same method as a previous study [21] that adopted two minutes to investigate the baseline degree of human emotion.

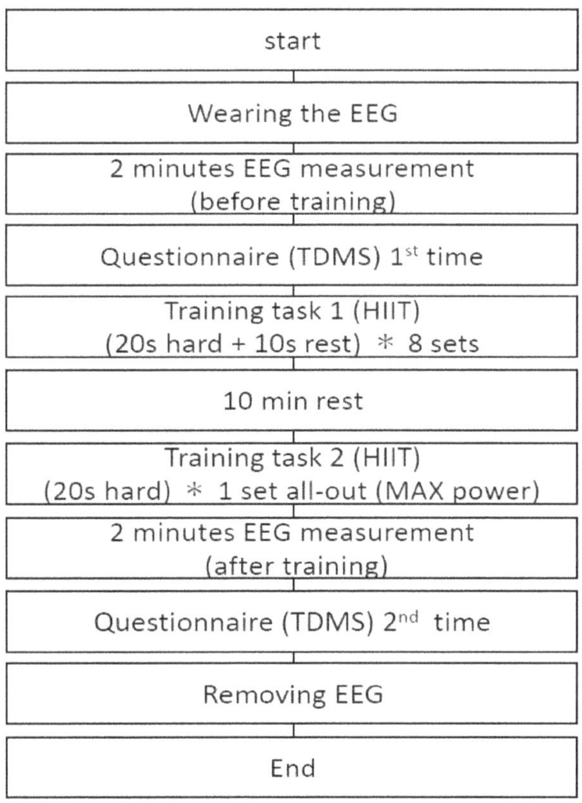
start
Wearing the EEG
2 minutes EEG measurement
(before training)
Questionnaire (TDMS) 1st time
Training task 1 (HIIT)
(20s hard + 10s rest) * 8 sets
10 min rest
Training task 2 (HIIT)
(20s hard) * 1 set all-out (MAX power)
2 minutes EEG measurement
(after training)
Questionnaire (TDMS) 2nd time
Removing EEG
End

Figure 1. Experimental procedure.

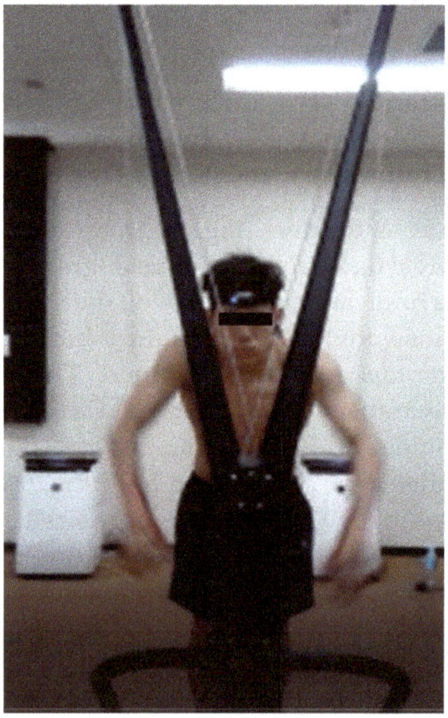

Figure 2. High Intensity Interval Training (HIIT) Training.

2.2. *Emotional Evaluation*

Subjective emotional evaluation was measured using a Two-Dimensional Mood Scale (TDMS) [22]. The TDMS is composed of eight items and four factors: activity, stability, comfort, and arousal. This study used the arousal score to evaluate the elite swimmers' emotional state.

A biological emotional evaluation in the form of an EEG was also conducted to assess the arousal state of the elite swimmers. In addition, the EEG measurement was used in this study because it is more easily measured in a daily living environment compared to other brain activity measurements. We adopted a simple band-type EEG device (NeuroSky Co., Ltd., Tokyo, Japan) that only measures the front polar area 1 (Fp1) lobe as defined by the international 10–20 system (Figure 3). Since Fp1 is located on the left frontal lobe, there is no need to worry about the possible noise interference caused by hair. The EEG obtained from Fp1 has been found to be suitable for obtaining data on people's psychological condition [23,24]. Thus, this study also assessed the Fp1 to estimate arousal level.

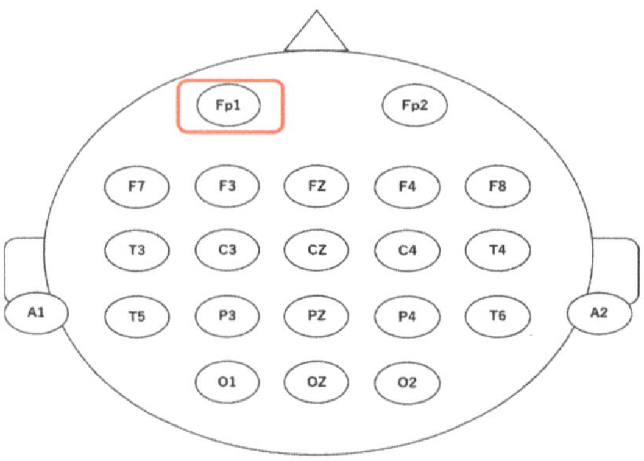

Figure 3. Measurement points of the international 10–20 system.

The electrical activity in the brain is often used as an objective evaluation index that employs biological data. Brainwaves are generally classified into four types according to their frequency range:

0.5–4 Hz: delta waves, 4–8 Hz: theta waves, 8–13 Hz: alpha waves, and 13–40 Hz: beta waves. Emotions are associated with each type [25] (Table 1).

Table 1. Type of brain wave and psychological state.

Type of Brain Wave	Frequency (Hz)	Psychological State
Delta wave	0.5–4 Hz	Non-REM sleep, unconscious
Theta wave	4–8 Hz	Sleep onset, illusion
Alpha wave	8–13 Hz	Relaxed mental state
Beta wave	13–40 Hz	Arousal

This study focused on the beta wave band. The EEG data obtained were recorded in a smartphone and the Kansei Module Logger [26]. This method produced the data output as sensitivity values were used. In addition, the Kansei Module Logger was set so that the occurrence ration of the beta wave band was defined as the arousal level, and the value was easily displayed as a value from 0 to 100. Hagiwara et al. [27] posited that the arousal level output by the Kansei Module Logger correlates with the subjective arousal level. The basic concept of Kansei Module Logger is that it calculates the power ratio between the beta wave bands. The potential difference obtained from the electrodes on the forehead and earlobe of the left Fp1 is amplified by the circuit inside the measuring instrument, digitized at 512 samples/sec, and subjected to the Hanning window processing. The power spectral analysis was then conducted using the fast Fourier transform. EEG data are analyzed every second by the fast Fourier transform, and the amplitude spectra can be obtained in the frequency range of 1–64 Hz. Thus, this study obtained delta, theta, alpha and beta waves. From the obtained power spectrum, the sum of each power in each frequency band was then calculated, and the ratio included in the total of the total power is shown as a relative numerical value. However, the sum of the power of each frequency cannot be used because the amplitude of each frequency band is different. Therefore, we took the average value of the power of each frequency band and obtained the representative value of that frequency band. The calculation method used the following Formula as a standard for analysis.

The average P_x of the x-wave power was calculated by Formula (1), where V_f is the power of the EEG at the frequency f [Hz]. Since this study concerns the beta wave band (13 Hz to 40 Hz), when $x = \beta$, it becomes (13, 40) [Hz], and the numerical value is applied to $(F^x{}_{max} - F^x{}_{min})$ in Formula (1). Next, the sum of the power averages (P_{sum}) in each frequency band is calculated by Formula (2). The ratio (R_x) included in the total power of the beta wave band was calculated in Formula (3).

$$P_x = \sum_{f=F^x_{\text{min}}}^{F^x_{\text{max}}} V_f / (F^x_{\text{max}} - F^x_{\text{min}} + 1) \tag{1}$$

$$P_{sum} = P_\delta + P_\theta + P_\alpha + P_\beta \tag{2}$$

$$R_x = P_x / P_{sum} \tag{3}$$

Based on the above calculation method, the Kansei Module Logger normalized the power ratio that can be taken in the beta band to the value of 0–100.

2.3. Analysis

For subjective data, the difference between the average value of arousal level by TDMS before and after training was used as the change value, and t-test was used to compare the PNI condition and control condition. For biological data, the difference between the average value of arousal measured before training and the average value of arousal measured after training was used as the amount of change. The paired t-test was then used to compare the difference between the PNI condition and the control condition. In the training data, the average load (W) for 8 sets of intervals and maximum power set of training load (W) after a 10-min rest were compared between the PNI condition and the control condition.

3. Results

3.1. Comparison of Changes in Arousal by TDMS before and after Training in PNI and Control Conditions

As a result of comparing the amount of change in arousal by TDMS before and after training in the PNI and the control conditions, the amount of change in the arousal level under PNI condition (M = +7.30, SD = 1.90) was found to be significantly higher than that in the control condition (M = +3.3, SD = 1.24) (t = 3.52, $p < 0.01$) (Figure 4).

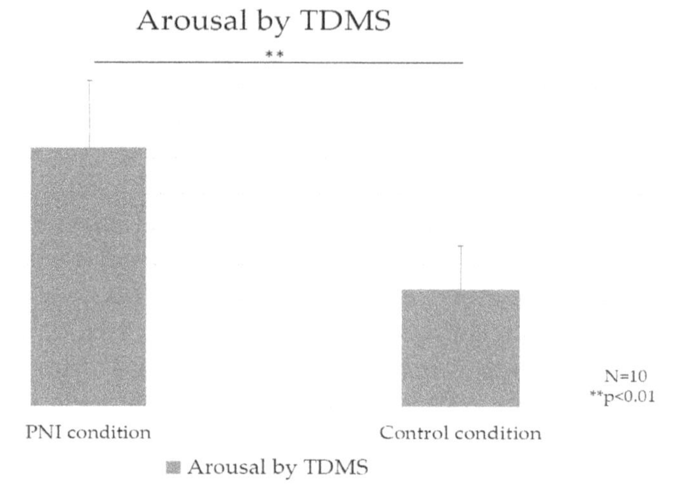

Figure 4. Comparing the amount of change in arousal by a Two-Dimensional Mood Scale (TDMS) in Positive-Negative Ions (PNI) and control conditions.

3.2. Comparison of Changes in Arousal by EEG before and after Training in the PNI and the Control Conditions

As a result of comparing the amount of change in arousal by EEG before and after training in the PNI and the control conditions, the amount of change in the arousal level under PNI condition (M = +8.16, SD = 2.14) was also found to be significantly higher than that in the control condition (M = +2.75, SD = 2.24) (t = 2.84, $p < 0.05$) (Figure 5).

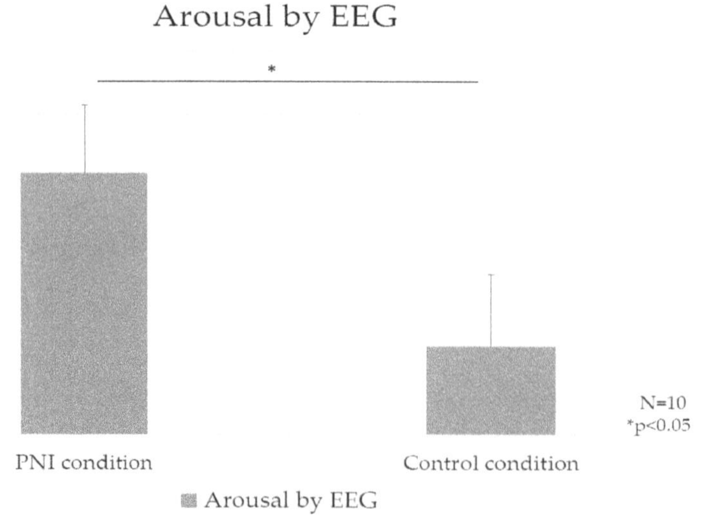

Figure 5. Comparing the amount of change in arousal by electroencephalogram (EEG) in PNI and control conditions.

3.3. Comparison of the Average Load (W) for Eight Sets of Interval Training in PNI and Control Conditions

As a result of comparing the average load (W) of interval training in the PNI and the control conditions, the average load (W) under PNI condition (M = 146.22, SD = 13.54) was shown to be significantly higher than that recorded in the control condition (M = 141.14, SD = 12.32) (t = 1.46, p < 0.10) (Figure 6).

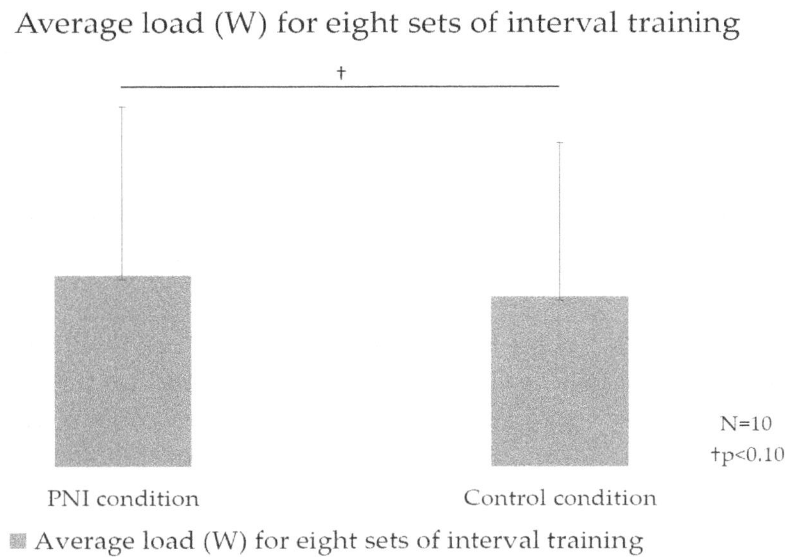

Figure 6. Comparing the average load (W) for 8 sets of interval training in PNI and control conditions.

3.4. Comparison of the Average of Training Load (W) during the Maximum Power Set in PNI and Control Conditions

As a result of comparing the average of training load (W) during the maximum power set in the PNI the and control conditions, the average load (W) under PNI condition (M = 192.78, SD = 19.36) was also found to be significantly higher than that in the control condition (M = 181.67, SD = 16.03) (t = 1.99, p < 0.05) (Figure 7).

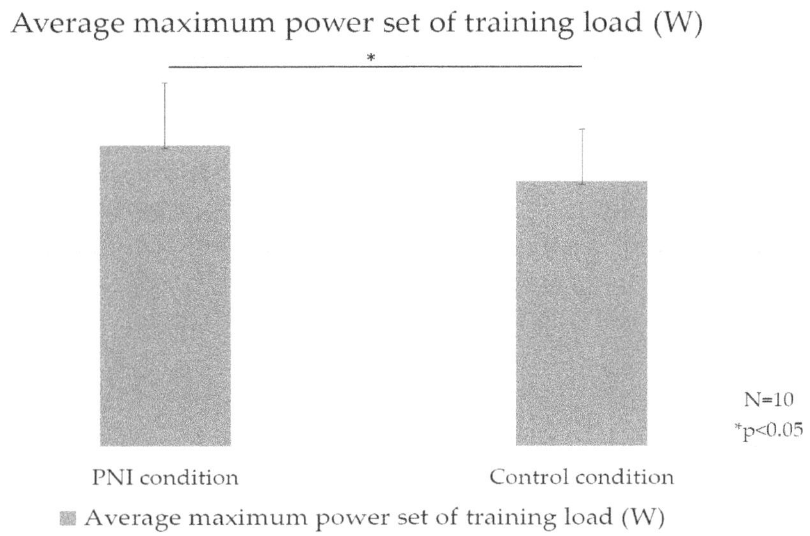

Figure 7. Comparing the average of training load (W) during the maximum power set in PNI and control conditions.

4. Discussion

This study aimed to investigate the psychological effects of both the subjective and objective arousal levels of elite Japanese swimmers during physical training under a positive and negative ion environment.

First, the results of the comparison of the subjective arousal level indicated that the PNI condition significantly improved the arousal level compared to the control condition. Previous studies [12–15] have clarified the relationship between negative ions and positive emotions by using subjective evaluation. In addition, subjective research has also shown the relationship between positive ions and emotions in previous studies [18,19]. In this study, as a result of verifying the subjective arousal level in an environment in which PNI are simultaneously generated, it is suggested that athletes may have a higher arousal level under the PNI condition. These results are considered to be new findings in the literature on PNI and emotions.

Second, the results of the comparison of the objective arousal levels obtained from EEG indicated that the PNI condition significantly improved the arousal level compared to the control condition. A few studies in the past [28,29] tried to clarify the relationship between negative ions and emotions using brain waves. Watanabe et al. [29] examined the effect of negative air ions on EEG, and the results indicated that the alpha wave tended to be higher in the negative ion condition than in the control condition. On the other hand, the results of this study indicated that the PNI condition demonstrated a significantly higher arousal level (beta band power level) than the control condition. Therefore, the results of this study differ from the previous studies that were mentioned earlier. A subjective evaluation study by Charry and Hawkinshire [19] showed that positive ions contribute to the improvement of tension. In this study, since the experiments were conducted in the environment in which positive ions were also generated, it is speculated that positive ions may affect the arousal level extracted from the EEG. As mentioned, it might demonstrate the existence of relationships between PNI conditions, and states of subjective and objective arousal. However, as mentioned previously, there is some skepticism in the study of ions; thus, it would be necessary to further study the relationships between air ions and athletes' emotions in the field of sports science.

Finally, the results of comparing the average load (W) of interval training under the PNI and the control conditions show the average load (W) under the PNI condition tended to be significantly higher than that recorded in the control condition. Moreover, the result of comparing the average of training load (W) during the maximum power set under the PNI condition was that it was recorded as significantly higher than under the control condition.

Several researches have examined the association between physical exercise and negative ions [30,31]. Ryushi et al. [30] demonstrated that, under the negative ion condition, the levels of serotonin and dopamine were decreased in the recovery period after moderate endurance exercise than those recorded under the control condition. Thus, it suggested that the negative ion condition might affect the feeling of relaxation after endurance training. This study also found that the load on the maximum power set after a 10-min rest was significantly higher, and that negative ion effects reduced dopamine and serotonin during the rest which led to a more relaxed state. There is a possibility that the PNI condition might have affected the maximum power set results for the participants.

5. Conclusions

This study suggests that the PNI condition may have a positive effect on sports training. However, there are limitations to this study. We conducted the experiments on 10 elite swimmers, but it is necessary to expand the sample size in order to generalize this study. It is thus necessary that future studies be conducted with more participants. In addition, although this study conducted the experiment twice in an environment in which the athletes were randomly switched, it is recognized that emotions may change depending on the condition of the athlete on that day. Therefore, it is suggested that conducting a longitudinal experiment on the same participants might shed more accurate findings on the matter.

Author Contributions: Conceptualization, G.H. and H.M.; methodology, G.H., H.M., and T.T.; investigation, M.M., H.F., and T.T.; writing—original draft preparation, G.H.; writing—review and editing, H.M. and T.T. All authors have read and agreed to the published version of the manuscript.

References

1. Perkins, D.; Wilson, G.V.; Kerr, J.H. The effects of elevated arousal and mood on maximal strength performance in athletes. *J. Appl. Sport Psychol.* **2001**, *13*, 239–259. [CrossRef]
2. Oxendine, J.B. Emotional arousal and motor performance. *Quest* **1970**, *13*, 23–30. [CrossRef]
3. Gould, D.; Krane, V. The arousal-performance relationship: Current status and future directions. In *Advances in Sport Psychology*; Horn, T.S., Ed.; Human Kinetics: Champaign, IL, USA, 1992; pp. 119–141.
4. Yamazaki, M.; Sugiyama, Y. Intervention effect of a motivation video for badminton athletes: Examination from watching the motivation video one hour before. *Res. J. Sport Perform.* **2009**, *1*, 275–288.
5. Fronso, S.d.; Robazza, C.; Filho, E.; Bortoli, L.; Comani, S.; Bertollo, M. Neural markers of performance states in an Olympic athlete: A EEG case study in air-pistol shooting. *J. Sports Sci. Med.* **2016**, *15*, 214–222. [PubMed]
6. Nagao, Y.; Sugiyama, Y. Influence on a collective efficacy of viewing a motivational video of a game in relation to type of video. *Res. J. Sport Perform.* **2013**, *5*, 352–368.
7. Jiang, S.Y.; Ma, A.; Ramachangran, S. Negative air ions and their effects on human health and air quality improvement. *Int. J. Mol. Sci.* **2018**, *19*, 2966. [CrossRef]
8. Yamamoto, D.; Wako, Y.; Kumabe, S.; Wako, K.; Sato, Y.; Fujishiro, M.; Yashimasa, Y.; Matsuura, I.; Ohnishi, Y. Positive and negative ions by air purifier have no effects on reproductive function or postnatal growth and development in rats. *Fundam. Toxicol. Sci.* **2015**, *2*, 101–110. [CrossRef]
9. Nishikawa, K. Air purification technology of positively and negatively charged cluster ions by plasma discharge at atmospheric pressure. *J. Plasma Fusion Res.* **2013**, *89*, 164–168.
10. Perez, V.; Alexander, D.D.; Bailey, W.H. Air ions and mood outcomes: A review and meta-analysis. *BMC Psychiatry.* **2013**, *13*, 29. [CrossRef]
11. Flory, R.; Ametepe, J.; Bowers, B. A randomized, placebo-controlled trial of bright light and high-density negative air ions for treatment of Seasonal Affective Disorder. *Psychiatry Res.* **2010**, *177*, 101–108. [CrossRef]
12. Goel, N.; Etwaroo, G.R. Bright light, negative air ions and auditory stimuli produce rapid mood changes in a student population: A placebo-controlled study. *Psychol. Med.* **2006**, *36*, 1253–1263. [CrossRef]
13. Terman, M.; Terman, J.S. Treatment of seasonal affective disorder with a high-output negative ionizer. *J. Altern. Complement Med.* **1995**, *1*, 87–92. [CrossRef]
14. Terman, M.; Terman, J.S. Controlled trial of naturalistic dawn simulation and negative air ionization for seasonal affective disorder. *Am. J. Psychiatry.* **2006**, *163*, 2126–2133. [CrossRef] [PubMed]
15. Terman, M.; Terman, J.S.; Ross, D.C. A controlled trial of timed bright light and negative air ionization for treatment of winter depression. *Arch. Gen. Psychiatry.* **1998**, *55*, 875–882. [CrossRef] [PubMed]
16. Malik, M.; Singh, K.; Singh, M. Effect of negative air ions on physiological and perceived psychological stress during computer operation. *Int. J. Environ. Health.* **2010**, *4*, 67–77. [CrossRef]
17. Lips, R.; Salawu, J.T.; Kember, P.; Probert, S.D. Intermittent exposures to enhanced air-ion concentrations for improved comfort and increased productivity? *Appl. Energy* **1987**, *28*, 83–94. [CrossRef]
18. Giannini, A.J.; Jones, B.T.; Loiselle, R.H. Reversibility of serotonin irritation syndrome with atmospheric anions. *J. Clin. Psychiatry* **1986**, *47*, 141–143.
19. Charry, J.M.; Hawkinshire, F.B. Effects of atmospheric electricity on some substrates of disordered social behavior. *J. Pers. Soc. Psychol.* **1981**, *41*, 185–197. [CrossRef]
20. Nishikawa, K.; Nojima, H. Air purification effect of positively and negatively charged ions generated by discharge plasma at atmospheric pressure. *Jpn. J. Appl. Phys.* **2001**, *40*, 835–837. [CrossRef]
21. Kanamaru, S.; Yokota, Y.; Naruse, Y.; Yairi, I. A research on quantification of the fear using EEG. In Proceedings of the 33rd Annual Conference of the Japanese Society for Artificial Intelligence, Niigata, Japan, 4–7 June 2019; pp. 1–4. [CrossRef]

22. Sakairi, Y.; Nakatsuka, K.; Shimizu, T. Development of the Two-Dimensional Mood Scale for self-monitoring and self-regulation of momentary mood states. *Jpn. Psychol. Res.* **2013**, *55*, 338–349. [CrossRef]
23. Mitsukura, Y. KANSEI Analyzing by EEG. *J. Inst. Electr. Eng. Jpn.* **2016**, *136*, 687–690. [CrossRef]
24. Hotta, M.; Kohata, Y. The evaluation of usability of EC site using electroencephalogram (EEG). In Proceedings of the 19th Japan Society of Kansei Engineering, University of Tsukuba, Tokyo, Japan, 11–13 September 2017; pp. 1–5.
25. Okubo, T.; Tamamaru, K.; Koshimizu, S. Development of the Impression Detection System by using a Portable EEG Device for Tourist Impression Analysis. *Trans. Jpn. Soc. Kansei Eng.* **2018**, *17*, 285–291. [CrossRef]
26. Littlesoftware Inc. Available online: https://hp.littlesoftware.jp (accessed on 10 May 2018).
27. Hagiwara, G.; Akiyama, D.; Tsunokawa, T.; Mankyu, H. Effectiveness of motivational videos for elite swimmers: Subjective and biological evaluations. *J. Hum. Sport Exerc.* **2019**, *14*, 178–188. [CrossRef]
28. Assael, M.; Pfeifer, Y.; Sulman, F.G. Influence of artificial air ionisation on the human electroencephalogram. *Int. J. Biometeorol.* **1974**, *18*, 306–372. [CrossRef] [PubMed]
29. Watanabe, I.; Mano, Y.; Noro, H. Effect of negative air ion in human electroencephalogram. *J. Jpn. Soc. Balneol. Climatol. Phys. Med.* **1998**, *61*, 121–126. [CrossRef]
30. Ryushi, T.; Kita, I.; Sakurai, T.; Yasumatsu, M.; Isokawa, M.; Aihara, Y.; Hama, K. The effect of exposure to negative air ions on the recovery of physiological responses after moderate endurance exercise. *Int. J. Biometeorol.* **1998**, *41*, 132–136. [CrossRef]
31. Nimmericher, A.; Holdhaus, J.; Mehnen, L.; Vidotto, C.; Loidl, M.; Barker, A.R. Effects of negative air ions on oxygen uptake kinetics, recovery and performance in exercise: A randomized, double-blinded study. *Int. J. Biometeorol.* **2014**, *58*, 1503–1512. [CrossRef]

9

Nutritional Intake, Sports Nutrition Knowledge and Energy Availability in Female Australian Rules Football Players

Dominique Condo [1,2,3,*], Rachel Lohman [1], Monica Kelly [3] and Amelia Carr [1]

1 Centre for Sport Research, School of Exercise and Nutrition Sciences, Faculty of Health, Deakin University, 221 Burwood Highway, Burwood, Melbourne, VIC 3125, Australia; rlohma@deakin.edu.au (R.L.); amelia.carr@deakin.edu.au (A.C.)
2 Institute for Physical Activity and Nutrition, School of Exercise and Nutrition Sciences, Faculty of Health, Deakin University, 221 Burwood Highway, Burwood, Melbourne, VIC 3125, Australia
3 Geelong Football Club, GMHBA Stadium, Geelong, VIC 3125, Australia; mkelly@geelongcats.com.au
* Correspondence: dominique.condo@deakin.edu

Abstract: This study aimed to assess nutritional intake, sports nutrition knowledge and risk of Low Energy Availability (LEA) in female Australian rules football players. Victorian Football League Women's competition (VFLW) players (n = 30) aged 18–35 (weight: 64.5 kg ± 8.0; height: 168.2 cm ± 7.6) were recruited from Victoria, Australia. Nutritional intake was quantified on training days using the Automated 24 h Dietary Assessment Tool (ASA24-Australia), and sports nutrition knowledge was measured by the 88-item Sports Nutrition Knowledge Questionnaire (SNKQ). The risk of LEA was assessed using the Low Energy Availability in Females Questionnaire (LEAF-Q). Daily mean carbohydrate intake in the current investigation was 3 $g{\cdot}kg^{-1}{\cdot}d^{-1}$, therefore, below the minimum carbohydrate recommendation for moderate exercise of approximately one hour per day (5–7 $g{\cdot}kg^{-1}{\cdot}d^{-1}$) and for moderate to intense exercise for 1–3 h per day (6–10 $g{\cdot}kg^{-1}{\cdot}d^{-1}$) for 96.3% and 100% of players, respectively. Daily mean protein intake was 1.5 $g{\cdot}kg^{-1}{\cdot}d^{-1}$, therefore, consistent with recommendations (1.2–2.0 $g{\cdot}kg^{-1}{\cdot}d^{-1}$) for 77.8% of players. Daily mean calcium intake was 924.8 $mg{\cdot}d^{-1}$, therefore, below recommendations (1000 $mg{\cdot}d^{-1}$) for 65.5% of players, while mean iron intake was 12.2 $mg{\cdot}d^{-1}$, also below recommendations (18 $mg{\cdot}d^{-1}$) for 100% of players. Players answered 54.5% of SNKQ questions correctly, with the lowest scores observed in the section on supplements. Risk of LEA was evident in 30% of players, with no differences in carbohydrate (p = 0.238), protein (p = 0.296), fat (p = 0.490) or energy (p = 0.971) intakes between players at risk of LEA and those not at risk. The results suggest that female Australian rules football players have an inadequate intake of carbohydrate and calcium and low sports nutrition knowledge. Further investigation to assess the risk of LEA using direct measures is required.

Keywords: carbohydrate intake; team sports; female athletes; nutritional recommendations; nutrition knowledge

---

1. Introduction

In 2017, the Australian Football League Women's (AFLW) competition commenced. In addition to the elite AFL competition, Australian rules football is comprised of numerous sub-elite competitions including the Victorian Football League (VFL) and regional leagues [1,2]. Prior to the initiation of the AFLW, there was no elite-level competition available to female Australian rules football players, and, therefore, many current players have transferred from other sports, including basketball and soccer [3]. Although AFLW in Australia is rapidly evolving, many AFLW and Victorian Football

League Women's (VFLW) players have experienced minimal elite sport experience within a structured training program [3]. It has been established that differences exist between the male elite AFL and sub-elite VFL competition, in terms of increased match intensity, greater running distance and overall game speeds for AFL players [2,4]. However, these differences may not exist between AFLW and VFLW players because the competitions are similar, both characterised by shorter quarters (up to 20 min), no limit on the number of rotations, and players' part-time status [3].

The nutritional requirements of Australian rules football players vary throughout the season [5], which may impact on macronutrient consumption, including appropriate carbohydrate, protein and total energy intake. Current daily carbohydrate recommendations for moderate- to high-intensity exercise (1–4 h duration) range between 5 and 12 $g{\cdot}k^{-1}$ body mass (BM) [6]. In the context of Australian rules football, moderate- to high-intensity exercise between 1 and 3 h is performed during pre-season training, in-season main training sessions and during a match. Carbohydrate requirements are reduced during low-intensity exercise of up to one hour (3–5 $g{\cdot}k^{-1}{\cdot}d^{-1}$ BM) [6]. Contrary to recommendations, previous studies have reported relatively low carbohydrate intakes in male AFL players (<5 $g{\cdot}kg^{-1}{\cdot}d^{-1}$) [5,7,8], and similar intakes have been identified in Australian female athletes from a range of individual and team sports [9]. While the recommended carbohydrate intake for high-intensity exercise is well established, the consistently reported low carbohydrate intake in team sport athletes may suggest that the physical demands of these sports require less carbohydrate than current recommendations. In contrast, athletes tend to exceed the recommended protein intake [9]. Protein requirements for athletes are higher than those for the general population (0.8–1.0 $g{\cdot}kg^{-1}{\cdot}d^{-1}$ [10]) to assist with muscle protein synthesis and recovery, with the current recommendations specifying that athletes consume 1.2–2 $g{\cdot}kg^{-1}{\cdot}d^{-1}$, depending on training program goals and overall energy budgets [6]. The average reported protein intake for Australian female athletes is 1.6 $g{\cdot}kg^{-1}{\cdot}d^{-1}$ [9]. At present, recommendations for micronutrient intake in athletes are consistent with general population health guidelines [10]. However, it is likely that certain athletes may have an increased requirement for specific micronutrients, including vitamins B for athletes who restrict their energy intake, which is common in female athletes [9], iron for endurance athletes and calcium and vitamin D for amenorrheic females [6,9]. The current literature assessing micronutrient intake in female athletes is limited, with one Australian study reporting that mean micronutrient intake met the relevant Australian Nutrient Reference Values [10]. Despite this, a significant proportion of individual athletes in this study failed to meet the general population health recommendations, in particular for folate (44%), calcium (22%), iron (19%) and magnesium (15%) [9].

Nutrition education is one strategy used to assist athletes to consume an adequate diet [11]. Athletes with higher nutrition knowledge are more likely to consume more fruit, vegetables and carbohydrate-rich foods than those with low nutritional understanding [12], which suggests that sports nutrition knowledge may be associated with appropriate dietary intake. Women have been reported to have a higher level of nutrition knowledge than men, with a recent study reporting that Australian female athletes had a higher total knowledge score than other participants [13]. In male Australian rules footballers, three studies have reported poor sports nutrition knowledge, with only approximately half of the questions being answered correctly [7,8,14]. Currently, sports nutrition knowledge in female football players who have not been training within an elite program or had regular exposure to nutrition support is unknown.

Energy availability (EA) is defined as the ingested energy remaining for all other metabolic processes after the energy cost of training has been subtracted [15]. Low EA (LEA) occurs when the amount of energy available for basic physiological functions becomes insufficient, which, if continued, may lead to a significant health risk for female athletes [16]. LEA may be present with or without a clinical eating disorder, with the causes often being unintentional and due to increased energy expenditure without an increase in energy intake [17]. Directly measuring EA can be challenging as it requires the quantification of 24 h energy intake and expenditure over a period of time, which is often impractical and burdensome for athletes. Furthermore, there is currently no gold standard approach for the measurement of exercise energy expenditure, as many tools used in an applied context, including accelerometers, underestimate energy expenditure at high exercise intensities [18]. Because of the challenges associated with directly measuring EA, the validated Low Energy Availability in Females Questionnaire (LEAF-Q) has been used to assess the risk of LEA in athletes, with the prevalence reported to range between 33 and 46% [19,20]. However, most of the existing literature has focused on endurance athletes, and little is known about team sport athletes. Furthermore, female Australian rules football players may be at an increased risk of low EA due to an increase in energy expenditure after joining a professional program. Thus, screening for the risk of LEA in this group of athletes may have important long-term implications for health and performance and may determine the need for further education to ensure appropriate dietary intake to meet the demands of the sport.

To date, no previous studies have assessed dietary intake, nutritional knowledge or risk of low energy availability in female Australian rules football players. Further, data assessing nutritional adequacy in Australian female athletes, in particular team sport athletes, are limited. As the AFLW league is new and rapidly growing, this information will be beneficial for coaches, fitness trainers, medical staff, nutritionists and dietitians working with these female athletes. Thus, the aims of the current investigation were to: (a) quantify energy, macronutrient and micronutrient intake in female Australian rules football players and compare these to current recommendations, (b) quantify sports nutrition knowledge in female Australian rules football players, and (c) quantify the risk of low EA in female Australian rules football players and compare nutrient intake between players who are at risk of low EA and those not at risk.

2. Materials and Methods

2.1. Subjects and Study Design

This study followed a cross-sectional design, involving VFLW players (n = 30) aged 18–35 years. Players were recruited in Victoria from one elite-level professional AFL club. Data collection was performed during the 2017 VFLW preseason (March–April). The study was conducted in accordance with the Declaration of Helsinki, and the Deakin University Human Research Ethics Committee approved the study (Project Approval Code: EC00213). All players provided their written informed consent prior to their involvement in the study.

2.2. Data Collection

2.2.1. Anthropometry

Height (cm) was measured using a portable stadiometer (Seca, 213, Hamburg, Germany), and body mass (kg) was measured using electronic scales (A&D Australasia, HW-PW200, Adelaide, South Australia) by a qualified research assistant.

2.2.2. Nutritional Intake

The Automated Self-Administered 24 Hour (ASA24) Dietary Assessment Tool [21], based on an Australian-based food and beverage database, was used to assess the previous 24 h (midnight to midnight) nutritional intake on three non-consecutive training days within a seven-day period. The data entered were checked via a follow-up interview with a qualified nutritionist. The mean daily intake of energy, macronutrients and micronutrients over the three 24 h recalls was calculated. The mean daily protein and carbohydrate intake was compared with the values reported in the current American College of Sports Medicine (ACSM) sports nutrition guidelines [6,22] and were expressed in grams (g), relative to BM ($g{\cdot}kg{\cdot}BM^{-1}$). Carbohydrate intake was compared to relevant recommended values (5–7 $g{\cdot}kg{\cdot}BM^{-1}$ and 6–10 $g{\cdot}kg{\cdot}BM^{-1}$) [6], given the physical demands and duration of pre-season training. Daily fat intake, expressed as a percentage of total daily energy intake, and micronutrient intake, expressed as milligrams (mg) or micrograms (μg), was compared with those established by the Australian general population health recommendations [10] as there are currently no guidelines specific to athletes. The current type of supplement use was captured via an online software program (Qualtrics, Provo, UT, USA).

2.2.3. Sports Nutrition Knowledge

Players completed the 88-item Sports Nutrition Knowledge Questionnaire (SNKQ) [23] via an online software program (Qualtrics, Provo, UT, USA). The SNKQ has been assessed for validity (content and construct) and reliability (test–retest), with findings indicating a high construct validity and good test–retest concordance and therefore suitability to be used to determine sports nutrition knowledge. The SNKQ consists of five sub-sections (general nutrition concepts, fluid, recovery, weight control and supplements). One point was awarded for each correct answer, and an 'unsure' or incorrect response received zero points. The overall score (out of 88) was expressed as a percentage of correctly answered questions.

2.2.4. Energy Availability

The 25-item LEAF-Q was used to assess the risk of LEA considering three factors: gastrointestinal function, injuries and menstrual function. The LEAF-Q has been validated in female athletes aged 18–39 training ≥5 times/week, with findings producing an acceptable sensitivity (78%) and specificity (90%) to classify current energy availability [16]. Consistent with the original validation study [16], players completed a paper version of the LEAF-Q to ensure validity and reliability were maintained. Scoring was based on the original validation study, with those who scored ≤7 being classified as 'not at risk' of LEA, and those who scored ≥8 being classified as 'at risk' of LEA [16].

2.3. Statistical Analysis

All statistical analyses were conducted using the Statistical Package for Social Sciences (SPSS 24.0, Chicago, IL, USA). Results were reported as mean ± standard deviation (SD) for normally distributed variables and median and interquartile range (IQR) for non-normally distributed variables. Independent samples *t*-tests were used to compare energy and macronutrient intake between players who were deemed to be at risk of low EA (≥8) and those who were shown to be not at risk of low EA (≤7). Statistical significance was set to a level of $p \leq 0.05$.

3. Results

The demographic characteristics of players (n = 30) are provided in Table 1. The completion rate of the ASA-24 dietary recalls, SNKQ and LEAF-Q was 29 (97%), 30 (100%) and 27 (90%), respectively, for 30 participants.

Nutritional intake is presented in Table 2. Mean carbohydrate intake was below recommendations for training days (moderate- to high-intensity activity), while protein and fat intake met current recommendations (Table 2). In comparison with current sports nutrition guidelines, carbohydrate intake was less than the recommended value for moderate exercise of approximately one hour (5–7 $g{\cdot}kg^{-1}$) in 96.3% of players and for moderate to intense exercise (6–10 $g{\cdot}kg^{-1}$) for 1–3 h [6] in 100% of players.

Micronutrient intake was consistent with current general population guidelines, with the exception of iron and calcium, while sodium intake exceeded the current recommendations (Table 3). In comparison to the general population guidelines, 65.5% of players' calcium intake was below recommendations, while none of the players met the minimum requirement for iron. Despite the average intake recommendations, 38% of players' magnesium and 20.7% of players' zinc was below the general population guidelines.

The median score for total sports nutrition knowledge was 48 correct answers out of possible 88 (54.5%) [23]. The lowest median scores were observed in the sub-section on supplements (18% correctly answered) (Table 4).

Table 1. Demographic characteristic of VFLW players (n = 30).

	(n = 30)
(Mean ± SD)	
Age (years)	24.15 (±4.1)
Mass (kg)	64.5 (±8.0)
Height (cm)	168.2 (±7.6)
Birth Place [N, (%)]	
Australia	30 (100)
Relationship Status [N, (%)]	
Married	3 (10.0)
De facto	0 (0.0)
Committed dating/Engaged	13 (43.3)
Never married/Single	14 (46.7)
Level of Education [N, (%)]	
Year 12 or equivalent	13 (43.3)
Trade/apprenticeship	1 (3.3)
Certificate/diploma	4 (13.3)
University degree	9 (30.0)
Higher University degree	3 (10.0)

VFLW: Victorian Football League Women's; SD: standard deviation; N: number.

Table 2. Macronutrient intake of VFLW players (mean ± SD) and current recommendations.

Nutrient Intake	VFLW (n = 29)	Recommendation	Percent Meeting Minimum Recommendation
Energy, kJ Energy $kJ{\cdot}kg^{-1}{\cdot}d^{-1}$	7826 ± 2411.6 199.5 ± 37.4	NA	NA
Protein, g Protein, $g{\cdot}kg^{-1}{\cdot}d^{-1}$	98 ± 32.1 1.5 ± 0.5	NA 1.2–2.0 [a]	NA 77.8%
Carbohydrate, g Carbohydrate, $g{\cdot}kg^{-1}{\cdot}d^{-1}$	192.4 ± 51.8 3.0 ± 0.8	NA 5–7 [b] 6–10 [c]	NA 3.7% 0%
Sugar, g Sugar, % of E	86.2 ± 33.1 18.6 ± 4.4	NA NA	NA NA
Fibre, g	25.5 ± 8	25g [d]	43.8%
Total fat, g Total fat, % of E	72.2 ± 33.4 33.2 ± 6.5	NA 20–35 [d]	NA 96.4%
Saturated fat, g Saturated fat, % of E	25.7 ± 14.6 11.6 ± 3.2	NA <10 [d]	NA 34.4%
Monounsaturated fat, g	29 ± 14.1	NA	NA
Polyunsaturated fat, g	11.4 ± 4.8	NA	NA

% of E: percentage of total energy intake; NA: Not Applicable. [a] source: reference [6], [b] source: reference [6], up to 1 h of moderate exercise/day [c] source: reference [6], 1–3 h of moderate- to high-intensity exercise/day, [d] source: reference [10].

Table 3. Micronutrient intake of VFLW players (mean ± SD) and current recommendations.

Nutrient Intake	VFLW (n = 29)	Recommended Dietary Intake (RDI) or Adequate Intake (AI) [a]	Upper Limit	Percent Meeting Minimum Recommendation
Calcium, mg	924.8 ± 544.7	1000	2500	34.5%
Iron, mg	12.2 ± 3.2	18	45	0%
Magnesium, mg	367.5 ± 137.8	310	350 (as a supplement)	82.8%
Phosphorus, mg	1569.3 ± 549.4	1000	4000	96.6%
Potassium, mg	3109 ± 1173	2800	NA	58.6%
Sodium, mg	2063.3 ± 957	460–920	Not Determined	100%
Zinc, mg	11.7 ± 4	8	40	79.3%
Selenium, µg	98.1 ± 64.7	60	400	79.5%
Vitamin C, mg	106.8 ± 115.3	45	NA	82.8%
Thiamine, mg	1.9 ± 1.9	1.1	NA	69.0%
Riboflavin, mg	2.8 ± 2.2	1.1	NA	96.6%
Niacin, mg	25.5 ± 8.9	14	35	96.7%
Folate, µg	484.6 ± 149.8	400	1000	69.0%
Vitamin B12, µg	13.7 ± 46.8	2.4	NA	93.1%

[a] source: reference [10].

Table 4. Nutrition knowledge scores in VFLW players (median (IQR), percent (%) of correct answers).

Sections (No. Questions)	VFLW (n = 30)
	Median (IQR), %
General Nutrition Concepts (46)	28 (7), 60.8%
Fluid (9)	6 (7), 66.7%
Recovery (7)	4 (3), 57.1%
Weight Control (15)	7 (3), 46.7%
Supplements (11)	2 (3), 18.2%
Total Nutrition Knowledge (88)	48 (12), 54.5%

IQR: Interquartile range.

The median score on the LEAF-Q was 7, with 8 out of 27 players (30%) scoring above 8, indicating a risk of LEA [16]. Energy and macronutrient intake did not differ ($p > 0.05$) between players who were classified as at risk of LEA and players who were classified as not at risk of LEA (Table 5). Table 6 highlights the key LEAF-Q responses. Many players reported injuries in the previous year, the most common being ankle- or foot-related. Nine of the 27 players (33%) reported exercise-induced changes to menstrual function. Gastrointestinal symptoms not related to menstruation were less frequent.

The most common forms of supplementation used by players were protein supplementation (65%) and vitamins and minerals supplementation (70%) (Figure 1). Performance-enhancing supplements such as creatine, B-alanine, caffeine and nitrates were not used by any player (Figure 1).

Table 5. Energy and macronutrient intake (mean ± SD) in VFLW players at risk of LEA and in players not at risk of LEA (n = 27).

	Not at Risk of LEA (LEAF-Q ≤ 7) (n = 19)	At Risk of LEA (LEAF-Q ≤ 8) (n = 8)	*p*-Value
Energy (kJ)	7734.7 ± 2192.4	7699.3 ± 2552.6	0.971
Protein ($g \cdot kg^{-1} \cdot d^{-1}$)	1.5 ± 0.4	1.7 ± 0.8	0.296
Carbohydrate ($g \cdot kg^{-1} \cdot d^{-1}$)	2.9 ± 0.8	3.4 ± 1.1	0.248
Fat (g)	73.1 ± 30.1	63.9 ± 31.7	0.490

LEA: Low Energy Availability; LEAF-Q: LEA in females Questionnaire.

Table 6. Responses to key components of the LEAF-Q (n = 27).

Leaf Questionnaire Component	Frequency (N)	Percent (%)
1. Injury history		
Number of days lost from participation due to injury in past year:		
0	11	40.7
1–7	6	22.2
8–14	4	14.8
15–21	3	11.1
≥22	3	11.1
Most common injuries reported (respondents could choose more than one)		
Back injury	3	11.1
Knee injury	2	7.4
Head injury/concussion	4	14.8
Groin injury	2	7.4
Shin splints/calf tightness	4	14.8
Ligament/tendon injury of the thumb	4	14.8
Rolled ankle/Achilles soreness/broken foot	6	22.2
Illness	2	7.4
Hamstring strain	1	3.7
Hip injury	1	3.7
Shoulder injury strained ac joint	2	7.4
2. Menstrual function exercise-related menstrual changes:		
Bleed less	3	11.1
Menstruation stops	4	14.8
Increased bleeding	2	7.4
Number of periods in the last year (n = 21) (if still menstruating)		
≥9	19	90.5
5–8	0	0
0–2	2	9.5
3. Gastrointestinal disturbances abdominal bloated/gaseous when not having periods:		
Daily-weekly	2	7.4
Seldom	12	44.4
Rarely or never	13	48.1
Cramps/stomach ache not related to your menstruation:		
Daily-weekly	1	3.6
Seldom	8	28.6
Rarely or never	19	67.9

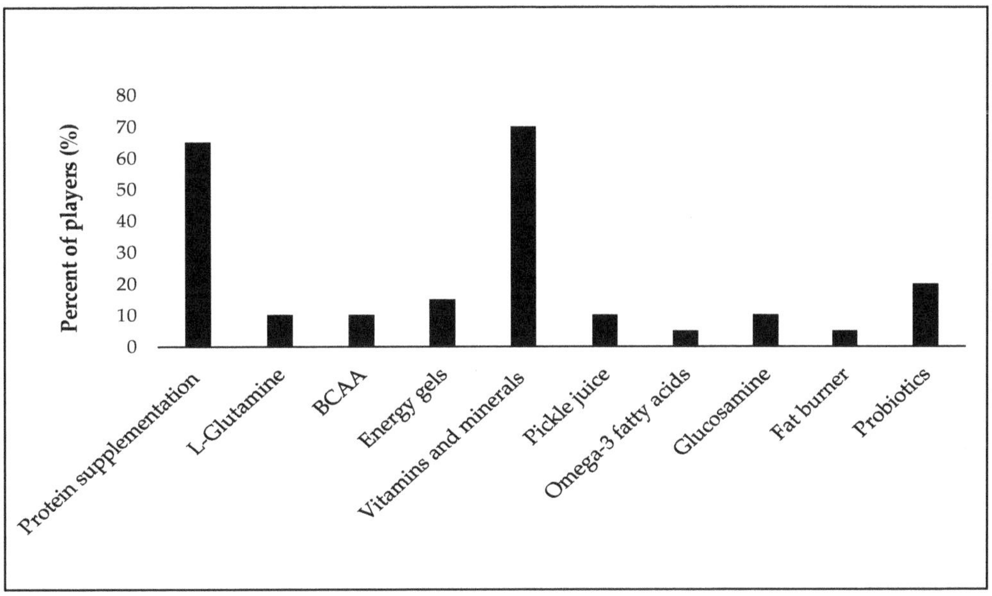

Figure 1. Current supplement use in VFLW players (n = 30). BCAA: branched-chain amino acids

4. Discussion

This is the first study to assess nutrient intake, sports nutrition knowledge and risk of LEA within female Australian rules football players. The key findings from this study were that carbohydrate intake on training days was below recommendations for players performing moderate training of approximately one hour per day (5–7 $g \cdot kg^{-1} \cdot d^{-1}$) and moderate- to high-intensity training of 1–3 h per day (6–10 $g \cdot kg^{-1} \cdot d^{-1}$) [6]. Protein intake was consistent with current recommendations (1.2–2 $g \cdot kg^{-1} \cdot d^{-1}$) [6] and consistent with previous findings [5,7,8]. The assessment of micronutrient intake showed that the average intake of calcium and iron was below the general population recommendations for females (1000 $mg \cdot d^{-1}$ and 18 $mg \cdot d^{-1}$, respectively), while other micronutrients were in line with recommendations. Sodium intake exceeded the recommended daily intake for the general population (460–920 $mg \cdot d^{-1}$). The overall sports nutrition knowledge scores were low, with the lowest level of knowledge related to supplementation (18% correctly answered). Furthermore, 30% of players were deemed to be at risk of LEA, which is similar to previously reported rates in female athletes [19,20].

Mean energy intake in this group of female Australian rules football players was 7826 ± 2411 $kJ \cdot kg^{-1}$, which is slightly below that reported in previous studies in Australian female athletes, with mean energy intakes ranging from 8674 kJ to 10,511 $kJ \cdot kg^{-1}$ [9,24,25]. The lower energy intake in the current investigation may be due to the nature of Australian rules football. Endurance athletes (such as cyclists and triathletes) have been reported to have higher energy intakes (11,850 kJ per day) than team sport athletes such as softball players (8959 kJ per day) and power sport athletes within individual sports such as track and field (8951 kJ per day) [9]. Furthermore, the method of estimating energy intake may also contribute to the differences in results, with previous studies using food frequency questionnaires (FFQ), which can overestimate energy intake [9], or 24 h recalls, which can underestimate energy intake [24]. In the current study, the repeated online 24 h recalls may have underestimated energy intake, since the ASA-24 is a self-administered tool. The estimation of energy requirements in football players is challenging, as requirements can increase or decrease depending on age, athlete caliber, overall daily activity levels and body composition [26]. Objective measures of energy expenditure such as those obtained by using accelerometers can provide a more accurate representation of energy requirements; however, there are limitations to their use in high-intensity sport as well as when performing resistance training [18,27]. To overcome differences in exercise modes, the use of weighed food diaries has been suggested as the gold standard for assessing dietary intake in athletes [9]. Therefore, further research is required to estimate energy expenditure and intake using the most accurate tools currently available, in order to more comprehensively determine whether energy intake within this population is sufficient.

Carbohydrate intake assessed on training days (involving a minimum of one hour of moderate exercise) in this group of VFLW players was below the minimum recommended 5 $g \cdot kg^{-1} \cdot d^{-1}$ [6]. This finding is consistent with previous findings in both Australian female athletes [9,24] and male AFL players [5,7,8]. Furthermore, the majority of players (96.3%) did not meet the recommendations for athletes performing moderate exercise for approximately 1 h per day (5–7 $g \cdot kg^{-1}$), while no players (0%) met the recommendation for moderate- to high-intensity exercise for 1–3 h per day (6–10 $g \cdot kg^{-1}$) [6], consistently with previous reports of carbohydrate intake during pre-season training [5,28]. Female athletes from a range of different sports have previously been reported to have a similar daily intake of carbohydrate to that of the current investigation (4.5 $g \cdot kg^{-1} \cdot d^{-1}$), with the lowest intakes in softball players (3.3 $g \cdot kg^{-1} \cdot d^{-1}$) [9]. Furthermore, it was reported that female endurance athletes' carbohydrate intake was 6.7 $g \cdot kg^{-1} \cdot d^{-1}$, higher than that for other female athletes [9], a result which may have been due to either a higher training demand or a greater knowledge of the importance of carbohydrate for performance in this sport [9]. Low-carbohydrate diets have become popular amongst the general public as well as female athletes, as they are often perceived to be a tool for weight or fat loss [29]. In athletes, a sustained low-carbohydrate intake may be insufficient to support the training demands, possibly impacting on performance and long-term health [29]. The carbohydrate intakes observed in the current investigation, however, are consistent with those previously reported for both male and female team sport athletes [30]. Furthermore, in the current study, there was no significant difference in carbohydrate intake between players who were at risk of LEA and those not at risk, suggesting that the carbohydrate intake in this group may be sufficient to meet the training demands. The current carbohydrate intake recommendations are based on the outcomes of studies that include athletes from varied populations, with a large proportion from endurance sport [6], and therefore it should be considered whether they are applicable to team-based sports, which often involve intermittent and skill-based training [31]. Thus, further research in female team sport athletes' habitual carbohydrate intake, glycogen depletion rates and optimal carbohydrate periodization interventions [32,33] is required to provide evidence for guidelines specific to a female team sport athlete population.

The mean intake of most micronutrients in the current investigation was above the Australian RDI for the general population. Only one other Australian study has measured micronutrient intake in female athletes, reporting similar findings [9], the key differences being that within the current study, calcium (924.8 mg·d^{-1}) and iron (12.2 mg·d^{-1}) intakes were below the RDI, and a higher proportion of athletes did not meet the RDI for calcium (65%) and iron (100%). Adequate intakes of calcium, which plays a vital role in bone health and injury risk [34,35], and iron, essential to carry oxygen and maintaining energy release [36], are important for females, in particular when performing high-intensity contact sport. The main sources of calcium in the diet are dairy foods, including milk, cheese and yoghurt [10], while the main sources of iron include meat products, in particular red meat [10]. In the current investigation, the mean intake of dairy food per day was 1.2 serves, which is below the recommended 2.5 serves for the age group of the participants [10]. Furthermore, 17% of players did not consume any dairy food, and only 53% of players reported drinking milk, while only 50% consumed red meat 2–4 times per week. A low intake of dairy [37] and meat [36] foods is commonly reported in young Australian females and may be a result of the perception that these foods can contribute to weight gain [38,39]. Furthermore, intolerances to dairy food and lactose products have become more common [40], and veganism has become more visible and accepted in the sports industry [41], possibly contributing to the low intakes of these minerals. Nonetheless, there is a need for further education focused on the importance of calcium intake and the appropriate dietary sources for female football players.

Sodium intake in the current investigation was substantially higher than the recommended intake for the Australian general population. In the current study, 20% of players reported consumption of sports drinks, which are typically high in sodium, on a daily basis, which may therefore have contributed to the overall sodium intake [42]. There is limited available evidence on the required sodium intake in an athletic population, as there is a high degree of inter-variability between athletes, often dependent on individual sweat sodium concentrations and sweat rates [43]. Furthermore, the current recommendations are aimed at reducing the risk of chronic disease [10], and a recent study found that the general health recommendations of a low-sodium diet may not be appropriate for athletes, especially in warm conditions [44]. Overall, there is limited understanding of the micronutrient requirements of athletes and whether their training demands can be adequately met by intakes that match the general population guidelines. For female athletes, menstruation may affect micronutrient status, especially that of iron, vitamin B12 and zinc, which is another consideration that warrants further investigation.

The results of the current investigation suggest that female Australian football players do not have a high level of sports nutrition knowledge. This is the first study to investigate sports nutrition knowledge within the female population of Australian rules football players; however, the median score for overall sports nutrition knowledge (54.4%) was similar to that previously reported in male Australian football players [7,14]. The aforementioned similarity in sports nutrition knowledge was found despite the previous studies' use of a different sports nutrition knowledge questionnaire [45]. In a recent study from our group using the same sports nutrition knowledge questionnaire as that used in the current investigation [46], we found scores to be 51% in both elite and sub elite male

Australian football players [8]. These observations collectively suggest that sports nutrition knowledge levels may be similar between male and female Australian rules football players. Improving upon low sports nutrition knowledge could be beneficial to male and female Australian rules football players, as it has recently been suggested that for team sport athletes, an increased level of sports nutrition knowledge might facilitate improvements in performance [47]. Furthermore, in the current investigation, knowledge specific to supplements elicited in the lowest median scores (18%), which is consistent with the result reported for male sub-elite players in our recent investigation [8], suggesting that deficits in specific areas of sports nutrition knowledge may affect both males and female Australian rules football players similarly.

In the current study, 30% of players were deemed to be at risk of LEA. This is the first investigation to explore the risk of low energy availability for female Australian rules football players. However, recent investigations have reported an incidence of LEA of 33.3% in a similar participant population and stage of the training year (competitive female soccer players in either their pre-season or competitive season) [48,49]. In the current study, energy and macronutrient intake did not differ between players who were classified as at risk of LEA and players who were classified as not at risk of LEA. This observation contrasts with the result of a previous investigation [45] which reported significantly lower daily energy intake in females with LEA. The aforementioned study, however, directly measured energy availability, whereas only the risk of LEA was quantified in the current investigation, highlighting the need for the further investigation and direct measurement of EA in female Australian football players. It has been conclusively determined that LEA can induce adverse health effects such as increased injury rates and menstrual dysfunction [50], and indeed, in the current investigation, players who were identified as "at-risk" of LEA reported injuries in the past year. Furthermore, exercise-induced changes to menstrual function were reported in one-third of players in the current investigation. There is at least some positive association between knowledge of appropriate nutritional practices and nutritional intake [51]. Therefore, the implementation of nutritional education programs that incorporate specific information about the potentially deleterious health effects of long-term LEA may assist to improve health outcomes for female Australian rules football players.

Several limitations need to be addressed in the current study. Firstly, the players in this study were recruited from one professional sporting club, and thus the sample size was limited by the number of players in the VFLW team. As a result, additional analysis investigating the correlation between nutritional intake and knowledge could not be included within the current investigation. This data would have provided insight into the potential factors influencing nutritional intake, forming the basis of targeted education programs. However, the aim of this study was to gather detailed dietary information in an emerging athlete population, which future studies can build upon. Furthermore, the findings may be specific to players from this club. However, given that this study was conducted during the early phase of the pre-season, in the inaugural year of the VFLW competition, it is unlikely that the club's philosophies, training or education programs would have impacted on the players. Although dietary intake data were captured on training days, training logs were not kept, which limited the detail of records in terms of training session duration and intensity. The dietary assessment tool also has limitations, as, although it is validated [21], the online ASA-24 is self-administered and, therefore, subject to memory bias and underreporting. Finally, the LEAF-Q used in this study can only assess the risk of LEA. To objectively and accurately investigate energy availability, gold standard methods to assess energy availability include doubly labelled water, portable metabolic carts and weighed food diaries over numerous days. However, these methods are costly, burdensome on athletes and often impractical in field-based studies. Other methods to assess energy expenditure such as the use of accelerometers and weighed food diaries (used for a limited number of days) may be more realistic to implement for athletes and would provide further information on the status of energy availability.

5. Conclusions

The results of the current investigation suggest that the female population of Australian rules football players exhibits inadequate carbohydrate, iron and calcium intake with respect to the current recommendations for athletes. Almost one-third of players may be at risk of LEA, and therefore the prevalence of LEA within this population may be similar to that reported for other female athletes. Protein intake was in line with athlete recommendations, while sodium intake within this athlete population appeared to exceed the recommended intake for general populations. Overall, sports nutrition knowledge was found to be low for female Australian football players, especially regarding supplementation. Female football players may benefit from education programs that provide details of the deleterious effects of prolonged LEA.

Author Contributions: All authors conceived and designed the experiments; R.L. and D.C. analysed the data; All authors wrote the paper.

Acknowledgments: The authors acknowledge the participants for their involvement in the study.

References

1. Gray, A.; Jenkins, D. Match analysis and the physiological demands of Australian Football. *Sports Med.* **2010**, *40*, 347–360. [CrossRef] [PubMed]
2. Johnston, R.D.; Black, G.M.; Harrison, P.W.; Murray, N.B.; Austin, D.J. Applied sport science of Australian football: A systematic review. *Sports Med.* **2018**, *48*, 1673–1694. [PubMed]
3. Clarke, A.C.; Ryan, S.; Couvalias, G.; Dascombe, B.J.; Coutts, A.J.; Kempton, T. Physical demands and technical performance in Australian Football League Women's (AFLW) competition match-play. *J. Sci. Med. Sport* **2018**, *21*, 748–752. [CrossRef] [PubMed]
4. Aughey, R.J. Widening margin in activity profile between elite and sub-elite Australian football: A case study. *J. Sci. Med. Sport.* **2013**, *16*, 382–386. [CrossRef]
5. Bilsborough, J.C.; Greenway, K.; Livingston, S.; Cordy, J.; Coutts, A.J. Changes in anthropometry, upper-body strength and nutrient intake in professional Australian Football players during a season. *Int. J. Sports Physiol. Perform.* **2016**, *11*, 290–300. [CrossRef] [PubMed]
6. Thomas, T.; Erdman, K.; Burke, L. American college of sports medicine joint position statement nutrition and athletic performance. *Med. Sci. Sports Exerc.* **2016**, *48*, 543–568. [PubMed]
7. Devlin, B.; Leveritt, M.; Kingsley, M.; Belski, R. Dietary intake, body composition, and nutrition knowledge of Australian Football and soccer players: Implications for sports nutrition professionals in practice. *Int. J. Sport Nutr. Exerc. Metab.* **2017**, *27*, 130–138.
8. Lohman, R.; Carr, A.; Condo, D. Nutritional intake in Australian football players: Sports nutrition knowledge, macronutrient and micronutrient intake. *Int. J. Sport Nutr. Exerc. Metab.* **2018**, in press. [CrossRef] [PubMed]
9. Heaney, S.; O'Connor, H.; Gifford, J.; Naughton, G. Comparison of strategies for assessing nutritional adequacy in elite female athletes' dietary intake. *Int. J. Sport Nutr. Exerc. Metab.* **2010**, *20*, 245–256. [CrossRef]
10. National Health and Medical Research Council (NHMRC). *Nutrient Reference Values for Australian and New Zealand*; NHMRC: Canberra, Australia, 2017.
11. Birkenhead, K.; Slater, G. A review of factors influencing athletes' food choices. *Sports Med.* **2015**, *45*, 1511–1522. [CrossRef]
12. Alaunyte, I.; Perry, J.L.; Aubrey, T. Nutritional knowledge and eating habits of professional rugby league players: Does knowledge translate into practice? *J. Int. Soc. Sports Nutr.* **2015**, *12*, 18. [CrossRef]
13. Spendlove, J.K.; Heaney, S.E.; Gifford, J.A.; Prvan, T.; Denyer, G.S.; O'Connor, H.T. Evaluation of general nutrition knowledge in elite Australian athletes. *Br. J. Nutr.* **2012**, *107*, 1871–1880. [CrossRef]
14. Devlin, B.; Belski, R. Exploring general and sports nutrition and food knowledge in elite male Australian athletes. *Int. J. Sport Nutr. Exerc. Metab.* **2015**, *25*, 225–232. [CrossRef]
15. Marquez, S.; Molinero, O. Energy availability, menstrual dysfunction and bone health in sports; an overview of the female athlete triad. *Nutr. Hosp.* **2013**, *28*, 1010–1017.

16. Melin, A.; Tornberg, A.B.; Skouby, S.; Faber, J.; Ritz, C.; Sjodin, A.; Sundgot-Borgen, J. The LEAF questionnaire: A screening tool for the identification of female athletes at risk for the female athlete triad. *Br. J. Sports Med.* **2014**, *48*, 540–545. [CrossRef] [PubMed]
17. Logue, D.; Madigan, S.M.; Delahunt, E.; Heinen, M.; Mc Donnell, S.J.; Corish, C.A. Low energy availability in athletes: A review of prevalence, dietary patterns, physiological health, and sports performance. *Sports Med.* **2018**, *48*, 73–96. [CrossRef]
18. Crouter, S.E.; Churilla, J.R.; Bassett, D.R., Jr. Estimating energy expenditure using accelerometers. *Eur. J. Appl. Physiol.* **2006**, *98*, 601–612. [CrossRef] [PubMed]
19. Folscher, L.L.; Grant, C.C.; Fletcher, L.; Janse van Rensberg, D.C. Ultra-marathon athletes at risk for the female athlete triad. *Sports Med. Open* **2015**, *1*, 29. [CrossRef] [PubMed]
20. Slater, J.; McLay-Cooke, R.; Brown, R.; Black, K. Female recreational exercisers at risk for low energy availability. *Int. J. Sport Nutr. Exerc. Metab.* **2016**, *26*, 421–427. [CrossRef]
21. Subar, A.; Kirkpatrick, S.; Mittl, B.; Zimmermanm, T.; Thompson, F.; Bingley, C.; Willis, G.; Islam, N.; Baranowski, T.; McNutt, S.; et al. The automated self-administered 24-hour dietary recall (ASA24): A resource for researchers, clinicians, and educators from the National Cancer Institute. *J. Acad. Nutr. Diet.* **2012**, *112*, 1134–1137. [CrossRef]
22. Campbell, B.; Kreider, R.; Ziegenfuss, T.; Bounty, P.; Roberts, M.; Burke, D.; Landis, J.; Lopez, H.; Antonio, J. International society of sports nutrition position stand: Protein and exercise. *J. Int. Soc. Sports Nutr.* **2007**, *4*, 8. [CrossRef] [PubMed]
23. Zinn, C.; Schofield, G.; Wall, C. Development of a psychometrically valid and reliable sports nutrition knowledge questionnaire. *J. Sci. Med. Sport* **2005**, *8*, 346–351. [CrossRef]
24. Baker, L.; Heaton, L.; Nuccio, R.; Stein, K. Dietitian-observed macronutrient intakes of young skill and team-sport athletes: Adequacy of pre, during and postexercise nutrition. *Int. J. Sport Nutr. Exerc. Metab.* **2014**, *24*, 166–176. [CrossRef] [PubMed]
25. Burkhart, S.J.; Pelly, F.E. Dietary intake of athletes seeking nutrition advice at a major international competition. *Nutrients* **2016**, *8*, 638. [CrossRef]
26. Mielgo-Ayuso, J.; Maroto-Sanchez, B.; Luzardo-Socorro, R.; Palacios, G.; Palacios Gil-Antunano, N.; Gonzalez-Gross, M. Evaluation of nutritional status and energy expenditure in athletes. *Nutr. Hosp.* **2015**, *31*, 227–236.
27. Rawson, E.S.; Walsh, T.M. Estimation of resistance exercise energy expenditure using accelerometry. *Med. Sci. Sports Exerc.* **2010**, *42*, 622–628. [CrossRef]
28. Walker, E.; McAinch, A.; Sweeting, A.; Aughey, R. Inertial sensors to estimate the energy expenditure of team-sport athletes. *J. Sci. Med. Sport* **2016**, *19*, 177–181. [CrossRef]
29. Burke, L.M.; Hawley, J.A.; Wong, S.H.; Jeukendrup, A.E. Carbohydrates for training and competition. *J. Sports Sci.* **2011**, *29*, S17–S27. [CrossRef]
30. Holway, F.; Spriet, L. Sport-specific nutrition: Practical strategies for team sports. *J. Sports Sci. Med.* **2011**, *29*, S115–S125. [CrossRef]
31. Bishop, D.; Spencer, M. Determinants of repeated-sprint ability in well-trained team-sport athletes and endurance-trained athletes. *J. Sports Med. Phys. Fit.* **2004**, *44*, 1–7.
32. Krustrup, P.; Mohr, M.; Steensberg, A.; Bencke, J.; Kjær, M.; Bangsbo, K. Muscle and blood metabolites during a soccer game: Implications for sprint performance. *Med. Sci. Sports Exerc.* **2006**, *38*, 1165–1174. [CrossRef] [PubMed]
33. Balsom, P.; Wood, K.; Olsson, P.; Ekblom, B. Carbohydrate intake and multiple sprint sports: With special reference to football (soccer). *J. Sci. Med. Sport* **1999**, *20*, 48–52. [CrossRef]
34. Warden, S.J.; Davis, I.S.; Fredericson, M. Management and prevention of bone stress injuries in long-distance runners. *J. Orthop. Sports Phys. Ther.* **2014**, *44*, 749–765. [CrossRef] [PubMed]
35. Goolsby, M.A.; Boniquit, N. Bone Health in Athletes. *Sports Health* **2017**, *9*, 108–117. [CrossRef] [PubMed]
36. Hinton, P.S. Iron and the endurance athlete. *Appl. Physiol. Nutr. Metab.* **2014**, *39*, 1012–1018. [CrossRef] [PubMed]
37. Parker, C.E.; Vivian, W.J.; Oddy, W.H.; Beilin, L.J.; Mori, T.A.; O'Sullivan, T.A. Changes in dairy food and nutrient intakes in Australian adolescents. *Nutrients* **2012**, *4*, 1794–1811. [CrossRef] [PubMed]
38. Barr, S.I. Dieting attitudes and behavior in urban high school students: Implications for calcium intake. *J. Adolesc. Health* **1995**, *16*, 458–464. [CrossRef]

39. Askovic, B.; Kirchengast, S. Gender differences in nutritional behavior and weight status during early and late adolescence. *Anthropol. Anz.* **2012**, *69*, 289–304. [CrossRef] [PubMed]
40. Lukito, W.; Malik, S.G.; Surono, I.S.; Wahlqvist, M.L. From 'lactose intolerance' to 'lactose nutrition'. *Asia Pac. J. Clin. Nutr.* **2015**, *24*, S1–S8.
41. Rogerson, D. Vegan diets: Practical advice for athletes and exercisers. *J. Int. Soc. Sports Nutr.* **2017**, *14*, 36. [CrossRef]
42. Valentine, V. The importance of salt in the athlete's diet. *Curr. Sports Med. Rep.* **2007**, *6*, 237–240. [CrossRef]
43. Baker, L.B. Sweating rate and sweat sodium concentration in athletes: A review of methodology and intra/interindividual variability. *Sports Med.* **2017**, *47*, 111–128. [CrossRef] [PubMed]
44. Holmes, N.; Miller, V.; Bates, G.; Zheo, Y. The effect of exercise intensity on sweat rate and sweat sodium loss in well trained athletes. *J. Sci. Med. Sport* **2011**, *14*, e112. [CrossRef]
45. Shifflett, B.; Timm, C.; Kananov, L. Understanding athletes' nutritional needs among athletes, coaches and athletic trainers. *Res. Quart. Exerc. Sport.* **2002**, *73*, 357–362. [CrossRef] [PubMed]
46. National Cancer Institute. ASA24-Australia: National Cancer Institute 2018. Available online: https://epi.grants.cancer.gov/asa24/respondent/australia.html (accessed on 10 February 2017).
47. Nikolaidis, P.T.; Theodoropoulou, E. Relationship between nutrition knowledge and physical fitness in semiprofessional soccer players. *Scientifica* **2014**, *2014*, 180353. [CrossRef] [PubMed]
48. Reed, J.; De Souza, M.; Williams, N. Changes in energy availability across the season in Division I female soccer players. *J. Sports Sci. Med.* **2013**, *31*, 314–324. [CrossRef] [PubMed]
49. Reed, J.; De Souza, M.; Kindler, J.; Williams, N. Nutritional practices associated with low energy availability in Division I female soccer players. *J. Sports Sci. Med.* **2014**, *32*, 1499–1509. [CrossRef] [PubMed]
50. Mountjoy, M.; Sundgot-Borgen, J.; Burke, L.; Ackerman, K.; Blauwet, C.; Constantini, N.; Lebrun, C.; Lundy, B.; Melin, A.; Meyer, N. IOC consensus statement on relative energy deficiency in sport (RED-S): 2018 update. *Br. J. Sports Med.* **2018**, *52*, 687–697. [CrossRef]
51. Spronk, I.; Heaney, S.E.; Prvan, T.; O'Connor, H.T. Relationship between general nutrition knowledge and dietary quality in elite athletes. *Int. J. Sport Nutr. Exerc. Metab.* **2015**, *25*, 243–251. [CrossRef]

10

Analysis of Serve and Serve-Return Strategies in Elite Male and Female Padel

Bernardino J. Sánchez-Alcaraz [1], Diego Muñoz [2,*], Francisco Pradas [3], Jesús Ramón-Llin [4], Jerónimo Cañas [5] and Alejandro Sánchez-Pay [1]

1 Department of Physical Activity and Sport, Faculty of Sport Sciences, University of Murcia, C/Argentina, s/n, 30720 San Javier, Murcia, Spain; bjavier.sanchez@um.es (B.J.S.-A.); aspay@um.es (A.S.-P.)
2 Department of Didactic of Musical, Plastic and Corporal Expression, Faculty of Sports Science, University of Extremadura, Avda de la Universidad, s/n, 10003 Cáceres, Spain
3 Department of Musical, Plastic and Corporal Expression, Faculty of Human Sciences and Education, University of Zaragoza, C/Pedro Cerbuna, 12, 50009 Zaragoza, Spain; franprad@unizar.es
4 Department of Musical, Plastic and Corporal Expression, Faculty of Education, University of Valencia, Av. Dels Tarongers, 4, 46022 Valencia, Spain; jesus.ramon@uv.es
5 Department of Physical Education and Sport, Faculty of Sport Sciences, University of Granada, Carretera de Alfacar, 21, 18071 Granada, Spain; jerocanias@yahoo.com
* Correspondence: diegomun@unex.es

Abstract: This aim of this study was to analyze serve and return statistics in elite padel players regarding courtside and gender. The sample contained 668 serves and 600 returns of serves from 14 matches (7 male and 7 female) of the 2019 Masters Finals World Padel Tour. Variables pertaining to serve (number, direction, court side and effectiveness), return of serve (direction, height, stroke type and effectiveness) and point outcome were registered through systematic observation. The main results showed that the serving pair had an advantage in rallies, under 8 shots in women and under 12 shots in men. Statistical differences according to gender and court side were found. Female players execute more backhand and cross-court returns and use more lobs than men. On the right court, serves are more frequently aimed at the "T" and more down the line returns are executed when compared to the left side. Such knowledge could be useful to develop appropriate game strategies and to design specific training exercises based on actual competition context.

Keywords: racket sports; performance analysis; game-actions; strokes

---

1. Introduction

Padel is a racket sport played in pairs (2 vs. 2). The court is characterized by its completely closed girth, as a small-sized grass court (20 × 10 m) surrounded by glass and metallic mesh areas on which the ball can bounce [1]. It has become a mass phenomenon in some countries, such as Spain, and is practiced in more than 35 countries around the world [2]. A professional padel circuit has been created (World Padel Tour), with tournaments in several countries. This development can be attributed to a high interaction between players and a low intensity of actions in a low level of competition [3,4]. Accordingly, the enjoyment and motivation of the players increases, inducing a greater adherence to practice [5–7].

Investigations in padel have increased in the past few years [8]. Research on padel has been mainly focused on describing the match activity and detecting effective performance indicators [9–11]. These investigations have provided primary information such as the rally length (10 to 15 s), the most common actions in offence (volley and smash) and defense (lob), and have highlighted the advantage of the net game. In addition, padel player performance has been characterized by the ratio between winning shots and errors [12]. Furthermore, previous researches have shown gender-related differences during competition [13,14]. Higher values have been observed in play time and total time in women over men players, as well as in the number and types of strokes [10]. Therefore, the players constantly try to play in offensive positions; for which they use different behaviors and technical-tactical actions, which define different styles of play [12]. The distribution of the different types of strokes, their trajectories and their efficacy stand out among these behaviours [3–5]. The results of the studies have shown that these variables may also differ depending on the gender or the side of the court on which the padel player plays [10,11]. Hence, different performance profiles of padel could exist related to gender and game-side on court [15].

However, there is an alarming lack of investigations examining players' serve and return statistics [16]. One of the most important performance indicators in racket sports is the serve [17]. In tennis, a serve directly wins the point through an ace or indirectly because of the advantage coming from the opponent's imbalance after a great serve [18]. Thus, tennis players win about 70% of points with the first serve, this percentage being higher in men's singles than in women's [17,19]. Previous studies found that serve was more determinant in tennis doubles, likely due to the presence of the server's partner covering the net [20]. Furthermore, the serve situation could influence point or game outcome in padel, since it allows players to adopt an offensive position. In this way, winners scored about 34% more points from the net than losers [9]. However, the serve in padel is different to other racket sports, because of the rules of game. In padel, the ball cannot be beaten as hard as in tennis, and the serve must be an underhand shot from a bouncing ball hit from below waist level. In addition, the effect and the side wall can affect the serve-return shot [16]. The receiver must play an accurate shot to avoid the serving pair hitting the ball into a tactically advantageous area, so they should vary the direction and height of their return of serve [15,16].

A better knowledge of players' behavior when serving or receiving is extremely useful for developing appropriate game strategies and to design specific training exercises [21]. However, at present little is known about the relationship between the serve and return of serve in padel, other than the fact that the server tends to maintain the tactical advantage until around shot five, when the advantage has dissipated [16,22]. In addition, Zhang and Zhou [23] differentiated specific serve tactics in table tennis that were associated with higher scoring rates. Furthermore, some studies highlighted the difference between first and second serves in terms of how aggressive the return could be [24]. Given that serve and return of serve are two of the most important shots in padel, the purpose of this study was to analyze serve and return statistics in elite padel players regarding court side and gender. This information could help coaches to better understand player strategies and their efficiency in padel games.

2. Materials and Methods

2.1. Sample and Variables

The study was reviewed and approved by the Ethical Committee of the University of Murcia. The sample contained 668 serves and 600 returns of serves from 14 professional matches (7 male and 7 female) of the 2019 Finals World Padel Tour. These tournaments gathered the best pairs in the world, ensuring the highest competitive level in all the matches. A total of 32 players, 16 men (mean (SD) age: 31.18 (7.27) years; height: 181.3 (4.1) cm) and 16 women (mean (SD) age: 28.66 (6.7) years; height: 168.4 (3.7) cm) performed the matches. Variables pertaining to serve and return statistics and point outcome were included in the analysis, following the methodology adopted in other similar studies [25]:

- Serve shots were analyzed regarding the serve number (1st and 2nd serve), court side (right and left), serve direction (side wall, middle and T) and effectiveness indicator (winner, error and continuity) (Figure 1).

- Return statistics were analyzed regarding the court side (right and left), stroke direction (down the line, middle and cross court), stroke height (straight and lob), stroke type (forehand and backhand) and effectiveness indicator (winner, error and continuity) (Figure 1).
- Point outcome: strokes were classified according to the winning or losing pair of the point (serving players win and returning players win).
- Total shots: number of total shots in the points were counted.

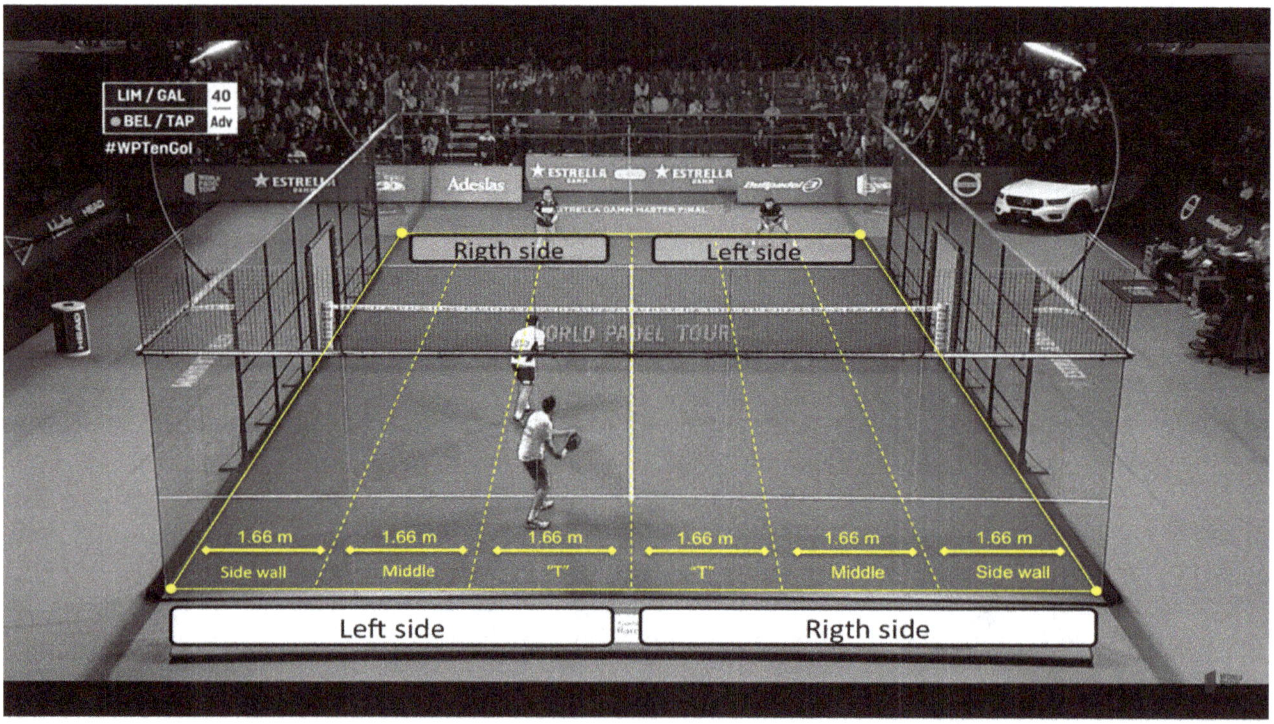

Figure 1. Illustration of court side and serve and return directions.

2.2. Procedure

The matches were downloaded from the official channel of the World Padel Tour [26]. Lince video analysis software was used to collect and register the data [27]. The Kinovea software [28] was used to place a visual grid over the video image for the serve and return directions data recording (Figure 1) and to register the feet of the serving player when impacting the ball, the place where the ball bounced after a successful serve and the direction of the ball after the returner hit it. Four observers specializing in padel (over 5 years of experience) were specifically trained to perform the recording. Observers were specifically trained in the use of the observational instrument for two weeks. The training focused on the clear identification of the variables (serve and return statistics, point outcome and total shots) and the use of the observational instrument software (Lince and Kinovea). Having completed the training process, each observer registered a training set not included in the final sample (n = 72 serves; n = 68 returns), to calculate inter-rater reliability. Consistency of records was analyzed using the free-marginal multirater Kappa [29] and the weighted Kappa [30]. The minimum score obtained was k = 0.87. Finally, intra-observer evaluation was done at the end of the observation process by Cohen's Kappa calculation, yielding a very good strength of agreement with scores over 0.92 [31].

2.3. Data Analysis

Descriptive analysis included means, standard deviations and frequencies. Assumptions of normality and homogeneity of variances were verified using the Kolmogorov–Smirnov test and Levene's test. Due to data not following a normal distribution, non-parametric tests were implemented [32].

Chi square analysis was performed to identify differences in serve and return statistics and point outcome between gender and court side. Column proportions were compared using Z tests on serve and return statistics according to the gender of the players and court side. A significance level of $p < 0.05$ was established which was adjusted according to Bonferroni in the Z tests. The associations among the categories of the variables were performed with corrected standardized residuals (CSR). The effect size was calculated using Cramer's V [33]. Rho Spearmen was used to know the relationship between serving point won and the number of strokes per point. IBM SPSS 25.0 Statistics for Macintosh (Armonk, NY: IBM Corp.) was used to process the data.

3. Results

3.1. Serve and Return Performances of Professional Padel Players Regarding Gender

Table 1 shows differences in serve and return statistics in relation to players' gender. With regards to serve performance, the players' gender determined the percentage of first and second serves ($\chi^2 = 5.05$; gL = 1; CRS = 2.2; $p < 0.05$). Thus, men obtained a significantly higher percentage of successful first serves than women. Furthermore, both men and women aimed more than 60% of their serves towards the side wall. Regarding return statistics, significant differences between men and women were found with regards to direction ($\chi^2 = 9.647$; gL = 2; CRS = 3.2; $p < 0.01$), height ($\chi^2 = 9.354$; gL = 2; CRS = 2.9; $p < 0.01$) and stroke type ($\chi^2 = 4.230$; gL = 1; CRS = 2.1; $p < 0.05$). Thus, women played a significantly higher proportion of backhand or cross-court returns and used the lob more when returning than men did. Finally, the point-result variable showed how men won a significantly higher percentage of points in a serve situation than women ($\chi^2 = 11.435$; gL = 1; CRS = 3.4; $p < 0.01$).

Figure 2 shows the relationship between the percentage of points won by the couple with the serve and the number of strokes per point, in relation to the players' gender. The correlation test results showed a significant relationship for male ($p < 0.001$; $r = 0.62$) and female ($p < 0.001$; $r = 0.54$) players between the percentage of points won in the serve and the number of strokes per point. Thus, the percentage of points won by the player with the serve went down as the number of strokes went up. Furthermore, with regards to gender, serving advantage was lost after the 12th stroke for men, while for women it was after the seventh stroke.

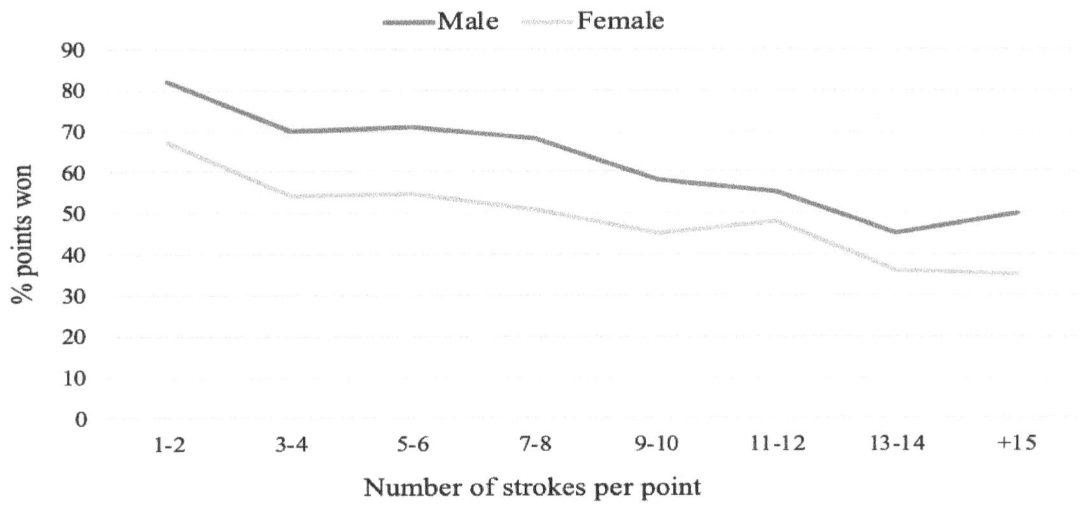

Figure 2. Percentage of points won by the serving couple with relation to the number of strokes per points: gender differences.

Table 1. Percentages for the serve and serve–return performances of the professional male and female padel players.

		Male *n* (%)	Female *n* (%)	Sig.
Serve statistics				
Serve Number				
	1st serve	378 (92.9)a	229 (87.7)b	0.025 *
	2nd serve	29 (7.1)a	32 (12.3)b	
Court side				
	Right	211 (51.8)	133 (51.0)	0.823
	Left	196 (48.2)	128 (49.0)	
Serve direction				
	Side wall	263 (64.6)	163 (62.5)	0.101
	Middle	45 (11.1)	19 (7.3)	
	T	99 (24.3)	79 (30.3)	
Effectiveness				
	Winner	0 (0.0)	0 (0.00)	0.085
	Error	36 (8.8)	34 (13.0)	
	Continuity	371 (91.2)	227 (87.0)	
Return statistics				
Stroke direction				
	Down the line	213 (57.4)a	103 (45.0)b	0.008 **
	Middle	95 (25.6)	69 (30.1)	
	Cross court	63 (17.0)a	57 (24.9)b	
Stroke height				
	Straight	242 (65.2)a	122 (53.3)b	0.009 **
	Lob	129 (34.7)a	107 (46.7)b	
Stroke type				
	Forehand	156 (42.0)a	77 (33.6)b	0.040 *
	Backhand	215 (58.0)a	152 (64.4)b	
Effectiveness				
	Winner	0 (0.0)	1 (0.4)	0.323
	Error	20 (5.4)	9 (3.9)	
	Continuity	351 (94.96)	219 (95.6)	
Point outcome				
	Serve pair win	232 (62.5)a	111 (48.5)b	0.001 **
	Returner pair win	139 (37.5)a	118 (51.5)b	

Note: n = Number; % = Percentage; * = $p < 0.05$; a, b = significant differences indicated in the Z tests for comparison of column proportions from $p < 0.05$, adjusted according to Bonferroni.

3.2. Serve and Return Performances of Professional Padel Players Regarding Court Side

Figure 3 shows serve statistics with regard to court side where said serve was played. As may be observed in the court shown above, court side significantly determined serve direction ($\chi^2 = 18.202$; gL = 2; CRS = 3.3; $p < 0.01$). It may be observed that most serves went towards the side wall, followed by the "T" and, in smaller proportion, the middle of the court. Furthermore, on the left side (ad court) players executed 12% more serves towards the side wall, whereas on the right side (deuce court) players served 14% more towards the "T." On the other hand, no significant differences were found with regards to court side for effectiveness ($\chi^2 = 1.047$; gL = 1; $p > 0.05$) and serve number ($\chi^2 = 2.972$; gL = 1; $p > 0.05$).

Figure 4 shows return statistics with regards to the player's side of the court. As may be observed, players executed around 60% of straight returns, with no significant differences regarding court side ($\chi^2 = 2.048$; gL = 2; $p > 0.05$). Furthermore, players obtained a high percentage of return effectiveness, with more than 90% of successful returns, and no difference between the right and left sides ($\chi^2 = 4.444$; gL = 2; CRS = 3.0; $p > 0.05$). Playing side significantly determined the return's direction ($\chi^2 = 28.711$; gL = 2; CRS = 7.6; $p < 0.01$). Thus, players returning from the left side executed almost 15% more down the line returns than players on the right side. Furthermore, the kind of returning stroke also showed significant differences regarding court side. Left side players executed more than 75% of their returns backhand, whereas right side players registered more balanced values, although they did execute more forehand returns. Finally, there were no significant differences between return statistics and stroke type, height or direction ($p < 0.005$).

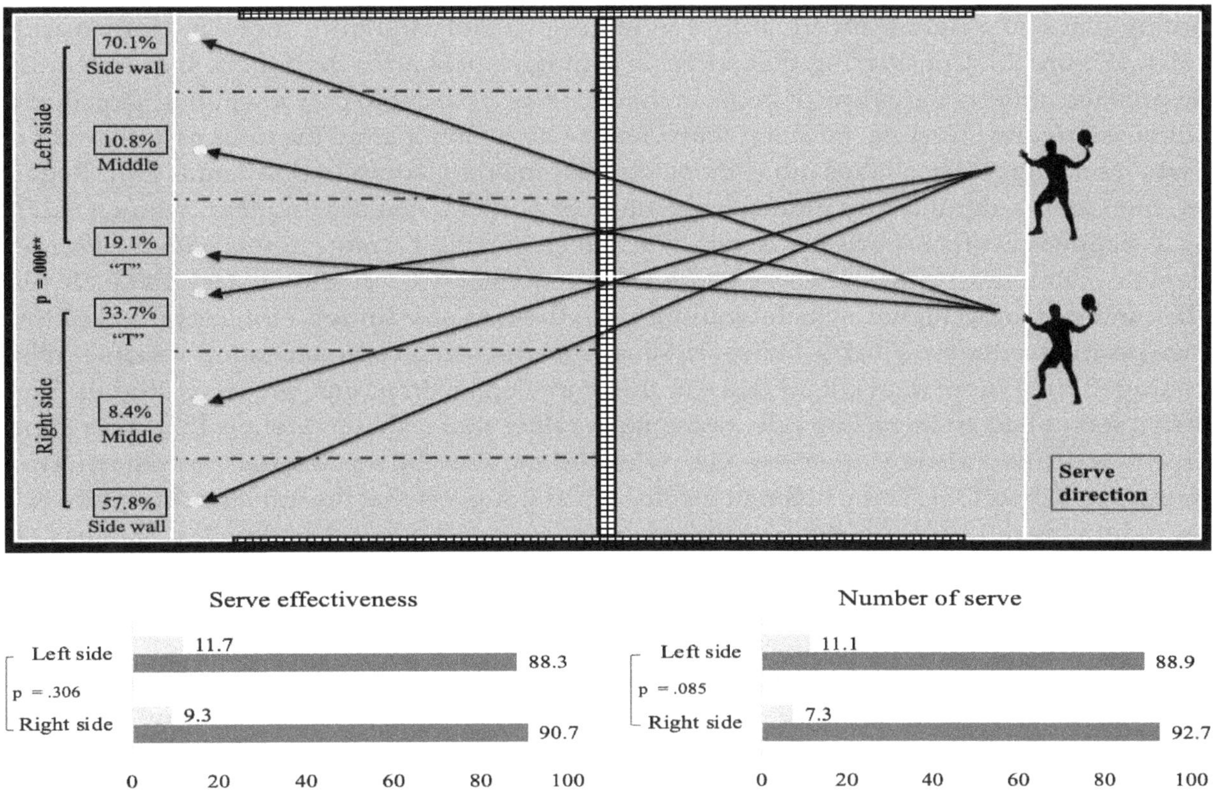

Figure 3. Serve statistics regarding court side.

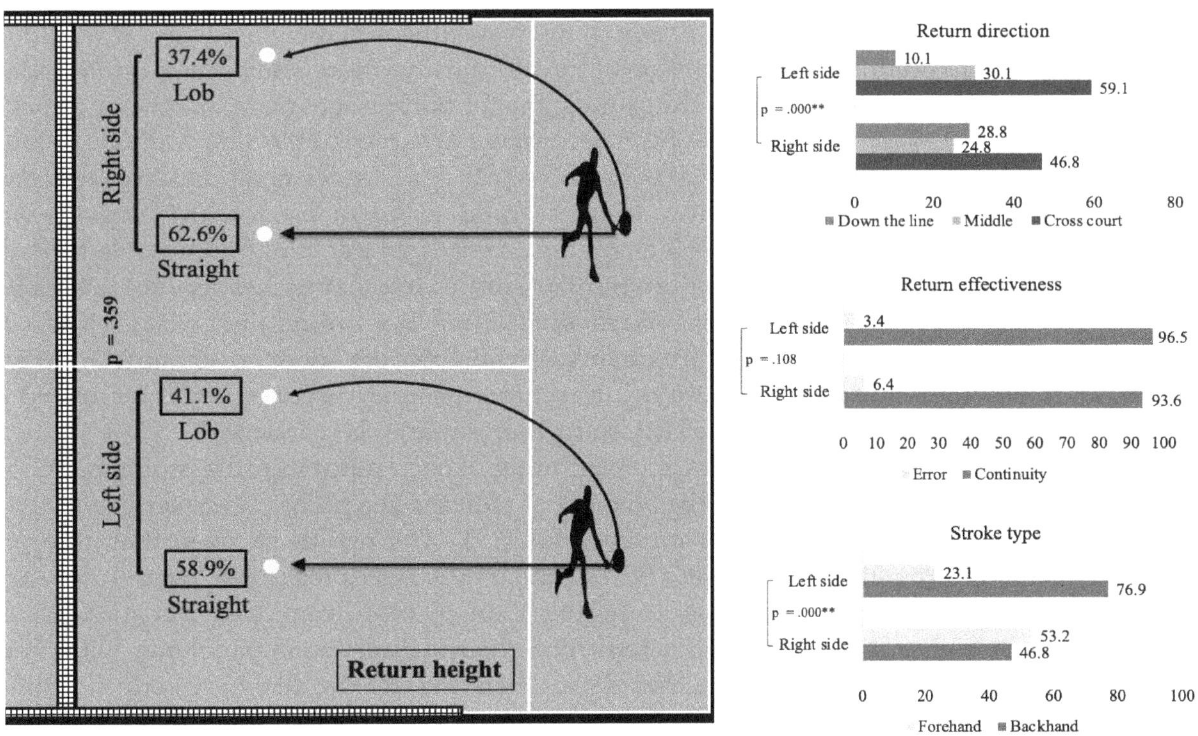

Figure 4. Serve return statistics regarding court side.

4. Discussion

This aim of this study was to evaluate the serve and return statistics in elite padel players regarding courtside and gender. The notational analysis of this research is one of the most important contributions because of the lack of previous research regarding this aspect in padel. The main results showed that the serving pair had a significant advantage in rallies, which lasted until shot 7 in women and shot 12 in men (Figure 2). Considering that serve advantage is lost after the fourth shot in tennis, this finding probably reflects the nature of padel in that it is much harder to play a winning shot, due to the court dimensions and structure, meaning that when a pair is dominating the rally, as at the start of the point when serving, it often takes more shots to finish the rally compared to tennis [16]. Regarding gender, men won a significantly higher percentage of points when serving than women (62.5% vs. 48.5%), as happens in other sports like tennis, where men obtain 14% more points with their serve than their female counterparts [34,35]. These gender differences may be due to the fact that male players are taller and can jump higher, which would enable them to sustain for a longer period of time an offensive position at the net [36,37]. However, deeper analysis and complementary variable collection is encouraged for a more relevant advance in this knowledge. In tennis, previous studies reported that men's serves had an impact on rally outcome in rallies that lasted four shots [22]. This impact of the serve was corroborated by other research, which found that the serving pair won the most rallies containing 1 to 4 shots [38]. These different results in padel suggest that the influence of service extends some way into the rally in padel because the predominance of the "serve and volley" strategy allows the serving pair to move close to the net first and adopt an offensive position [9,39]. Despite serve advantage being lost when the return players use technical actions that facilitate a change of position, such as lobs, this transition from offensive to defensive position only appears in 37% of points [40]. On the other hand, the results showed first serve effectiveness as being close to 90%. Even though there were no gender significant differences, the higher occurrence of first service faults reported by women could be due to a higher predisposition to obtain a direct point by forcing the first service [15].

With regards to serve direction, the results of this study showed how players served primarily towards the side wall, increasing that percentage on the left side (advantage), which is usually the place where more decisive points are fought. The greater distance covered by the player serving during the point [39] could explain this crossed direction of the serve towards the glass, since it would allow him to buy more time to occupy a better position at the net. Furthermore, the bounce on the side wall may complicate the return stroke, which could cause a greater number of errors, as other authors have claimed [15]. Other studies reported that the high percentage of serves to the side wall on the left side could be explained by the hand-dominance of the players [12]. Thus, since most padel players playing on the left side of the court are right-handed, servers would seek to serve towards the side wall to seek both the backhand of the return as well as the uncertainty of the wall bounce. No differences between genders were found in serve direction. Similar studies in other racket sports, such as tennis, showed that the serve aimed at the "T" was the most effective in winning the point [41]. However, on the left side of the court, better results are obtained when players serve cross-court or open [42]. It is important to highlight that some of these results regarding serve direction could be related more to players' hand dominance than court side [12], so further research is warranted.

The results of this study confirmed that the beginning of each point in professional padel seems very important and decisive for increasing the chances of winning the point. Then, serve effectiveness is directly related to the opponent's serve-return skills [17]. The results showed that a very high percentages of serve returns stayed in (around 90%), but no differences regarding gender or courtside were found. This effectiveness percentage is higher than in other racket sports such as tennis, where serve power is higher [43]. Furthermore, return height and direction in padel may allow couples in the defensive position to execute a stroke that allows them to send the attacking couple to the back of the court [11]. Previous authors showed how sending deep lobs to the corners and close to the walls will keep the rivals far from the net. However, the results of our study showed that players hit about 60% straight and 40% lob shots. These data are confirmed by a previous analysis in a national padel competition, and reflect the importance for the player serving to run toward the net and be able to approach the net to make the straight return more advantageous [16]. Furthermore, the return's height and direction showed significant differences with regards to players' gender and the side of the court. Thus, women executed more lobs and cross-court returns than men. This higher use of lobs by female players has been confirmed in previous studies that suggest a more defensive playing style among women [10,44,45]. Thus, because over-head strokes (smash and tray) are the most successful shots during a match, with a significantly higher percentage in the male category [10,46], players returning the serve have to use the lob only in comfortable positions to overcome their opponents at the net, since a poorly executed lobbed return could have as a response a winning smash from the serving players. At the national level, the lob return of serve achieved long rallies 48.8% of the time for good depth (around 5.5 m beyond the net) off first serves and 61.8% of the time off second serves, and 79.8% of the time for excellent depth (around 8.5 m beyond the net) irrespective of serve [16].

With regards to playing side, players returning the serve on the left side stroke more with their backhand than forehand, and play more straight and down the line strokes than players on the right side, corroborating the findings of Torres-Luque et al. [10], who found that about 75% of serves were directed to the backhand of players. This fact could be due to a higher game aggression of players when resting in the left side, not allowing serving players to take the lead in the point [9,47]. Furthermore, these differences in return with regards to playing side are especially important considering that 75% of the decisive points are played on the left side of the court [35].

Although this is the first study addressing serve and return statistics in professional padel, the study presents some limitations. First, contextual variables such as match status were not registered. Given the influence of situational variables on game performance [48], it would be very interesting to include such information in future research on padel. On the other hand, other variables that may affect serve and return statistics, such as serve speed or spin and players' hand dominance [12,22,43], have not been taken into account. Finally, the sample was limited, so future studies should analyze a greater number and tournaments and padel players.

5. Conclusions

The current investigation has described the advantage of serving in padel by comparing points won by servers and receiving players after a different number of shots within rallies. Given the server has a significant advantage, the aim of the return is to avoid the serving pair winning the rally quickly. This could be best achieved by good depth on lobs, regardless of the direction, and pace on straight shots, predominately aimed toward the server [16]. Statistical differences according to gender and court side were found. Female players execute more backhand and cross-court returns and use more lobs than men. On the right court, serves are more frequently aimed at the "T" and more down the line returns are executed when compared to the left side. Such knowledge may have implications for accuracy and the quality of training drills based on specific technical–tactical demands.

Author Contributions: Conceptualization, B.J.S.-A., D.M. and J.C.; methodology, B.J.S.-A., J.R.-L., F.P., A.S.-P. and D.M.; software, B.J.S.-A. and F.P.; validation, B.J.S.-A., F.P., J.R.-L. and D.M.; formal analysis, B.J.S.-A., J.C. and A.S.-P.; investigation, B.J.S.-A., J.C., J.R.-L., D.M. and A.S.-P.; resources, B.J.S.-A., J.R.-L., A.S.-P. and D.M.; data curation, B.J.S.-A., J.R.-L., A.S.-P. and D.M.; writing—original draft preparation, B.J.S.-A., J.C. and D.M.; writing—review and editing, B.J.S.-A., F.P., J.R.-L., A.S.-P. and D.M.; visualization, B.J.S.-A., J.C., F.P., J.R.-L., A.S.-P. and D.M.; supervision, B.J.S.-A., F.P., J.R.-L., A.S.-P. and D.M. All authors have read and agreed to the published version of the manuscript.

References

1. International Padel Federation. Rules of Padel. FIP, V.D. Available online: https://www.padelfip.com/wp-content/uploads/2017/06/Rules-of-Padel.pdf (accessed on 1 July 2020).
2. Courel-Ibáñez, J.; Sánchez-Alcaraz, B.J.; García, S.; Echegaray, M. Evolution of padel in spain according to practitioners' gender and age [Evolución del pádel en España en función del género y edad de los practicantes]. *Cult. Cienc. Deporte* **2017**, *12*, 39–46. [CrossRef]
3. Carrasco, L.; Romero, S.; Sañudo, B.; de Hoyo, M. Game analysis and energy requirements of paddle tennis competition. *Sci. Sports* **2011**, *26*, 338–344. [CrossRef]
4. Courel-Ibáñez, J.; Sánchez-Alcaraz, B.J.; Cañas, J. Game performance and length of rally in professional padel players. *J. Hum. Kinet.* **2017**, *55*, 161–169. [CrossRef]
5. Castillo-Rodríguez, A.; Alvero-Cruz, J.R.; Hernández-Mendo, A.; Fernández-García, J.C. Physical and physiological responses in paddle tennis competition. *Int. J. Perform. Anal. Sport* **2014**, *14*, 524–534. [CrossRef]
6. Duda, J.L. Motivation in Sport: The relevance of competence and achievement goals. In *Handbook of Competence and Motivation*; Elliot, A., Dweck, C., Eds.; Guildford Publications: New York, NY, USA, 2005; pp. 311–330.
7. Courel-Ibáñez, J.; Sánchez-Alcaraz, B.J.; Muñoz, D.; Grijota, F.J.; Chaparro, R.; Díaz, J. Gender reasons for practicing paddle tennis [Motivos de género para la práctica de pádel]. *Apunt. Educ. Fis. y Deportes.* **2018**, *133*, 116–125. [CrossRef]
8. Sánchez-Alcaraz, B.J.; Courel-Ibáñez, J.; Cañas, J. Temporal structure, court movements and game actions in padel: A systematic review [Estructura temporal, movimientos en pista y acciones de juego en pádel: Revisión sistemática]. *Retos, Nuevas Tend. Deport Educ. Física Recreación* **2018**, *33*, 221–225.
9. Courel-Ibáñez, J.; Sánchez-Alcaraz, B.J.; Cañas, J. Effectiveness at the net as a predictor of final match outcome in professional padel players. *Int. J. Perform. Anal. Sport* **2015**, *15*, 632–640. [CrossRef]
10. Torres-Luque, G.; Ramirez, A.; Cabello-Manrique, D.; Nikolaidis, P.T.; Alvero-Cruz, J.R. Match analysis of elite players during paddle tennis competition. *Int. J. Perform. Anal. Sport* **2015**, *15*, 1135–1144. [CrossRef]
11. Courel-Ibáñez, J.; Sánchez-Alcaraz, B.J.; Muñoz, D. Exploring game dynamics in padel: Implications for assessment and training. *J. Strength Cond. Res.* **2019**, *33*, 1971–1977. [CrossRef]
12. Courel-Ibáñez, J.; Sánchez-Alcaraz, B.J. The role of hand dominance in padel: Performance profiles of professional players. *Motricidade* **2018**, *14*, 33–41. [CrossRef]
13. García-Benítez, S.; Pérez-Bilbao, T.; Echegaray, M.; Felipe, J.L. The influence of gender on temporal structure and match activity patterns of professional padel tournaments. *Cult. Cienc. Deport* **2016**, *33*, 241–247. [CrossRef]
14. Sánchez-Alcaraz, B.J. Game actions and temporal structure diferences between male and female professional paddle players [Diferencias en las acciones de juego y la estructura temporal entre el pádel masculino y femenino profesional]. *Acción Mot.* **2014**, *12*, 17–22.
15. Lupo, C.; Condello, G.; Courel-Ibáñez, J.; Gallo, C.; Conte, D.; Tessitore, A. Effect of gender and match outcome on professional padel competition. *RICYDE Rev. Int. Cienc. Deport* **2018**, *51*, 29–41. [CrossRef]
16. Ramón-Llin, J.; Guzmán, J.F.; Llana, S.; Martínez-Gallego, R.; James, N.; Vučković, G. The effect of the return of serve on the server pair's movement parameters and rally outcome in padel using cluster analysis. *Front. Psychol.* **2019**, *10*, 1–8. [CrossRef] [PubMed]
17. Gillet, E.; Leroy, D.; Thouvarecq, R.; Stein, J.F. A notational analysis of elite tennis serve and serve-return strategies on slow surface. *J. Strength Cond. Res.* **2009**, *23*, 532–539. [CrossRef]
18. Reid, M.; McMurtrie, D.; Crespo, M. The relationship between match statistics and top 100 ranking in professional men's tennis. *Int. J. Perform. Anal. Sport* **2010**, *10*, 131–138. [CrossRef]
19. O'Donoghue, P. The most important points in grand slam singles tennis. *Res. Q. Exerc. Sport* **2001**, *72*, 125–131. [CrossRef]
20. Furlong, J. The service in lawn tennis: How important is it? In *Science and Racket Sports I*; Reilly, T., Hughes, M.D., Lees, A., Eds.; E &FN Spon: London, UK, 1995.
21. McGarry, T. Applied and theoretical perspectives of performance analysis in sport: Scientific issues and challenges. *Int. J. Perform. Anal. Sport* **2009**, *9*, 128–140. [CrossRef]

22. O'Donoghue, P.; Brown, E. The importance of service in Grand Slam singles tennis. *Int. J. Perform. Anal. Sport* **2008**, *8*, 70–78. [CrossRef]
23. Zhang, H.; Zhou, Z. An analytical model of the two basic situation strategies in table tennis. *Int. J. Perform. Anal. Sport* **2017**, *17*, 970–985. [CrossRef]
24. Vernon, G.; Farrow, D.; Reid, M. Returning serve in Tennis: A qualitative examination of the interaction of anticipatory information sources used by professional tennis players. *Front. Psychol.* **2018**, *9*, 1–11. [CrossRef] [PubMed]
25. Hizan, H.; Whipp, P.; Reid, M. Gender differences in the spatial distributions of the tennis serve. *Int. J. Sport Sci. Coach.* **2015**, *10*, 87–96. [CrossRef]
26. World Padel Tour Youtube Chanel. Available online: https://www.youtube.com/user/WorldPadelTourAJPP (accessed on 1 February 2020).
27. Gabin, B.; Camerino, O.; Anguera, M.T.; Castañer, M. Lince: Multiplatform sport analysis software. *Procedia-Soc. Behav. Sci.* **2012**, *46*, 4692–4694. [CrossRef]
28. Kinovea Sofware (V.08.26,). Available online: https://www.kinovea.org. (accessed on 1 February 2020).
29. Randolph, J.J. *Free-Marginal Multirater Kappa: An Alternative to Fleiss' Fixed-Marginal Multirater Kappa*; Joensuu University Learning and Instruction Symposium: Joensuu, Finlandia, 2005.
30. Robinson, G.; O'Donoghue, P.G. A weighted kappa statistic for reliability testing in performance analysis of sport. *Int. J. Perform. Anal. Sport* **2007**, *7*, 12–19. [CrossRef]
31. Altman, D.G. *Practical Statistics for Medical Research*; Chapman and Hall: London, UK, 1991.
32. Pallant, J. *SPSS Survival Manual: A Step by Step Guide to Data Analysis Using SPSS Program*; Alen & Unwin: Crows Nest, Australia, 2011.
33. Cohen, J. Statistical Power Analysis for the Behavioural Science (2nd Edition). In *Statistical Power Anaylsis for the Behavioral Sciences*; Lawrence Erlbaum: Hillsdale, NJ, USA, 1988.
34. Reid, M.; Morgan, S.; Whiteside, D. Matchplay characteristics of Grand Slam tennis: Implications for training and conditioning. *J. Sport Sci.* **2016**, *34*, 1791–1798. [CrossRef]
35. Sim, M.K.; Choi, D.G. The winning probability of a game and the importance of points in tennis matches. *Res. Q. Exerc. Sport* **2020**, *91*, 361–372. [CrossRef]
36. Sánchez-Muñoz, C.; Muros, J.J.; Cañas, J.; Courel-Ibáñez, J.; Sánchez-Alcaraz, B.J.; Zabala, M. Anthropometric and physical fitness profiles of world-class male padel players. *Int. J. Environ. Res. Public Health* **2020**, *17*, 508. [CrossRef]
37. Castillo-Rodríguez, A.; Hernández-Mendo, A.; Alvero-Cruz, J.R. Morphology of the elite paddle player—Comparison with other racket sports. *Int. J. Morphol.* **2014**, *32*, 177–182. [CrossRef]
38. Fitzpatrick, A.; Stone, J.A.; Choppin, S.; Kelley, J. A simple new method for identifying performance characteristics associated with success in elite tennis. *Int. J. Sport Sci. Coach.* **2019**, *14*, 43–50. [CrossRef]
39. Ramón-Llin, J.; Guzmán, J.F.; Belloch, S.L.; Vučković, G.; James, N. Comparison of distance covered in paddle in the serve team according to performance level. *J. Hum. Sport Exerc.* **2013**, *8*, 738–742. [CrossRef]
40. Escudero-Tena, A.; Fernández-Cortes, J.; García-Rubio, J.; Ibáñez, S.J. Use and efficacy of the lob to achieve the offensive position in women's professional padel. Analysis of the 2018 WPT finals. *Int. J. Environ. Res. Public Health* **2020**, *17*, 4061. [CrossRef]
41. Unierzyski, P.; Wieczorek, A. Comparison of tactical solutions and game patterns in the finals of two grand slam tournaments in tennis. In *Science and Racket Sports III*; Kahn, J., Lees, A., Maynard, I., Eds.; Routledge: London, UK, 2004; pp. 169–174.
42. Cui, Y.; Gómez, M.Á.; Gonçalves, B.; Sampaio, J. Performance profiles of professional female tennis players in grand slams. *PLoS ONE* **2018**, *13*, e0200591. [CrossRef]
43. O'Donoghue, P.; Ballantyne, A. The impact of speed of service in Grand Slam singles tennis. In *Science and Racket Sports III*; Lees, A., Kahn, J., Maynard, I., Eds.; Routledge: London, UK, 2008; pp. 179–184.
44. García-Benítez, S.; Courel-Ibáñez, J.; Pérez-Bilbao, T.; Felipe, J.L. Game responses during young padel match play: Age and sex comparisons. *J. Strength Cond. Res.* **2018**, *32*, 1144–1149. [CrossRef] [PubMed]
45. Muñoz, D.; Courel-Ibáñez, J.; Sánchez-Alcaraz, B.J.; Díaz, J.; Grijota, F.J.; Munoz, J. Analysis of the use and effectiveness of lobs to recover the net in the context of padel [Análisis del uso y eficacia del globo para recuperar la red en función del contexto de juego en pádel]. *Retos Nuevas Tend. Deport Educ. Física Recreación* **2017**, *31*, 19–22.

46. Priego, J.I.; Olaso, J.; Llana, S.; Pérez, P.; Gonález, J.C.; Sanchís, M. Padel: A quantitative study of the shots and movements in the high-performance. *J. Hum. Sport Exerc.* **2013**, *8*, 925–931. [CrossRef]
47. Martínez-Gallego, R.; Guzmán Luján, J.F.; James, N.; Pers, J.; Ramón-Llin, J.; Vučković, G. Movement characteristics of elite tennis players on hard courts with respect to the direction of ground strokes. *J. Sport Sci. Med.* **2013**, *12*, 275–281.
48. Gómez, M.Á.; Lago-Peñas, C.; Pollard, G. Situational variables. In *Routledge Handbook of Sports Performance Analysis*; McGarry, T., O'Donoghue, P., Sampaio, J., Eds.; Routledge: London, UK, 2003; pp. 259–269.

11

Honey Supplementation and Exercise

Samuel P. Hills, Peter Mitchell, Christine Wells and Mark Russell *

School of Social and Health Sciences, Leeds Trinity University, Horsforth, Leeds LS18 5HD, UK
* Correspondence: m.russell@leedstrinity.ac.uk

Abstract: Honey is a natural substance formed primarily of carbohydrates (~80%) which also contains a number of other compounds purported to confer health benefits when consumed. Due to its carbohydrate composition (low glycaemic index, mostly fructose and glucose), honey may theoretically exert positive effects when consumed before, during or after exercise. This review therefore appraised research examining the effects of honey consumption in combination with exercise in humans. Online database (PubMed, MEDLINE, SPORTDiscus) searches were performed, yielding 273 results. Following duplicate removal and application of exclusion criteria, nine articles were reviewed. Large methodological differences existed in terms of exercise stimulus, population, and the nutritional interventions examined. All nine studies reported biochemical variables, with four examining the effects of honey on exercise performance, whilst five described perceptual responses. Acute supplementation around a single exercise session appeared to elicit similar performance, perceptual, and immunological responses compared with other carbohydrate sources, although some performance benefit has been observed relative to carbohydrate-free comparators. When consumed over a number of weeks, honey may dampen immunological perturbations arising from exercise and possibly improve markers of bone formation. More well-controlled research is required to better understand the role for honey in a food-first approach to exercise nutrition.

Keywords: carbohydrate; antioxidant; immune function; endurance; intermittent exercise; glucose; fructose

---

1. Introduction

Honey is defined by European Communities legislation as "the natural sweet substance produced by *Apis mellifera* bees from the nectar of plants or from secretions of living parts of plants or excretions of plant-sucking insects on the living parts of plants, which the bees collect, transform by combining with specific substances of their own, deposit, dehydrate, store and leave in honeycombs to ripen and mature" and is categorised primarily according to origin and mode of production or presentation [1]. A popular foodstuff, honey is comprised of ~80% carbohydrate, and ~19% water [2], and typically contains a wide variety of other components such as organic acids, proteins, amino acids, minerals, polyphenols, vitamins, aroma compounds, and approximately 500 enzymes [2,3]. This diverse profile has seen honey being used for a variety of different health and medicinal purposes [2–7]. For example, amongst numerous other proposed health benefits, honey is espoused to have antioxidant, antimicrobial, and anti-inflammatory properties [3–6,8]. Such effects may be at least partially attributable to honey's high osmolarity inhibiting bacterial growth, the antimicrobial effects of glucose oxidase and resultant hydrogen peroxide production, and/or the presence of antibacterial substances such as polyphenols [2]. Notably, there exists over 320 different varieties of honey, and the composition of this substance can vary substantially depending upon the variety of plant from which nectar is derived, in addition to the environmental conditions within which the plants grow [2,3,6,9,10].

The primary carbohydrates present in honey are the monosaccharides glucose (~30–35%) and fructose (~35–40%). However, ~5–10% of honey's volume may consist of up to 25 additional di- and trisaccharides in varying quantities [2,3,6,7]. In keeping with the natural variation in composition, the glycaemic index (GI) of honey (and thus potentially the postprandial insulinaemic response) also appears to differ between varieties. Depending upon botanical source, GI values ranging from ~32–85 have been reported [3], with the GI of any given honey appearing to depend largely upon its relative concentration of fructose. Indeed, a higher fructose to glucose ratio is associated with a lower GI value [3,11], and a number of studies have identified fructose-rich varieties of honey, such as Acacia honey, with "low" (i.e., values ≤ 55 [12]) or "moderate" (i.e., values of 55–69 [12]) GI ratings [3,11–13].

Carbohydrate has been recognised as an important fuel for exercise since the early 1900s [14], and it is now well established that commencing activity with high concentrations of muscle glycogen may enhance physical performance during exercise of >60–90 min in duration [15–18]. Moreover, consuming carbohydrates immediately prior to, and during, exercise can help to maintain performance throughout both prolonged endurance events [14,16,19–21] and intermittent exercise representative of team sports [14,22,23]. Indeed, carbohydrate ingestion may augment exercise capacity via a sparing of endogenous fuel stores (i.e., muscle and liver glycogen, and blood glucose concentrations), and/or by acting directly on the central nervous system. This latter suggestion is supported by increases in short-term (i.e., events lasting ≤60 min) exercise performance when carbohydrate solutions are simply swilled around the mouth [14,24].

The American College of Sports Medicine have provided broad recommendations for carbohydrate consumption during exercise, and therein suggest intakes of ~30–60 $g \cdot h^{-1}$ [25]. However, whilst it was traditionally believed that ~60 $g \cdot h^{-1}$ represented the upper limit of carbohydrate (i.e., glucose) oxidation during endurance exercise, more recent evidence suggests that simultaneously ingesting carbohydrates from multiple sources (e.g., glucose and fructose) may increase oxidation capacity by up to ~75% [15,21]. Notably, consuming a combination of glucose and fructose at a rate of 108–144 $g \cdot h^{-1}$ has improved performance during prolonged cycling exercise when compared with the equivalent dose of glucose alone [14,26,27]. Such developments may be important for athletes engaged in prolonged endurance events (i.e., events of ≥2.5 h in duration) in which fuel availability is likely to be a substantial performance-limiting factor [14]. Given its multiple-carbohydrate composition, there may be a theoretical basis to suggest that honey supplementation could offer a viable and natural alternative to traditional forms of exogenous carbohydrate provision.

In team sports such as soccer, players experience limited opportunities to consume carbohydrates outside of scheduled stoppages in play (i.e., half-time). For this reason, research designs based around a regular feeding pattern throughout exercise (i.e., every 15 min) may be limited in their ecological validity. Moreover, when high GI carbohydrates, including those contained within most commercially available sports drinks, are ingested before and during team sport specific exercise, including at half-time, sharp declines in blood glucose concentrations are typically observed during the early stages of the second half [28–31]. Given the likely mechanisms involved (for a review of this topic, please see [29]), it has been proposed that altering the GI of carbohydrates consumed pre-match and at half-time, may help to counteract these responses in team sports athletes [29]. Theoretically, low GI carbohydrates produce a lower insulinaemic response and a slower delivery of glucose into the systemic circulation, thus helping to maintain blood glucose concentrations throughout the second half [29,31]. In support, Stevenson et al. [31] observed better maintenance of blood glucose concentrations during the second half of simulated soccer match-play when an 8% solution of low GI isomaltulose (GI: 32) was consumed during the pre-exercise warm-up and at half-time, when compared with an equivalent volume of high GI maltodextrin (GI: 90–100). Whilst no between-trial differences were observed for any performance measure, these findings appear to suggest a potential role for low GI carbohydrate sources for athletes engaged in intermittent team sports when ecologically valid feeding patterns are used.

It is well established that a heavy schedule of prolonged and/or intense exercise can lead to immunity impairment [32,33], and an increased risk of sustaining upper respiratory tract infections [34,35]. An in-depth discussion on the relationship between nutritional strategies and immune responses to exercise is beyond the scope of this article (interested readers please see [33,34,36]), but it is noteworthy that, whilst a viable short term approach for augmentation of endurance training adaptations [15,19,37], exercising in a carbohydrate-depleted state (i.e., following days of low carbohydrate intake and/or prior glycogen depleting exercise) elicits greater elevations in circulating stress hormones and further disruption of several markers of immune function (e.g., interleukin-6; IL-6, interleukin-1 receptor antagonist; IL-1ra and interleukin-10; IL-10), compared with when carbohydrate availability is greater [34]. In addition, consuming ~30–60 $g \cdot h^{-1}$ of carbohydrates during exercise, particularly throughout prolonged endurance exercise, may also attenuate many of these negative responses through better maintenance of blood glucose concentrations and a concomitant blunting of stress hormone release [33,34,36,38].

In addition to carbohydrates, supplementing with antioxidants may have the potential to somewhat counter the immune disturbances experienced following exercise. Whilst evidence for the efficacy of this strategy is at best mixed (see [33]), a 60 day program of antioxidant supplementation attenuated the cytokine (i.e., tumor necrosis factor alpha; TNF-α, interleukin-1 beta; IL-1β, and IL-6) response to a 45 min cycling bout, compared with when the same exercise was completed pre-supplementation [39]. It should be noted that homeostatic disruption may represent a key driver of cellular adaptations to training, and some evidence suggests that interventions aiming to artificially reduce oxidative stress (e.g., supplementing with high doses of antioxidants), have the potential to interfere with molecular signalling [15,33,40]. Although the impact on long-term training adaptations remains unclear, athletes seeking to maintain immune function may wish to initially consider a food-first approach, which prioritises consumption of a range of antioxidant- and phytochemical-rich foods [33].

It has been suggested that honey, due to its high carbohydrate content, may be a suitable energy source for athletes or exercising populations [3]. While possible gastric tolerance issues remain to be confirmed, when consumed around exercise, honey may provide multiple transportable carbohydrates as recommended for endurance athletes, whilst the lower GI of honey compared with that of most commercially available sports drinks has potential applications for athletes engaged in intermittent sports [29,31]. Moreover, honey exhibits natural antioxidant properties that may provide an appropriate balance between controlling the immunosuppressive response to exercise, and maintaining the signalling pathways necessary for positive training adaptation. To this end, a small body of research is beginning to surface surrounding the potential application of honey as a strategy to either enhance athletic performance, improve recovery, or otherwise influence responses to exercise. With this in mind, the aim of the current review was to systematically identify and appraise the current body of research that has examined the effects of honey supplementation in combination with exercise in humans.

2. Materials and Methods

This review was undertaken in accordance with the Preferred Reporting Items for Systematic Reviews and Meta-Analyses (PRISMA) guidelines [41]. Computerised searches were run in the online databases PubMed, Medline, and SPORTDiscus during May 2019, thus articles published up until this time were considered. The search strategy incorporated the terms (honey) AND (exercis* OR soccer OR football OR rugby OR cycling OR resistance-exercis* OR sport* OR dancer OR dancing OR cyclist* OR running OR runner* OR hockey OR basketball OR handball OR swim* OR "team sport*" OR team-sport* OR endurance OR performance OR rowing OR rower* OR sprint OR jump OR power

OR strength OR training OR hurling OR weightlift*), and the filters applied were: English language, humans, clinical trial, journal article, and peer-reviewed. References listed within bibliographies of the retrieved records, in addition to articles already known to the authors, were also considered for inclusion.

2.1. Study Selection

Based upon the specific aims of this review, studies identified from the original search strategy were systematically excluded according to the following criteria: (A) studies not conducted with living human participants; (B) studies which involved either no exercise stimulus, no nutritional intervention which included honey, or both; or (C) studies that were review articles.

2.2. Quality Assessment

After application of the pre-defined exclusion criteria, the remaining full text articles were assessed for methodological quality via the Physiotherapy Evidence Database (PEDro) scale. This assessment scores experimental studies out of a maximum of 10 points, based upon satisfaction of a range of criteria. Eight of these criteria evaluated a study's internal validity, and a further two criteria related to whether sufficient statistical information was presented. The PEDro scale has previously been identified as a valid and reliable indicator of methodological quality [42,43]. As per previous review papers in this field, only articles with a PEDro score of at least five out of 10 were included in order to improve the credibility of the analyses [44].

3. Results

A total of 273 records were identified through the original search strategy (including one record previously known to the authors). Following removal of 129 duplicates, 144 records were screened according to the pre-defined exclusion criteria. Of the 133 records excluded at this stage, 56 studies were not conducted with living human participants (exclusion criteria A); 71 involved either no exercise stimulus, no nutritional intervention which included honey, or both (exclusion criteria B); whilst six records were excluded on the basis that they were review articles (exclusion criteria C). When the remaining 11 full text articles were assessed for eligibility and quality, a further two records were excluded on the basis of scoring <5 out of 10 on the PEDro scale. Therefore, a total of nine articles were retained and included in this review (Figure 1).

In the nine eligible articles, outcomes were presented for 186 participants (individual study sample sizes ranging from nine to 40 participants), being mostly amateur athletes, of whom 125 were male and 61 were female. Four studies reported crossover, repeated measures designs, whilst five studies assigned participants to independent groups. Exercise modalities included team sport simulations, running, cycling, rowing, resistance exercise, and dance. Considerable methodological variation also existed with regards to the patterns and dosages of honey supplementation, with some studies feeding honey either before, during or after a single exercise session, and others investigating the effects of honey supplementation over several weeks (e.g., through a training 'block'). Articles were pooled according to three broad themes and two sub-themes (Tables 1–4), which are presented in turn below. Studies have examined the effects of honey supplementation (either acutely or over multiple weeks) on (a) biochemical markers, (b) physical and skilled performance, and (c) perceptual responses. A number of articles investigated multiple constructs and were therefore included within more than one theme.

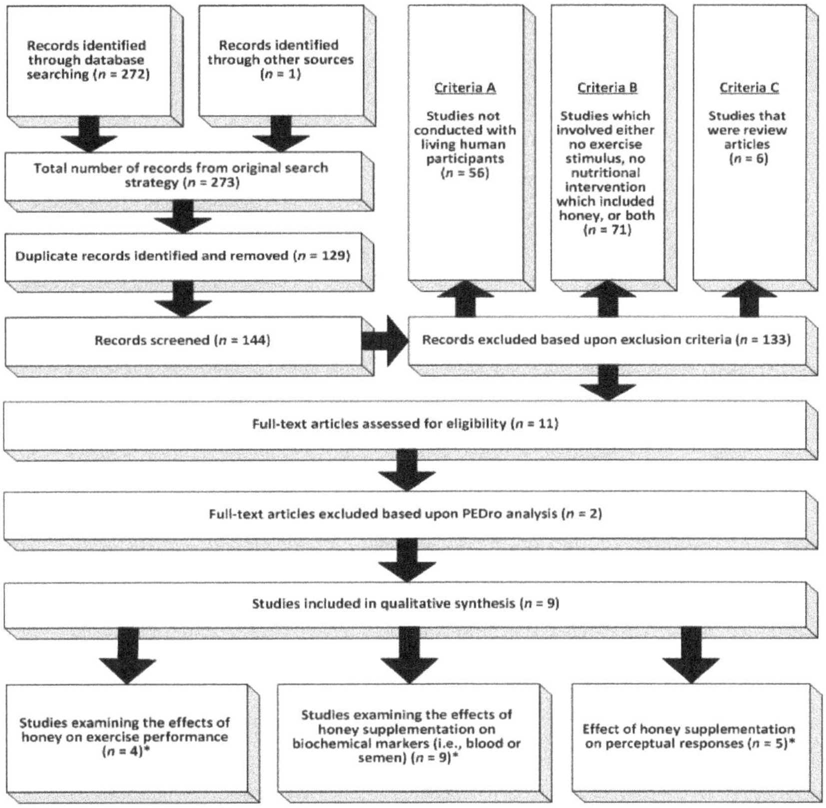

Figure 1. Selection process for articles included in the systematic review. * denotes that some studies examined multiple constructs, thus are included in more than one category.

3.1. *Effect of Honey Supplementation on Biochemical Markers (i.e., Blood or Semen)*

All nine eligible studies included at least one outcome variable derived from bodily fluid. Blood samples (venous or capillary) were taken in eight of these instances, whilst the remaining study derived indices of immune status from markers present within semen. As substantial methodological variation was observed, results are separated into (a) studies investigating the acute effects of honey consumption around a single exercise session (Table 1) and (b) those in which honey supplementation occurred over multiple weeks (Table 2).

3.1.1. Acute Honey Consumption around a Single Exercise Session

Five of the nine studies concerned the acute effects of honey supplementation (Table 1). In 59 males and 21 females, honey was administered in various doses, frequencies and forms (i.e., solution, gel, or powder) during rowing [45], cycling [46], and soccer specific exercise [47], as well as between running bouts in hot conditions [48], and immediately following resistance exercise [49]. Partly due to the inherent difficulty in consolidating findings from such different methodological approaches, the influence of acute honey supplementation on blood glucose concentrations and insulin responses during and following exercise remains inconclusive. In addition, consuming honey around a single exercise session appears to produce similar immune and hormonal (e.g., testosterone and cortisol concentrations) responses when compared with consumption of other carbohydrate sources.

3.1.2. Honey Supplementation over Multiple Weeks

The remaining four articles (involving a total of 76 males and 40 females) investigated biochemical changes when honey was consumed over periods ranging from 31 days to 16 weeks (Table 2). Three studies investigated immunological markers, two via blood samples, and one via semen analysis [50–52], whilst one study assessed whether honey supplementation combined with aerobic dance exercise influenced markers of bone formation and/or resorption [53]. Consuming 70 g honey prior to each training session over periods of eight to 16 weeks attenuated the negative immune response to a programme of moderate to intense cycling exercise when compared with no nutritional supplement [50,51]. Although potential benefits have been observed, the influence of daily honey supplementation is less clear with respect to markers of bone formation/resorption [53], and when consumed in smaller quantities (i.e., 3 × 10 mL of a honey and yeast product per day) over 31 days of running training [52]. Unfortunately, in each of these four studies it is unclear whether the groups used as comparators were energy or carbohydrate-matched compared with those consuming honey.

3.2. Effect of Honey Supplementation on Physical or Skilled Performance

Four eligible studies (Table 3) have assessed the influence of honey supplementation on at least one measure of physical or skilled performance in a total of 53 males. Three studies investigated the acute effects of honey consumption during team sport [47], running [48], or cycling [46] exercise, whilst one study used various cycling ergometer tests to assess the influence of consuming 70 g of honey 90 min prior to each training session on adaptations throughout a 16 week period of training [51]. Whilst benefits were observed when honey was compared to consuming no carbohydrate at all [46,48], findings have been largely inconsistent with regards to the influence of honey supplementation on exercise performance (Table 3).

3.3. Effect of Honey Supplementation on Perceptual Responses

Five articles have reported perceptual responses from a total of 59 males and 21 females, when honey was consumed before, during, or immediately after exercise (Table 4). A variety of Likert scales were employed to measure constructs relating to taste, texture, gut comfort, and perceived fatigue [45–49]. Although honey may elicit a sweeter taste compared with water [48], no differences in ratings of perceived exertion or perceptions of fatigue, either during or after exercise, were reported with honey as opposed to water or other forms of carbohydrate.

Table 1. Studies examining the effect of acute honey supplementation on biochemical responses to a single exercise session.

Study	Participants	Design	Exercise Stimulus	Nutritional Intervention	Data Collection Method and Time-Points	Outcome Variables	Main Results
Abbey and Rankin [47]	Male soccer players of NCAA Division I, post collegiate, and club standard (n = 10).	Randomised, single blind, crossover.	Soccer specific exercise (5 × 15 min blocks, plus 10 min half-time), followed by progressive 20 m shuttle run to fatigue.	6% CHO-electrolyte solution (honey, commercial sports drink, or placebo). 8.8 $mL{\cdot}kg^{-1}$ (0.5 g·kg·body $mass^{-1}$) CHO consumed 30 min pre-exercise and at half-time.	Blood samples at 30 min pre-exercise (T1), immediately post-exercise (T2), 60 min post-exercise (T3).	Blood glucose, insulin, cortisol, plasma volume, IL-1ra, IL-6 and IL-10, total ORAC, and plasma ORAC.	Plasma IL-1ra was ↓ at T2 for honey vs. sports drink, and ↓ at T3 for honey vs. placebo. ↔ between trials for glucose, insulin, cortisol, plasma volume, IL-6, IL-10, total or plasma ORAC.
Ahmad et al. [48]	Male runners of recreational standard (n = 10).	Randomised, single blind, crossover.	60 min run at ~65% $\dot{V}O_2$ max, followed by 2 h 'rehydration phase' and 20 min treadmill running test.	6.8% CHO solution (honey) or water to recover 150% of body mass lost during run one. Fluid consumed 0 min (60% of mass loss), 30 min (50%), and 60 min (40%) after run one.	Blood samples at pre (T1), immediately post (T2), 30 min post (T3), 60 min post (T4), 90 min post (T5), and 120 min post (T6) 60 min run, and immediately post 20 min run (T7).	Blood glucose, serum insulin, haematocrit, and serum osmolality.	Serum insulin was ↑ at T3-T6 for honey vs. water. Serum osmolality was ↑ at T4 for honey vs. water. ↔ between trials for glucose or haematocrit.
Earnest et al. [46]	Amateur male cyclists (n = 9).	Randomised, double blind, counterbalanced, crossover.	64 km time trial on cycling ergometer.	15 g of gel (honey, dextrose, or placebo) with 250 mL H_2O consumed every 16 km (5 × 15 g total) plus an additional 250 mL of water every 3.2 km.	Blood samples at pre-exercise (T1), 16 km (T2), 32 km (T3), 48 km (T4), and 64 km (T5).	Blood glucose and insulin concentrations.	↔ between trials for glucose or insulin. In dextrose, glucose at T4 was ↓ vs. T1 (not the case for honey or placebo).

Table 1. *Cont.*

Study	Participants	Design	Exercise Stimulus	Nutritional Intervention	Data Collection Method and Time-Points	Outcome Variables	Main Results
Kreider et al. [49]	Resistance trained individuals (n = 40; males: n = 19, females: n = 21).	Randomised, four independent groups.	3 sets of 10 repetitions at approximately 70% of 1RM on chest press, seated row, shoulder press, lat pulldown, leg extension, leg curl, biceps curl, triceps extension, and leg press.	40 g of whey protein with 120 g of either sucrose, powdered honey, or maltodextrin consumed within 5 min post-exercise. Other group consumed no supplement.	Blood samples at pre-exercise (T1), post exercise (T2), and 30 min (T3), 60 min (T4), 90 min (T5), and 120 min (T6) post-feeding.	Glucose, insulin, testosterone, cortisol, testosterone: cortisol ratio, WBC, neutrophils, total neutrophils: total lymphocytes ratio, creatinine, BUN, BUN: creatinine ratio, CK, LDH, AST, and ALT.	Glucose at T4 was ↑ for honey vs sucrose, and at T3 was ↑ for honey vs. sucrose, maltodextrin, and no CHO. Insulin at T3-T6 was ↑ for honey, sucrose, and maltodextrin vs. no CHO. ↔ between groups for testosterone, cortisol, testosterone:cortisol, WBC, neutrophils, total neutrophils, total lymphocytes, LDH, AST, or ALT. BUN: creatinine at T5, was ↑ for honey and maltodextrin, and at T6 was ↑ for honey and sucrose vs. no CHO.
Łagowska et al. [45]	Trained male rowers (n = 11).	Randomised, crossover.	Rowing ergometer: 2 × 40 min with a 5 min break, performed at an intensity corresponding to ~75% of the onset of blood lactate accumulation.	150 mL of CHO solution (either commercial sports drink; 7.8% CHO, or 'natural' drink containing banana, fruit juice, and honey; 6.7% CHO), consumed immediately pre-exercise and every 15 min during exercise (6 × 150 mL total).	Blood samples at pre-exercise (T1), and 3 min post-exercise (T2).	Blood glucose, lactate, chemical antioxidants, urea, CK, haematocrit, leukocytes, WBC, lymphocytes, monocytes, and granulocytes.	Glucose was ↓ at T2, for natural vs. commercial drink. Glucose at T2, was ↓ for natural, but ↑ for commercial drink vs. T1. Chemical antioxidant level at T2, was ↓ for natural vs. commercial drink. ↔ between trials for lactate, urea, CK, haematocrit, leukocytes, WBC, lymphocytes, monocytes, or granulocytes.

ALT: alanine aminotransaminase, AST: aspartate aminotransaminase, BUN: blood urea nitrogen, CHO: carbohydrate, CK: creatine kinase, IL-1ra: interleukin-1 receptor antagonist, IL-6: interleukin-6, IL-10: interleukin-10, LDH: lactate dehydrogenase, NCAA: National Collegiate Athletic Association, ORAC: oxygen radical absorbance capacity, WBC: white blood cell counts, 1RM: one repetition maximum, ↑: increased/higher, ↓: decreased/lower, ↔: no difference.

Table 2. Studies examining the effect of honey supplementation over the course of multiple weeks on biochemical responses to exercise.

Study	Participants	Design	Exercise Stimulus	Nutritional Intervention	Data Collection Method and Time-Points	Outcome Variables	Main Results
Gmunder et al. [52]	Long distance runners (n = 16: male: n = 13, female: n = 3). Standard not specified.	Randomised, double blind, two independent groups.	27 day training period, followed by 21 km running time trial.	3 × 10 mL per day (30 mL per day for 31 days) of either a supplement comprised of herbal yeast, malt, honey, and orange juice, or a supplement comprised of sucrose and caramel.	Blood samples at day 0 (T1), pre 21 km run at day 27 (T2), immediately post run (T3), two days post run (T4).	WBC, leukocyte counts, lymphocyte counts, Con A, CD3, CD4, CD16, CD16/8, CD19, IgA, IgE, IgM, IgG subclasses 1-4, β2M, IL-2 receptors, neopterin, plasma proteins, cortisol, adrenaline, noradrenaline.	↔ between groups for any blood marker. In honey, natural killer/suppressor cells (CD8, CD16, and CD16/8), and IgG subclass 1 at T4 were ↓, whilst Con A, and IgG subclass 2 at T4 were ↑ vs. T3 (not the case for sucrose). In sucrose, neopterin and β2M at T4 were ↓ vs. T3 (not the case for honey).
Hajizadeh et al. [51]	Amateur male cyclists (n = 24).	Randomised, two independent groups.	16 week training period.	70 g honey dissolved in 250 mL distilled water. Consumed 90 min prior to each training session for 16 weeks. Other group consumed no supplement.	Blood samples at week 0 (T1), immediately (T2), 12 h (T3), and 24 h (T4) after the last training session in week 8, and immediately (T5), 12 h (T6), 24 h (T7), 7 days (T8), and 30 days (T9) after the last training session in week 16.	Lymphocyte counts, DNA damage, IL-1β, IL-6, IL-8, IL-10, TNF-a, glutathione, TAS, hydrogen peroxide, and lipid peroxide.	Hydrogen peroxide, and lipid peroxide, IL-1β, IL-6, IL-10, and TNF-a at T2-T8, were ↓ for honey vs. no supplement. Glutathione at T4-T7 was ↑ for honey vs. no supplement. T2-T7 was ↑ for honey vs. no supplement.

Table 2. *Cont.*

Study	Participants	Design	Exercise Stimulus	Nutritional Intervention	Data Collection Method and Time-Points	Outcome Variables	Main Results
Ooi et al. [53]	Females (*n* = 37).	Four (matched) independent groups.	Two groups: 3 aerobic dance sessions per week for 6 weeks. Other two groups: no exercise.	Two groups: 20 g honey with 300 mL water consumed daily for 6 weeks. Other two groups: no supplementation.	Blood samples at week 0 (T1) and after week 6 (T2).	ALP and 1CTP.	ALP at T2 for honey, and honey plus exercise was ↑ vs. T1 (not the case with no honey). ↔ between groups for ALP or 1CTP. ↔ between T1 and T2 for 1CTP.
Tartiban and Maleki [50]	Male amateur road cyclists (*n* = 39).	Randomised, double blind, two independent groups.	8 weeks intensified training period.	70 g of honey or 70 g CHO-free sweetener, with 250 mL water. Consumed 90 min prior to each training session for 8 weeks.	Semen samples at week 0 (T1), immediately (T2), 12 h (T3), and 24 h (T4) after the last training session in week 4, and immediately (T5), 12 h (T6), and 24 h (T7) after the last training session in week 8.	Semen volume, motility, morphology, concentration, and number of spermatozoa, plus IL-1β, IL-6, IL-8, TNF-α, ROS, malondialdehyde, and antioxidants superoxide dismutase, catalase, and TAC.	Semen volume at T6 was ↑ for honey vs. placebo. Semen motility, morphology and TAC at T6-T7, semen concentration at T4-T5, number of spermatozoa at T2-T3 and T5-T7, catalase at T4 and T5-T7, and superoxide dismutase at T2-T3 and T5-T7 were all ↑ for honey vs. placebo. IL-1β at T2 and T5-T7, IL-6 at It2-T7, IL-8 at T2-T3, TNF-α at T4, ROS at T4-T7, and malondialdehyde at T5-T7 were all ↓ for honey vs. placebo.

ALP: serum alkaline phosphatase, β2m: beta-2 microglobulin, CD3: cluster of differentiation 3, CD4: cluster of differentiation 4, CD16: cluster of differentiation 16, CD16/8: cluster of differentiation 16/8, CD19: cluster of differentiation 19, CHO: carbohydrate, Con A: concanavalin A, IgA: immunoglobulin A, IgE: immunoglobulin E, IgM: immunoglobulin M, IgG immunoglobulin G, IL-1β: interleukin-1 beta, IL1ra: interleukin-1 receptor antagonist, IL-2: interleukin 2, IL-6: interleukin-6, IL-8: interleukin-8, IL-10: interleukin-10, LDH: lactate dehydrogenase, ORAC: oxygen radical absorbance capacity, ROS: reactive oxygen species, TAC: total antioxidant capacity, TAS: total antioxidant status, TNF-α: tumor necrosis factor alpha, WBC: white blood cell counts, 1CTP: serum C-terminal telopeptide of type 1 collagen, ↑: increased/higher, ↓: decreased/lower, ↔: no difference.

Table 3. Studies examining the effect of honey supplementation on exercise (physical or skilled) performance.

Study	Participants	Design	Exercise Stimulus	Nutritional Intervention	Data Collection Method and Time-Points	Outcome Variables	Main results
Abbey and Rankin [47]	Male soccer players of NCAA Division I, post collegiate, and club standard ($n = 10$).	Randomised, single blind, crossover.	Soccer specific exercise (5 × 15 min blocks, plus 10 min half-time), followed by progressive 20 m shuttle run to fatigue.	6% CHO-electrolyte solution (either honey, commercial sports drink, or placebo). 8.8 mL·kg^{-1} (0.5 g·kg·body mass^{-1}) CHO consumed 30 min pre-exercise and at half-time.	220 m running time trial, dribbling/agility assessment, and soccer shooting test all performed every 15 min during exercise: 220 m running time trial Progressive 20 m shuttle run to fatigue performed following 75 min of exercise.	Time taken to complete (time trial, and dribbling/ agility test), number of targets hit (shooting assessment). Time to exhaustion.	↔ between trials for any performance measure.
Ahmad et al. [48]	Male runners of recreational standard ($n = 10$).	Randomised, single blind, crossover.	60 min run at ~65% $\dot{V}O_2$ max, followed by 2 h 'rehydration phase' and 20 min treadmill running test.	Either 6.8% CHO solution (honey) or water, to recover 150% of body mass lost during run one consumed at 0 min (60% of mass loss), 30 min (50%), and 60 min (40%) after run one.	20 min treadmill running test performed 120 min following completion of 60 min run	Total distance covered.	20 min running performance was ↑ for honey vs. water.
Earnest et al. [46]	Amateur male cyclists ($n = 9$).	Randomised, double blind, counterbalanced, crossover.	64 km time trial on cycling ergometer.	15 g of gel (honey, dextrose, or placebo) with 250 mL water consumed every 16 km (5 × 15 g total). Plus an additional 250 mL of water every 3.2 km.	64 km cycling ergometer test.	Time taken to complete 64 km, and per 16 km. Mean power over 64 km, and per 16 km.	↔ between trials for time taken to complete, or mean power over 64 km. In honey and dextrose trials, mean power over 48–64 km was ↑ vs. 0–16 km, 16–32 km, and 32–48 km (not the case for placebo). In placebo, time taken for 48–64 km and 32–48 km was ↑ vs. 0–16 km, (not the case for honey or dextrose).

Table 3. *Cont.*

Study	Participants	Design	Exercise Stimulus	Nutritional Intervention	Data Collection Method and Time-Points	Outcome Variables	Main results
Hajizadeh et al. [51]	Amateur male road cyclists ($n = 24$).	Randomised, two independent groups.	16 week training period.	70 g honey dissolved in 250 mL distilled water. Consumed 90 min prior to each training session for 16 weeks. Other group consumed no supplement.	5 km, and 40 km cycling ergometer tests, and power assessment at week 0 (T1) and week 16 (T2).	Time taken to complete (5 km and 40 km tests), peak power output (power assessment).	↔ between groups for time taken to complete 5 km or 40 km, or peak power output at T2. For all measures, performance in both groups was ↑ at T2 vs. T1

CHO: carbohydrate, NCAA: National Collegiate Athletic Association, ↑: increased/higher, ↓: decreased/lower, ↔: no difference.

Table 4. Studies examining the effect of honey supplementation on perceptual responses around exercise.

Study	Participants	Design	Exercise Stimulus	Nutritional Intervention	Data collection Method and Time-Points	Outcome Variables	Main Results
Abbey and Rankin [47]	Male soccer players of NCAA Division I, post-collegiate, and club standard ($n = 10$).	Randomised, single blind crossover.	Soccer-specific exercise (5 × 15 min blocks, plus 10 min half-time), followed by progressive 20 m shuttle run to fatigue.	6% CHO-electrolyte solution (honey, commercial sports drink, or placebo). 8.8 mL·kg^{-1} (0.5 g·kg·body mass^{-1}) CHO consumed 30 min pre-exercise and at half-time.	Every 15 min during exercise, scale not reported.	RPE.	↔ between trials for RPE.
Ahmad et al. [48]	Male runners of recreational standard ($n = 10$).	Randomised, single blind crossover.	60 min run at ~65% $\dot{V}O_2$ max, followed by 2 h 'rehydration phase' and 20 min treadmill running test on.	6.8% CHO solution (honey) or H_2O to recover 150% of body mass lost during run one. Fluid consumed 0 min (60% of mass loss), 30 min (50%), and 60 min (40%) after run one.	Likert scale (1–5), 0 min (T1), 30 min (T2), and 60 min (T3) after run one.	Perceptions of thirst, sweetness, nausea, fullness and stomach upset.	Perceptions of sweetness at T1-T3 were ↑ for honey vs. for honey vs. water. ↔ between trials for perceptions of thirst nausea, fullness, or stomach upset between trials.

Table 4. *Cont.*

Study	Participants	Design	Exercise Stimulus	Nutritional Intervention	Data collection Method and Time-Points	Outcome Variables	Main Results
Earnest et al. [46]	Amateur male cyclists (n = 9).	Randomised, double blind, counterbalanced, crossover.	64 km time trial on cycling ergometer.	15 g of gel (honey, dextrose, or placebo) with 250 mL water consumed every 16 km. Plus an additional 250 mL of water every 3.2 km.	Likert scale (6–20) at pre-exercise, 16 km, 32 km, 48 km, and 64 km.	RPE.	↔ between trials for RPE.
Kreider et al. [49]	Resistance trained individuals (n = 40; males: n = 19, females: n = 21).	Randomised, four independent groups.	3 sets of 10 repetitions at approximately 70% of 1 RM on chest press, seated row, shoulder press, lat pulldown, leg extension, leg curl, biceps curl, triceps extension, and leg press.	40 g of whey protein with 120 g of either sucrose, powdered honey, or maltodextrin. Consumed within 5 min post-exercise. Other group consumed no supplement.	Likert scale (1–10) at pre-exercise (T1), post exercise (T2), and 30 min (T3), 60 min (t4), 90 min (T5), and 120 min (T6) post-feeding.	Severity of perceived hypoglycaemia, dizziness, fatigue, headache, and stomach upset.	↔ between groups for perceptions of hypoglycaemia, dizziness, fatigue, headache, or stomach upset.
Łagowska et al. [45]	Trained male rowers (n = 11).	Randomised, crossover.	Rowing ergometer: 2 × 40 min with a 5 min break, performed at an intensity corresponding to ~75% of the onset of blood lactate accumulation.	150 mL of CHO solution (either commercial sports drink; 7.8% CHO, or 'natural' drink containing banana, fruit juice, and honey; 6.7% CHO), consumed immediately pre-exercise and every 15 min during exercise (6 × 150 mL total).	Likert scale (1–5) at post-exercise:	Perceptions of taste, smell, thirst quenching ability, beverage consistency, and refreshment.	Satisfaction with beverage consistency was ↓ for natural vs. commercial drink. ↔ between trials for perceptions of taste, smell, thirst quenching ability, or refreshment.

CHO: carbohydrate, NCAA: National Collegiate Athletic Association, RPE: rating of perceived exertion, 1RM: one repetition maximum, ↑: increased/higher, ↓: decreased/lower, ↔: no difference.

4. Discussion

This review aimed to systematically evaluate the current body of research that has assessed the influence of honey supplementation on a number of physiological, performance, and perceptual responses to exercise. Whilst nine eligible articles were identified, substantial methodological variation exists between studies, thus making it difficult to draw firm conclusions with regards to the potential efficacy of honey supplementation for exercising populations. As is the case with many supplements, it seems likely that a number of factors, including but not limited to, the dose and timing of honey ingestion, individual responsiveness, and the type, duration, and/or intensity of exercise, modulate the responses observed [44].

4.1. Effect of Honey Supplementation on Biochemical Markers (i.e., Blood or Semen)

4.1.1. Acute Honey Consumption around a Single Exercise Session

One of the primary aims for athletes consuming carbohydrates before and during exercise is to maintain fuel availability (i.e., preserve glycogen stores and increase blood glucose concentrations) to help attenuate declines in performance as exercise progresses. With regards to honey consumption prior to and/or during an exercise bout, blood glucose responses have been largely inconsistent but notably the effects on glycogen degradation remain to be examined (Table 1).

Only one study has reported a statistically significant difference in blood glucose concentrations as a result of consuming a honey-containing supplement. Lagowska et al. [45] observed lower post-exercise blood glucose concentrations when a "natural" carbohydrate beverage containing honey, fruit juice, and banana was consumed during 80 min (2 × 40 min, separated by 5 min) of rowing exercise, compared with a commercially available carbohydrate solution. Whilst the reasons for these findings remain unclear, the differential responses may be attributable to the amount of carbohydrate consumed. Although both conditions entailed consumption of six boluses of 150 mL of solution (i.e., one every 15 min during exercise), the "natural" drink contained 6.7% carbohydrates, whereas the comparator was a 7.8% solution. It seems likely that differences in the absolute quantity of carbohydrate consumed, irrespective of source, may at least partly explain the differential blood glucose responses in favour of the higher amount. Unfortunately, because the precise quantity of each constituent within the two drinks was not reported, further speculation is rendered difficult.

Blood glucose concentration maintenance may be of particular interest to athletes engaged in sports which require high levels of technical skill (e.g., team sport athletes). Whist a definitive link between hypoglycaemia and reductions in sport-specific physical or skilled performance has not yet been established in exercising participants, the role of blood glucose in brain function is clear. Indeed, the brain is one of the few human organs that relies heavily on blood glucose to maintain optimal functioning [54]. Notably, exercise studies have indicated that the rate of cerebral glucose uptake begins to decline when blood glucose concentrations fall below ~3.6 mmol·L^{-1} [55], a concentration which has previously been observed in team sport players ~15–30 min following half-time [28]. Moreover, the link between blood glucose concentrations and cognitive functioning is highlighted by increased fine motor speed, psycho-motor speed, and visual discrimination speed accompanying increased glycaemia following soccer match-play in the heat [56]. As cognitive processes are likely to be vital, not only to the skilled actions involved in team sports but also to tactical and/or strategic decision making, nutritional strategies that help maintain or increase blood glucose concentrations could be of benefit to team sports players during the latter stages of a match [29]. Given its typical carbohydrate composition (i.e., containing primarily low GI fructose), there exists a theoretical basis to suggest honey as a potentially worthwhile intervention in this context [29].

When high GI carbohydrates are consumed during team sport specific exercise, a temporary lowering of blood glucose concentrations may be experienced during the early stages of the second half [28–31]. To date, only one study has combined honey supplementation with simulated soccer match-play, and no differences in insulin or blood glucose concentrations were observed immediately or one hour following exercise cessation when either a honey solution, a carbohydrate-matched commercially available sports drink, or an energy-free placebo were consumed [47]. However, because blood samples were not taken regularly throughout exercise, whether or not honey influenced transient changes in blood glucose responses as seen previously, remains unclear. Given the role of blood glucose concentrations in the maintenance of brain function, future research into the potential influence of honey supplementation on blood glucose concentrations, in addition to physical, skilled, and cognitive performance throughout intermittent exercise, would be worthwhile.

Other studies involving honey consumption prior to and/or during exercise have also reported no significant treatment effects for blood glucose concentrations [46,48]. Notwithstanding, blood glucose concentrations were maintained throughout a 64 km cycling time-trial when 15 g of either honey or dextrose were consumed every 16 km [46]. In contrast, in the placebo condition, blood glucose concentrations had declined after 48 km relative to the initial 16 km [46]. Although no differences between honey and dextrose were observed, it is unclear whether the honey and dextrose trials were carbohydrate- or energy-matched. Indeed, whilst the authors state that 15 g of gel was consumed in each condition, it should be considered that whereas dextrose is ~100% carbohydrate, honey in its natural form may be only ~80% carbohydrate or less [2]. The lack of information regarding whether carbohydrates were consumed in equivalent doses makes interpretation of the results difficult, but if discrepancies existed, the differences in absolute carbohydrate intake may have influenced the results in addition to the source of carbohydrates alone.

Alongside providing amino acids for muscle repair and fluid for rehydration, rapid replenishment of glycogen stores is of primary importance for facilitating recovery following exercise [17,57]. Moreover, co-ingesting carbohydrates and protein during the post-exercise period may help to promote an anabolic environment, offset the acute immunosuppressive effects of intense exercise, and facilitate glycogen restoration [17,19,33,57]. Krieder et al. [49] investigated the effects of consuming 40 g whey protein alongside 120 g of either sucrose, powdered honey, or maltodextrin within five minutes of completing a bout of resistance exercise. When compared with individuals taking no supplement, all three carbohydrate groups returned higher insulin concentrations at 30, 60, 90 and 120 min post-feeding. Although this may be expected given that carbohydrates and whey protein are insulinogenic [58], it is interesting to note that blood glucose concentrations in the honey group were higher after 30 min post-feeding compared with those in the sucrose group, and higher than all three other conditions at 60 min following consumption. In keeping with the lower GI of honey compared with the other sources of carbohydrate assessed, these patterns appear to suggest a more prolonged appearance of carbohydrate in the bloodstream when honey was consumed. Whilst no treatment effect was observed for testosterone or cortisol, these blood glucose and insulin responses may suggest potential for the use of honey when post-exercise recovery is required.

When honey is consumed prior to, and/or during, a single exercise session, limited effects have been observed with regards to immunological markers (Table 1). Although the plasma IL-1ra response to team sport specific exercise was dampened following honey supplementation (i.e., a 6% solution providing a total of 1 $g \cdot kg^{-1}$ body mass) compared with when a commercial sports drink or carbohydrate-free placebo were consumed, similar IL-6 responses were observed [47]. The authors thus proposed that the antioxidant and/or polyphenol content of the honey supplement may have somewhat interrupted the intracellular production or release of IL-1ra in response to exercise-induced elevations in IL-6. Conversely, previous carbohydrate research showed that ingesting a 6.4% glucose and maltodextrin solution before, and at 15 min intervals during, simulated soccer match-play attenuated a number of post-exercise immune disturbances (i.e., increases in plasma cortisol and IL-6, and inhibition of bacterially stimulated neutrophil degranulation), compared with a placebo [59]. Although comparisons are complicated by inconsistencies in the specific methods employed (i.e., length of exercise bout, pattern, dose, and type of carbohydrate provision, and the time-frame of measurement), it appears plausible that differences in blood glucose responses may at least partially explain the divergent findings. In support, increases in stress hormone concentrations during exercise may be attenuated when blood glucose is maintained via the feeding of exogenous carbohydrates [33,34,36,38]. That said, Abbey and Rankin [47] observed no differences in blood glucose concentrations between the honey, commercial beverage, and placebo conditions.

Although the evidence remains limited (Table 1), other studies have also shown that honey exhibits similar effects on immunological responses compared with other carbohydrate sources, at least where acute consumption around a single exercise session is concerned [45,49]. More well-controlled research is therefore required to determine whether honey has any ameliorating influence on immune markers, compared with that provided by other sources of carbohydrate.

4.1.2. Honey Supplementation over Multiple Weeks

In contrast to findings from acute honey supplementation studies, the literature available to date suggests that honey, consumed over the course of multiple weeks, may dampen the inflammatory response to periods of repeated exercise [50,51]. Indeed, ingesting 70 g of unprocessed honey ~90 min prior to each training session over 16 weeks of moderate-to-intense cycling training resulted in reduced plasma cytokine (i.e., IL-1β, IL-6, IL-10, and TNF-α) concentrations immediately, 12 h, and 24 h after the last training session in the eighth week, and immediately, 12 h, 24 h, and seven days after the last training session in week 16, compared with when no supplement was consumed [51]. Moreover, glutathione levels and total antioxidant status were higher with honey supplementation. Very similar patterns of cytokine and antioxidant responses were reported when Tartiban et al. [50] implemented the same supplementation and exercise strategy over an eight week period. This latter study, albeit investigating semen as opposed to blood markers, also noted reductions in indices of oxidative stress (i.e., reactive oxygen species and malondialdehyde) when honey was consumed throughout the eight week period. Whilst oxidative stress may play an important role in cellular adaptations to training [15,33,40], these studies in amateur male cyclists appear to demonstrate a potential application for honey supplementation during periods in which reductions in exercise-induced immune disturbances are desired. However, whilst it was stated that all participants were advised to maintain their normal diets for the duration of both investigations, and that diet diaries were completed to ensure compliance, neither articles provided detailed information outlining participants' overall energy, or macronutrient intake and/or distribution. As carbohydrate availability may influence immunological responses to exercise [34], it remains unclear whether the reported results stem from the inherent properties of honey itself, or simply reflect the outcome of an increased carbohydrate or energy intake in the honey group. In addition, more research, using ecologically valid and robust methods, is required to determine whether attenuation of acute immunological perturbations results in decreased incidences of infection.

In contrast to the above studies in cyclists [50,51], Gmunder et al. [52] reported no significant between-group differences in immunological responses to a 21 km run completed after 27 days of treatment when participants consumed 30 mL per day of either a supplement containing (a) herbal yeast, malt, honey, and orange juice, or (b) sucrose and caramel. Whilst definitive conclusions are difficult to draw, it seems plausible that the absolute quantity of honey consumed by runners in this study was insufficient to confer any antioxidant effect. Indeed, the primary health benefits of honey consumption have been demonstrated with intakes >50 g [3]. Considering the paucity of well-controlled studies published to date, further work is required to investigate the immunological effects of acute and longer term honey supplementation within exercising populations. In particular, research examining the effects of different variables which may influence the efficacy of supplementation; such as dose, duration and/or form of honey supplementation, different exercise modalities and/or intensities, different levels of athlete, and/or the role played by an individual's starting nutritional status, would be of particular interest [3,44]. From a practical perspective, the relationship between potential reductions in immunological perturbations as a result of honey supplementation and (a) the risk of developing an infection, (b) recovery and subsequent exercise performance, and (c) long-term training adaptations, must represent a research priority to help guide practitioners and athletes.

Ooi et al. [53] studied 37 females over the course of six weeks with an interest in markers of bone formation (i.e., serum alkaline phosphatase) and resorption (i.e., serum C-terminal telopeptide of type 1 collagen). Participants were assigned to one of four groups, whereby two groups performed aerobic dance exercises three times per week (with one group also consuming 20 g honey per day), whilst the remaining two groups remained sedentary (again with one group also consuming 20 g honey per day). Although there were no differences for either outcome variable when groups were directly compared, the two groups who consumed honey experienced significant increases in serum alkaline phosphatase, tentatively indicating greater bone formation over the six week period. In contrast, both non-supplemented groups maintained similar levels at week six compared with week zero [53]. Honey supplementation has previously shown potential to enhance markers of bone structure in rodent studies [60], and it could be the case that certain components such as vitamin K, and minerals such as calcium, phosphorus, iron, and magnesium found in honey contribute to improved bone health, especially when combined with an exercise programme.

4.2. Effect of Honey Supplementation on Physical or Skilled Performance

It is recommended that consuming carbohydrates prior to, and during, exercise may enhance indices of physical (i.e., time to exhaustion) and skilled (i.e., soccer passing and shooting accuracy) performance [14,16,19–23,44]. Moreover, combining different forms of carbohydrates may increase oxidation rates and allow for worthwhile ingestion of a greater overall total volume of exogenous energy during prolonged endurance exercise [14,26,27]. Given that honey contains multiple sources of carbohydrates (i.e., primarily fructose and glucose), this natural substance seems intuitively able to offer potential as a "food-first" approach to carbohydrate supplementation. However, studies investigating the influence of honey on physical or skilled performance have reported mixed results (Table 3), with only one investigation reporting a clear performance benefit [48].

When amateur runners used a 6.8% Acacia honey solution to restore ~150% of body mass losses following a 60 min run in the heat, improved running performance (i.e., distance covered) versus ingestion of an equivalent volume of water occurred during the 20 min treadmill test that followed 120 min later [48]. Given the established role of carbohydrate–electrolyte beverages in fuelling for, and recovering from, exercise, such findings are not unexpected. However, because no carbohydrate-matched alternative to honey was assessed, it cannot be determined whether the positive outcomes are linked the unique properties of honey, or a result of carbohydrate consumption (i.e., as opposed to water) per se.

Whilst no significant between-condition differences were observed for overall time taken to complete a 64 km time-trial, ingesting 15 g of either honey or dextrose in gel form every 16 km enabled cyclists to maintain average 16 km time throughout the duration of exercise, and to increase average power output during the final 16 km compared with the preceding 16 km segments [46]. In contrast, when an energy-free placebo was consumed, significant declines in performance were observed over 48–64 km compared with the opening 16 km of exercise. Although this investigation identified no differences between honey and dextrose for any performance measure, the rate of carbohydrate consumption may have been a factor. Indeed, because carbohydrates consumed from a single source (i.e., glucose) may be oxidised at up to ~60 $g{\cdot}h^{-1}$, the full benefits of consuming multiple transportable carbohydrates (i.e., in terms of increased oxidation rates) may not be realised until absolute carbohydrate intake exceeds this level [14]. Moreover, a clear dose-response relationship exists between carbohydrate intake and endurance performance [14,61,62]. As noted above in relation to blood glucose responses, it is unclear whether the honey and dextrose trials were carbohydrate- or energy-matched. Due to reporting being vague on this matter, there is the potential that discrepancies in absolute carbohydrate intake may have influenced the results in addition to the source of carbohydrates alone.

With regards to intermittent exercise, carbohydrate supplementation has previously demonstrated benefits in terms of maintaining physical and skilled performance during the latter stages of simulated team sport match-play, whether consumed frequently (i.e., every 15 min) during exercise [28,30] or in more ecologically valid feeding patterns (i.e., before exercise and at half-time) [23]. However, ingesting a honey solution containing 6% carbohydrates demonstrated no benefit to any measure of physical or skilled performance assessed either during, or immediately following, 75 min of soccer specific exercise, when compared with a carbohydrate-matched commercially available sports drink and an energy-free placebo [46]. Whilst it may appear surprising that neither carbohydrate intervention influenced performance, it has been suggested that when limited opportunities exist to ingest carbohydrates, consuming solutions containing upwards of 10% carbohydrates may enable ergogenic rates of energy intake (e.g., >50 $g{\cdot}h^{-1}$) to be achieved whilst minimising abdominal discomfort [29]. For example, Harper et al. [23] observed significant improvements in dribbling speed and self-paced exercise performance during the latter stages of simulated soccer match-play when a 12% carbohydrate–electrolyte solution was delivered in 250 mL boluses prior to the beginning of each half, compared with either water or an electrolyte placebo. Future research into the effects of consuming higher concentrations of honey (i.e., ≥10% carbohydrate) on physical, skilled, and cognitive performance during team sport specific exercise would be beneficial.

Whilst short periods of deliberately training with low endogenous and exogenous carbohydrate availability may promote positive training adaptations through increases in mitochondrial enzyme activity, increases in lipid oxidation, and potential improvements in exercise capacity [15,19,37], consuming a diet rich in carbohydrates may help athletes to fuel and recover from training and thus itself promote beneficial responses via an increase in training intensity [19]. In the only eligible study to have investigated the performance effects of honey supplementation over a period of multiple days, amateur male road cyclists who supplemented with 70 g of honey 90 min prior to each training session demonstrated no additional improvements in 5 km or 40 km cycling time-trial performance, or peak power output over a 16 week period compared with those taking no supplement [51]. Unfortunately, detailed dietary analysis was not provided, thus it is not possible to comment upon the adequacy of, or differences in, overall carbohydrate intake in either group over the 16 week duration. Well-controlled research to determine whether longer-term honey consumption translates into favourable performance adaptations will be difficult to conduct. Whilst longer-term consumption may have a number of other benefits for health and wellbeing [3,5,7], research into the performance effects of honey supplementation on an acute level (i.e., immediately prior to and/or during exercise) may have a more sound theoretical underpinning.

4.3. *Effect of Honey Supplementation on Perceptual Responses*

Honey has demonstrated similar effects on subjective ratings of effort, compared with when other sources of carbohydrates, energy free placebos, or water have been consumed (Table 4). Such findings reflect previous reports in relation to intermittent exercise, whereby nutritional interventions failed to influence perceived exertion [30,31]. Moreover, whilst possible reductions in ratings of perceived exertion have been observed during prolonged endurance cycling when a mixture of glucose and fructose were consumed versus glucose alone, these responses occurred at substantially higher rates of carbohydrate ingestion (i.e., 90 $g{\cdot}h^{-1}$) than those provided by the studies presented in this review [63]. Indeed, the only perceptual responses affected by honey consumption relate to flavour and texture as opposed to exertion or fatigue. Specifically, a honey solution elicited a sweeter taste compared with plain water [48], and a natural beverage based upon honey, banana, and fruit juice provided a less satisfying consistency than a commercially available sports drink [45]. Within tolerable limits, sweeter tasting beverages may promote increases in voluntary fluid intake during exercise [64], and such findings may suggest a potential application of honey to encourage a greater rate of carbohydrate consumption in individuals suffering from flavour fatigue.

The fact that a honey solution (6% carbohydrate) produced similar perceptions of thirst, nausea, fullness, and stomach upset compared with plain water [48], may be an important observation. One of the traditional concerns with recommending low GI carbohydrates around exercise has surrounded the risk of gastric distress when the time-frame for appearance of exogenous carbohydrate is prolonged [65].

Although Ahmad et al. [48] only assessed perceptual responses immediately after each carbohydrate feeding, and not during the 20 min exercise bout that followed, previous research incorporating soccer match simulation has shown similar abdominal discomfort values when an 8% isomaltulose solution was consumed, compared with an equivalent volume of high GI maltodextrin [31]. Taken together, these studies may provide food for thought for practitioners and athletes who may previously have been deterred from considering lower GI carbohydrates before and during exercise.

5. Conclusions and Future Research Recommendations

Due to the potential health benefits and to offset the risks posed by supplement contamination, many athletes, practitioners and researchers espouse a "food-first" approach to sports nutrition. As honey is a natural substance comprised of ~80% carbohydrate (primarily fructose and glucose), and is known to possess antioxidant, antimicrobial, and anti-inflammatory properties, there exists a theoretical basis for its use as a nutritional supplement in exercising populations. This review summarised the available literature which has investigated the effects of honey supplementation when combined with exercise over a number of different time-frames, dosages, and modalities. Whilst the large methodological differences within the studies represented a substantial limitation, information is presented which may inform worthwhile future research.

Compared with other forms of carbohydrate, honey ingestion has had a similar effect on exercise performance, perceptions of fatigue, blood glucose concentrations, and immunological responses when consumed immediately prior to and/or during exercise, although some positive influence has been observed. When routinely consumed over multiple weeks, honey may attenuate many of the immune perturbations typically associated with a programme of moderate-to-intense exercise. Unfortunately, the research designs employed and the level of detail with which the methods have been reported make it difficult to establish whether the observed responses are attributable to the intrinsic properties of honey itself, or reflect other factors such as discrepancies in carbohydrate intake between conditions. Similarly, the same limitations mean that honey may have had certain effects (either positive or negative) which could have been masked by "noise" from external influences. Despite the lack of conclusive evidence, theory supports the use of honey, particularly as a potential ergogenic aid when consumed around exercise. Future research should take a robust approach to assessing whether honey may offer benefits to physical, skilled, or cognitive performance during different modalities, durations, and intensities of exercise, when directly compared to equivalent volumes of carbohydrates delivered in traditional forms. From these authors' perspective, the application to skilled performance during team sports may be of particular interest. Moreover, studies directly comparing the responses of male and female athletes would be a valuable addition to the knowledge base.

Author Contributions: S.P.H., P.M., C.W., and M.R. contributed to the structure and writing of the article. All authors were also involved in reviewing the available literature, and highlighting opportunities for future research.

References

1. Council, E. Council Directive 2001/110/EC of 20 December 2001 relating to honey. *Off. J. Eur. Commun. L* **2002**, *10*, 47–52.
2. Schneider, M.; Coyle, S.; Warnock, M.; Gow, I.; Fyfe, L. Anti-microbial activity and composition of manuka and portobello honey. *Phytother. Res.* **2013**, *27*, 1162–1168. [CrossRef] [PubMed]
3. Bogdanov, S.; Jurendic, T.; Sieber, R.; Gallmann, P. Honey for nutrition and health: A review. *J. Am. Coll. Nutr.* **2008**, *27*, 677–689. [CrossRef] [PubMed]
4. Manyi-Loh, C.E.; Clarke, A.M.; Ndip, N. An overview of honey: Therapeutic properties and contribution in nutrition and human health. *Afr. J. Microbiol. Res.* **2011**, *5*, 844–852.

5. Erejuwa, O.O.; Sulaiman, S.A.; Ab Wahab, M.S. Honey: A novel antioxidant. *Molecules* **2012**, *17*, 4400–4423. [CrossRef]
6. Ahmed, S.; Othman, N.H. Review of the medicinal effects of tualang honey and a comparison with manuka honey. *Malays. J. Med. Sci.* **2013**, *20*, 6–13.
7. Samarghandian, S.; Farkhondeh, T.; Samini, F. Honey and health: A review of recent clinical research. *Pharmacogn. Res.* **2017**, *9*, 121.
8. Meo, S.A.; Al-Asiri, S.A.; Mahesar, A.L.; Ansari, M.J. Role of honey in modern medicine. *Saudi J. Biol. Sci.* **2017**, *24*, 975–978. [CrossRef]
9. Conti, M.E.; Stripeikis, J.; Campanella, L.; Cucina, D.; Tudino, M.B. Characterization of Italian honeys (Marche Region) on the basis of their mineral content and some typical quality parameters. *Chem. Cent. J.* **2007**, *1*, 14. [CrossRef]
10. Batista, B.; Da Silva, L.; Rocha, B.; Rodrigues, J.; Berretta-Silva, A.; Bonates, T.; Gomes, V.; Barbosa, R.; Barbosa, F. Multi-element determination in Brazilian honey samples by inductively coupled plasma mass spectrometry and estimation of geographic origin with data mining techniques. *Food Res. Int.* **2012**, *49*, 209–215. [CrossRef]
11. Deibert, P.; König, D.; Kloock, B.; Groenefeld, M.; Berg, A. Glycaemic and insulinaemic properties of some German honey varieties. *Eur. J. Clin. Nutr.* **2010**, *64*, 762–764. [CrossRef] [PubMed]
12. Atkinson, F.S.; Foster-Powell, K.; Brand-Miller, J.C. International tables of glycemic index and glycemic load values: 2008. *Diabetes Care* **2008**, *31*, 2281–2283. [CrossRef] [PubMed]
13. Robert, S.D.; Ismail, A. Two varieties of honey that are available in Malaysia gave intermediate glycemic index values when tested among healthy individuals. *Biomed. Pap. Med. Fac. Univ. Palacky Olomouc Czech. Repub.* **2009**, *153*, 145–147. [CrossRef] [PubMed]
14. Jeukendrup, A. A step towards personalized sports nutrition: Carbohydrate intake during exercise. *Sports Med.* **2014**, *44*, 25–33. [CrossRef]
15. Close, G.L.; Hamilton, D.L.; Philp, A.; Burke, L.M.; Morton, J.P. New strategies in sport nutrition to increase exercise performance. *Free Radic. Biol. Med.* **2016**, *98*, 144–158. [CrossRef] [PubMed]
16. Coyle, E.F.; Coggan, A.R.; Hemmert, M.; Ivy, J.L. Muscle glycogen utilization during prolonged strenuous exercise when fed carbohydrate. *J. Appl. Physiol.* **1986**, *61*, 165–172. [CrossRef] [PubMed]
17. Burke, L.M.; van Loon, L.J.; Hawley, J.A. Postexercise muscle glycogen resynthesis in humans. *J. Appl. Physiol.* **2016**, *122*, 1055–1067. [CrossRef] [PubMed]
18. Hawley, J.A.; Schabort, E.J.; Noakes, T.D.; Dennis, S.C. Carbohydrate-loading and exercise performance. *Sports Med.* **1997**, *24*, 73–81. [CrossRef]
19. Burke, L.M.; Hawley, J.A.; Wong, S.H.; Jeukendrup, A.E. Carbohydrates for training and competition. *J. Sports Sci.* **2011**, *29*, S17–S27. [CrossRef]
20. Jeukendrup, A.E. Carbohydrate intake during exercise and performance. *Nutrition* **2004**, *20*, 669–677. [CrossRef]
21. Jeukendrup, A.E. Carbohydrate feeding during exercise. *Eur. J. Sports Sci.* **2008**, *8*, 77–86. [CrossRef]
22. Nicholas, C.W.; Williams, C.; Lakomy, H.K.; Phillips, G.; Nowitz, A. Influence of ingesting a carbohydrate-electrolyte solution on endurance capacity during intermittent, high-intensity shuttle running. *J. Sports Sci.* **1995**, *13*, 283–290. [CrossRef] [PubMed]
23. Harper, L.D.; Stevenson, E.J.; Rollo, I.; Russell, M. The influence of a 12% carbohydrate-electrolyte beverage on self-paced soccer-specific exercise performance. *J. Sci. Med. Sport* **2017**, *20*, 1123–1129. [CrossRef] [PubMed]
24. Burke, L.M.; Maughan, R.J. The Governor has a sweet tooth–mouth sensing of nutrients to enhance sports performance. *Eur. J. Sports Sci.* **2015**, *15*, 29–40. [CrossRef] [PubMed]
25. Rodriguez, N.R.; Di, N.M.; Langley, S. American College of Sports Medicine position stand. Nutrition and athletic performance. *Med. Sci. Sport Exerc.* **2009**, *41*, 709–731.
26. Currell, K.; Jeukendrup, A. Superior endurance performance with ingestion of multiple transportable carbohydrates. *Med. Sci. Sport Exerc.* **2008**, *40*, 275. [CrossRef] [PubMed]
27. Triplett, D.; Doyle, J.A.; Rupp, J.C.; Benardot, D. An isocaloric glucose-fructose beverage's effect on simulated 100-km cycling performance compared with a glucose-only beverage. *Int. J. Sport Nutr. Exerc. Metab.* **2010**, *20*, 122–131. [CrossRef] [PubMed]

28. Kingsley, M.; Penas-Ruiz, C.; Terry, C.; Russell, M. Effects of carbohydrate-hydration strategies on glucose metabolism, sprint performance and hydration during a soccer match simulation in recreational players. *J. Sci. Med. Sport* **2014**, *17*, 239–243. [CrossRef] [PubMed]
29. Hills, S.; Russell, M. Carbohydrates for soccer: A focus on skilled actions and half-time practices. *Nutrients* **2017**, *10*, 22. [CrossRef] [PubMed]
30. Russell, M.; Benton, D.; Kingsley, M. Influence of carbohydrate supplementation on skill performance during a soccer match simulation. *J. Sci. Med. Sport* **2012**, *15*, 348–354. [CrossRef] [PubMed]
31. Stevenson, E.J.; Watson, A.; Theis, S.; Holz, A.; Harper, L.D.; Russell, M. A comparison of isomaltulose versus maltodextrin ingestion during soccer-specific exercise. *Eur. J. Appl. Physiol.* **2017**, *117*, 2321–2333. [CrossRef] [PubMed]
32. Walsh, N.P.; Gleeson, M.; Shephard, R.J.; Gleeson, M.; Woods, J.A.; Bishop, N.; Fleshner, M.; Green, C.; Pedersen, B.K.; Hoffman-Goete, L.; et al. Position statement part one: Immune function and exercise. *Exerc. Immunol. Rev.* **2011**, *17*, 6–63. [PubMed]
33. Peake, J.M.; Neubauer, O.; Walsh, N.P.; Simpson, R.J. Recovery of the immune system after exercise. *J. Appl. Physiol.* **2016**, *122*, 1077–1087. [CrossRef] [PubMed]
34. Gleeson, M.; Nieman, D.C.; Pedersen, B.K. Exercise, nutrition and immune function. *J. Sports Sci.* **2004**, *22*, 115–125. [CrossRef] [PubMed]
35. Nieman, D.C.; Johanssen, L.M.; Lee, J.W.; Arabatzis, K. Infectious episodes in runners before and after the Los Angeles Marathon. *J. Sports Med. Phys. Fitness* **1990**, *30*, 316–328. [PubMed]
36. Walsh, N.P.; Gleeson, M.; Pyne, D.B.; Nieman, D.C.; Dhabhar, F.S.; Shephard, R.J.; Oliver, S.J.; Bermon, S.; Kajeniene, A. Position statement part two: Maintaining immune health. *Exerc. Immunol. Rev.* **2011**, *17*, 64–103. [PubMed]
37. Bartlett, J.D.; Hawley, J.A.; Morton, J.P. Carbohydrate availability and exercise training adaptation: Too much of a good thing? *Eur. J. Sport Sci.* **2015**, *15*, 3–12. [CrossRef] [PubMed]
38. Nieman, D.C.; Nehlsen-Cannarella, S.L.; Fagoaga, O.R.; Henson, D.A.; Utter, A.; Davis, J.M.; Williams, F.; Butterworth, D.E. Influence of mode and carbohydrate on the cytokine response to heavy exertion. *Med. Sci. Sport Exerc.* **1998**, *30*, 671–678. [CrossRef]
39. Vassilakopoulos, T.; Karatza, M.-H.; Katsaounou, P.; Kollintza, A.; Zakynthinos, S.; Roussos, C. Antioxidants attenuate the plasma cytokine response to exercise in humans. *J. Appl. Physiol.* **2003**, *94*, 1025–1032. [CrossRef]
40. Morrison, D.; Hughes, J.; Della Gatta, P.A.; Mason, S.; Lamon, S.; Russell, A.P.; Wadley, G.D. Vitamin C and E supplementation prevents some of the cellular adaptations to endurance-training in humans. *Free Radic. Biol. Med.* **2015**, *89*, 852–862. [CrossRef]
41. Liberati, A.; Altman, D.G.; Tetzlaff, J.; Mulrow, C.; Gøtzsche, P.C.; Ioannidis, J.P.; Clarke, M.; Devereaux, P.J.; Kleijnen, J.; Moher, D. The PRISMA statement for reporting systematic reviews and meta-analyses of studies that evaluate health care interventions: Explanation and elaboration. *PLoS Med.* **2009**, *6*, e1000100. [CrossRef] [PubMed]
42. Maher, C.G.; Sherrington, C.; Herbert, R.D.; Moseley, A.M.; Elkins, M. Reliability of the PEDro scale for rating quality of randomized controlled trials. *Phys. Ther.* **2003**, *83*, 713–721. [PubMed]
43. De Morton, N.A. The PEDro scale is a valid measure of the methodological quality of clinical trials: A demographic study. *Aust. J. Physiother.* **2009**, *55*, 129–133. [CrossRef]
44. Russell, M.; Kingsley, M. The efficacy of acute nutritional interventions on soccer skill performance. *Sports Med.* **2014**, *44*, 957–970. [CrossRef] [PubMed]
45. Łagowska, K.; Podgórski, T.; Celińska, E.; Wiertel, Ł.; Kryściak, J. A comparison of the effectiveness of commercial and natural carbohydrate–electrolyte drinks. *Sci. Sports* **2017**, *32*, 160–164. [CrossRef]
46. Earnest, C.P.; Lancaster, S.L.; Rasmussen, C.J.; Kerksick, C.M.; Lucia, A.; Greenwood, M.C.; Almada, A.L.; Cowan, P.A.; Kreider, R.B. Low vs. high glycemic index carbohydrate gel ingestion during simulated 64-km cycling time trial performance. *J. Strength Cond. Res.* **2004**, *18*, 466–472. [PubMed]
47. Abbey, E.L.; Rankin, J.W. Effect of ingesting a honey-sweetened beverage on soccer performance and exercise-induced cytokine response. *Int. J. Sport Nutr. Exerc. Metab.* **2009**, *19*, 659–672. [CrossRef]
48. Ahmad, N.S.; Foong Kiew, O.; Ismail, M.S.; Mohamed, M. Effects of post-exercise honey drink ingestion on blood glucose and subsequent running performance in the heat. *Asian J. Sports Med.* **2015**, *6*, e24044. [CrossRef]

49. Kreider, R.B.; Earnest, C.P.; Lundberg, J.; Rasmussen, C.; Greenwood, M.; Cowan, P.; Almada, A.L. Effects of ingesting protein with various forms of carbohydrate following resistance-exercise on substrate availability and markers of anabolism, catabolism, and immunity. *J. Int. Soc. Sports Nutr.* **2007**, *4*, 18. [CrossRef]
50. Tartibian, B.; Maleki, B.H. The effects of honey supplementation on seminal plasma cytokines, oxidative stress biomarkers, and antioxidants during 8 weeks of intensive cycling training. *J. Androl.* **2012**, *33*, 449–461. [CrossRef]
51. Hajizadeh Maleki, B.; Tartibian, B.; Mooren, F.C.; Kruger, K.; FitzGerald, L.Z.; Chehrazi, M. A randomized controlled trial examining the effects of 16 weeks of moderate-to-intensive cycling and honey supplementation on lymphocyte oxidative DNA damage and cytokine changes in male road cyclists. *Cytokine* **2016**, *88*, 222–231. [CrossRef] [PubMed]
52. Gmünder, F.K.; Joller, P.W.; Joller-Jemelka, H.I.; Bechler, B.; Cogoli, M.; Ziegler, W.H.; Müller, J.; Aeppli, R.E.; Cogoli, A. Effect of a herbal yeast food supplement and long-distance running on immunological parameters. *Br. J. Sport Med.* **1990**, *24*, 103–112. [CrossRef] [PubMed]
53. Ooi, F.K. Effects of combined aerobic dance exercise and honey supplementation on bone turnover markers in young females. *Asian J. Exerc. Sports Sci.* **2011**, *8*, 53–63.
54. Schönfeld, P.; Reiser, G. Why does brain metabolism not favor burning of fatty acids to provide energy?-Reflections on disadvantages of the use of free fatty acids as fuel for brain. *J. Cereb. Blood Flow Metab.* **2013**, *33*, 1493–1499. [CrossRef] [PubMed]
55. Boyle, P.J.; Nagy, R.J.; O'Connor, A.M.; Kempers, S.F.; Yeo, R.A.; Qualls, C. Adaptation in brain glucose uptake following recurrent hypoglycemia. *Proc. Natl. Acad. Sci. USA* **1994**, *91*, 9352–9356. [CrossRef] [PubMed]
56. Bandelow, S.; Maughan, R.; Shirreffs, S.; Ozgünen, K.; Kurdak, S.; Ersöz, G.; Binnet, M.; Dvorak, J. The effects of exercise, heat, cooling and rehydration strategies on cognitive function in football players. *Scand. J. Med. Sci. Sports* **2010**, *20*, 148–160. [CrossRef] [PubMed]
57. Burke, L.M.; Kiens, B.; Ivy, J.L. Carbohydrates and fat for training and recovery. *J. Sports Sci.* **2004**, *22*, 15–30. [CrossRef]
58. Salehi, A.; Gunnerud, U.; Muhammed, S.J.; Östman, E.; Holst, J.J.; Björck, I.; Rorsman, P. The insulinogenic effect of whey protein is partially mediated by a direct effect of amino acids and GIP on β-cells. *Nutr. Metab.* **2012**, *9*, 48. [CrossRef]
59. Bishop, N.C.; Gleeson, M.; Nicholas, C.W.; Ali, A. Influence of carbohydrate supplementation on plasma cytokine and neutrophil degranulation responses to high intensity intermittent exercise. *Int. J. Sport Nutr. Exerc. Metab.* **2002**, *12*, 145–156. [CrossRef]
60. Zaid, S.S.M.; Sulaiman, S.A.; Othman, N.H.; Soelaiman, I.-N.; Shuid, A.N.; Mohamad, N.; Muhamad, N. Protective effects of Tualang honey on bone structure in experimental postmenopausal rats. *Clinics* **2012**, *67*, 779–784. [CrossRef]
61. Smith, J.W.; Zachwieja, J.J.; Péronnet, F.; Passe, D.H.; Massicotte, D.; Lavoie, C.; Pascoe, D.D. Fuel selection and cycling endurance performance with ingestion of [^{13}C] glucose: Evidence for a carbohydrate dose response. *J. Appl. Physiol.* **2010**, *108*, 1520–1529. [CrossRef] [PubMed]
62. Smith, J.W.; Pascoe, D.D.; Passe, D.H.; Ruby, B.C.; Stewart, L.K.; Baker, L.B.; Zachwieja, J.J. Curvilinear dose-response relationship of carbohydrate (0–120 gh $^{-1}$) and performance. *Med. Sci. Sports Exerc.* **2013**, *45*, 336–341. [CrossRef] [PubMed]
63. Jeukendrup, A.E.; Moseley, L.; Mainwaring, G.I.; Samuels, S.; Perry, S.; Mann, C.H. Exogenous carbohydrate oxidation during ultraendurance exercise. *J. Appl. Physiol.* **2006**, *100*, 1134–1141. [CrossRef] [PubMed]
64. Passe, D.; Horn, M.; Murray, R. Impact of beverage acceptability on fluid intake during exercise. *Appetite* **2000**, *35*, 219–229. [CrossRef] [PubMed]
65. Oosthuyse, T.; Carstens, M.; Millen, A.M. Ingesting isomaltulose versus fructose-maltodextrin during prolonged moderate-heavy exercise increases fat oxidation but impairs gastrointestinal comfort and cycling performance. *Int. J. Sport Nutr. Exerc. Metab.* **2015**, *25*, 427–438. [CrossRef] [PubMed]

12

Comparative Biomechanical Analysis of the Hurdle Clearance Technique of Colin Jackson and Dayron Robles

Milan Čoh [1], Nejc Bončina [1], Stanko Štuhec [1] and Krzysztof Mackala [2,*]

[1] Faculty of Sport, University of Ljubljana, Gortanova ul. 22, 1000 Ljubljana, Slovenia; Milan.Coh@fsp.uni-lj.si (M.Č.); nejc.boncina@gmail.com (N.B.); Stanko.Stuhec@fsp.uni-lj.si (S.Š.)

[2] Department of Track and Field, University School of Physical Education, Al. Ignacego Paderewskiego 35, 51-612 Wrocław, Poland

* Correspondence: krzysztof.mackala@awf.wroc.pl

Abstract: The purpose of the study was to compare the biomechanical parameters of the hurdle clearance technique of the fifth hurdle in the 110 m hurdle race of Colin Jackson of Great Britain (12.91 s world record was set in 1994) and Dayron Robles of Cuba (12.87 s world record was set in 2008), two world record holders. Despite the athletes having performed at different times, we used comparable biomechanical diagnostic technology for both hurdlers. Biomechanical measurements for both were performed by the Laboratory for Movement Control of the Institute of Sport, Faculty of Sport in Ljubljana. A three-dimensional video analysis of the fifth hurdle clearance technique was used. High standards of biomechanical measurements were taken into account, thus ensuring the high objectivity of the obtained results. The following program was used: the ARIEL kinematic program (Ariel Dynamics Inc., Trabuco Canyon, CA, USA). The results of the comparative analysis found minimal differences between the two athletes, which was expected given their excellence. Dayron Robles's hurdle clearance was more effective, as it was characterized by a smaller loss of horizontal center of mass (COM) velocity. Robles's hurdle clearance took 0.50 s: 0.10 s for the take-off, 0.33 s for the flight phase, and 0.07 s for the landing phase. Colin Jackson completed the hurdle clearance slightly slower, as it took him 0.54 s. Jackson's take-off phase also lasted 0.10 s, his flight phase 0.36 s, and his landing 0.08 s. The two athletes are quite different in their morphological constitution. Dayron Robles is 10 cm taller than Colin Jackson, resulting in a lower flight parabola of CM during hurdle clearance of the Cuban athlete. Dayron Robles has a more effective hurdle clearance technique compared to Jackson's achievement. It can be considered that their individual techniques of overcoming the hurdle, reached their individual highest efficiency at this time.

Keywords: hurdling; biomechanics; hurdle clearance; technique analysis

---

1. Introduction

The high hurdle race is one of the most technically demanding athletic events, and from a biomechanical standpoint, the hurdle race is a combination of a cyclic sprint and an acyclic clearance of ten 1.067 m high hurdles. According to Bruggemman [1], the high hurdle event can be divided into the following phases: approach run to the first hurdle, clearance of the hurdles and the rhythm between hurdles, and run-out from the last hurdle to the finishing line. Therefore, a proper hurdling technique is a complicated combination of various running and jumping kinematics [2]. Additionally the hurdler must show a high level of sprinting skill, excellent flexibility in the hip joint, coordination, balance, dynamic perception, elastic power, and a high level of technical knowledge [3,4]. Thus, athletes, coaches, and professionals are constantly looking for opportunities to improve the high hurdle performance, focusing on hurdling technique with particular emphasis on the kinematics and kinetics analysis. During the last three decades, there has been a considerable amount of references concerning the analysis of hurdling technique at different levels in order to improve performance [5–11].

One of the key elements that defines a competitive result in high hurdles is the hurdle clearance technique [11–17]. When clearing a hurdle, the loss of horizontal velocity should be minimized. This was confirmed by Amara et al. [17] and Coh et al. [18], who based on their hurdle clearance analyses, claimed that horizontal velocity is one of the most crucial factors, therefore losing it should be minimized; if not, the running time will be reduced. Additionally for the fastest possible and biomechanically effective clearance of the hurdle, the athlete's take-off distance and landing distance are essential. Furthermore, Salo and Grimshaw [19] determined the optimal ratio for an efficient hurdle clearance. The ratio applies to the dependency between the take-off of the trial leg and the landing of the lead leg and should be 60:40 in flight distance. The hurdle clearance depends on other factors, especially those that define the movement trajectory of the center of mass (COM). The correct positioning of these two points determines the optimal flight trajectory of the COM, which is reflected in the flight time, which should be as short as possible [5,9,12,20]. According to Coh et al. [18] and Bubaj et al. [21] these two situations is a prerequisite for an optimal flight path of the center of mass (COM). This optimal path results in a shorter flight time. In addition to the correct position, the kinematic–dynamic structure of the take-off and landing are important, as they directly affect the speed of hurdle clearance [7,10,16,22,23]. To sum up the above considerations after Lopez et al. [24], Li et al. [22], Park et al. [25], and Amara et al. [17], the main criteria of an optimal hurdle clearance technique include horizontal velocity, height of COM at take-off, velocity of the trail-leg, flight time, height of COM at landing, and contact time.

Over the years, with the development of technology, the ability to record and film competitions in track and field has increased significantly. There has been a considerable amount of biomechanical data concerning the kinematic analysis of hurdle races at a high level of performance such as the Olympic Games, World Championships, or international meetings [24–29]. These analyses of the specialized video recording are related to the technical aspects of single event observations where competition stress and adrenaline are imposed on athletes. There has been a limited number of studies where obtaining the kinematic parameters of 110-m male hurdlers on the basis of video techniques analyses has been carried out on two consecutive races with the same competitors–hurdlers. Therefore, researchers use various video recordings in their analyses, although sometimes there are methodological differences in data collection processes. A similar procedure was used for the analysis of hurdle races of Colin Jackson and Dayron Robles, who set high standards in this athletic discipline. They were both world record holders in their 110 m high hurdle race careers and won medals at every major international competition. Colin Jackson set the world record in the 60 m hurdle race in 1993 in Sindelfingen (Germany) with a time of 7.30 s. A year later, he improved the world record in the 110 m hurdles with a time of 12.91 s, still considered the seventh-best time in the history of this athletic discipline. Dayron Robles also improved the world record in the 110 m hurdle race (12.87 s) in 2008 in Ostrava (Czech Republic), which is considered to be the second-best result of all time in high hurdle races.

These studies were conducted to analyze comparable data held by the Laboratory for Movement Control of the Institute of Sport, Faculty of Sport in Ljubljana. Biomechanical measurements of both athletes were performed at different times, but under comparable conditions with similar measurement technologies. In both cases, a kinematic analysis of the fifth hurdle clearance technique was used. High standards of biomechanical measurements were taken into account, thus ensuring the high objectivity of the obtained results. We are aware that the study would have been even more valuable had we been able to analyze a greater number of obstacle clearances, but this was not possible due to organizational and technical constraints. The main aim of the study was to identify, analyze, and compare the essential kinematic parameters of the hurdle clearance technique at hurdle 5 of two athletes who have set the highest standards of biomechanical rationality of hurdle clearance in 110 m high hurdle races.

2. Materials and Methods

2.1. Participants

In this experiment, the participants were two world class hurdlers: Colin Jackson (body mass 75 kg, and height 182 cm) from Great Britain and Dayron Robles from Cuba (body mass 79 kg and height 191 cm). Both competitors specialized in 110 m hurdle, and were or are world record holders in 110 m hurdles. Some more personalized and anthropometric data of both athletes are shown in Table 1. The participants provided informed consent and were informed of the protocol and procedures for the study prior to the official video recording. The selection of athletes to conduct the experiment was specific and dependent on the possibility of making a video recording with its entire comprehensive procedure during an international meeting, and above all dependent on the level of participants in these competitions. Due to the fact that the experiment concerns the analysis of the hurdle technique for only two competitors, it can be qualified as a case study—the work reports scientifically sound experiments and provides a substantial amount of new information. The study was approved by the Human Ethics Committee of the University of Ljubljana.

Table 1. Basic anthropometric and biographical data of Colin Jackson (Great Britain) and Dayron Robles (Cuba).

Parameters	Colin Jackson	Dayron Robles
Date of birth	1967	1986
Body height (cm)	1.82	1.92
Body mass (kg)	75	79
Body Mass Index (BMI)	22.64	21.43
Best result (s)	12.91 *	12.87 **
Experimental result (s)	13.47	13.00
100 m best results (s)	10.29	10.71

BMI (Body Mass Index), * World Record in 1993, ** World record in 2008.

2.2. Experimental Design

The experiment design used was a comparison of dynamic and kinematic variables between two 110 m hurdles races at the segment between hurdles 4 and 5 and hurdle clearance of two world record holder. Both recordings of hurdles took place during regular international athletics competitions, although in two different places and two different years. These two conditions forced the experiment to match two different race recording methodologies. The hurdle races of Jackson and Robles were both recorded using two cameras each, although of different resolutions of 50 Hz frames per second and 100 Hz per second, respectively. From a methodological point of view, this may be a significant difference, but the conditions of variability were respected when processing data. In order to avoid the errors involved in analysis, real measurements were recalculated, taking into account the measurement error, which actually means that they corresponded (e.g., 50 Hz means 0.04 s between frames, so a hurdle clearance time of 0.5 s vs. 0.54 s represents a single frame). In both analyses the model of Dempster [30] was used for the calculation of the body's COM and the kinematic program ARIEL (Ariel Dynamics Inc., Trabuco Canyon, CA, USA) for the digitization was applied.

2.3. Procedure of Measurements—Colin Jackson

Colin Jackson's biomechanical analysis was carried out on 28 June 2002, at the International Meet in Velenje (EA Classic). His finish time was 13.47 s. The weather conditions were optimal; the outside temperature was 27 °C with a wind speed of + 0.2 m/s. Authorization to perform the experiment was approved by the Slovenian Track and Field Association. Biomechanical measurements were performed by a team of experts from the Laboratory for Movement Control of the Faculty of Sport in Ljubljana. Two synchronized cameras, namely Sony DSR-300-PK DVCAM Camcorders with Fujinon 17x lenses, were located at the main stands (the zone of hurdle 5) and operating at 50 Hz (shutter speed: 1/1000) were used to film the races. To record all kinematic parameters, the cameras were set at an angle of 120 to the direction of the moving hurdler in the segment between hurdles 4 and 5 (Figure 1). The zone of the 5th hurdle was calibrated with a calibration cube, one at the beginning of hurdle 4 and one at the end of hurdle 5. A 15-segment Dempster's model [30] and the ARIEL kinematic program (Ariel Dynamics Inc., Trabuco Canyon, CA, USA) were used to calculate the center of mass.

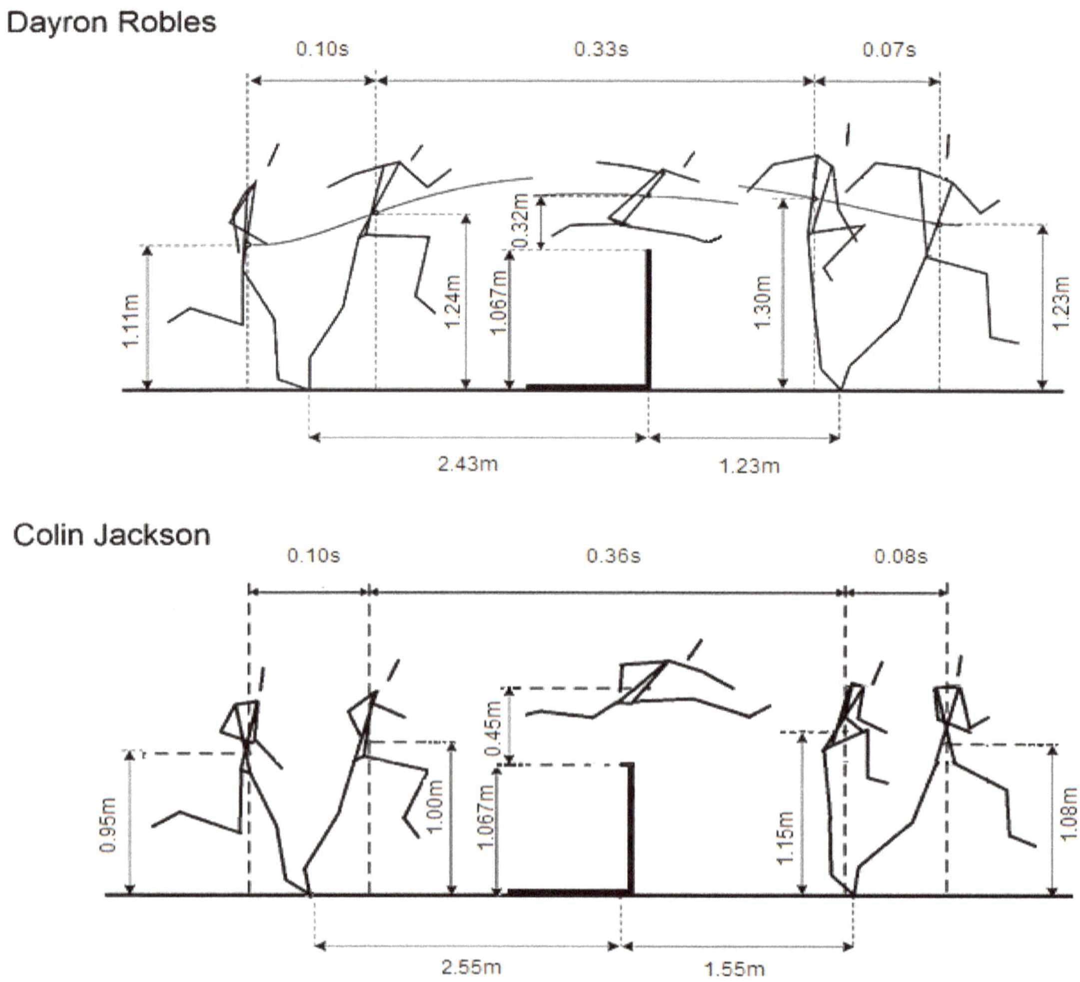

Figure 1. Comparison of biomechanical parameters of hurdle clearance.

2.4. Procedure of Measurements—Dayron Robles

Biomechanical analyses of Dayron Robles's 5th hurdle clearing technique was performed at the 2011 IAAF World Challenge—Zagreb International Race. Weather conditions were optimal; the outside temperature was 23 °C, and the wind speed was −0.2 m/s. Authorization to perform biomechanical measurements was obtained from the Technical Delegate of the European Athletics Federation and the Organizing Committee of the competition. The running track lane in the zone of the 5th hurdle was covered by two Casio high-frequency digital Casio EX-F1 512 × 384 (300 fps) sampled down to 100 fps cameras (Casio Computer Co., Ltd., Tokyo, Japan), which were interconnected and synchronized. The shutter speed of the Casio cameras was 1/300 s. The cameras were set perpendicular to the zone of the 5th hurdle (running hurdler) at an angle of 90°. The zone of the 5th hurdle was calibrated with a 2 m × 2 m × 2 m reference frame, within which eight points were measured. Data processing utilized an APAS computer system for 3D kinematic analysis (Ariel Performance Analysis System). Digitization of a 15-segment athlete body model was carried out, defined by 15 reference points [30] The point coordinates were smoothed with a 14 Hz digital filter. The center of mass (COM) was calculated from the digitized points based on Dempster's (1955) model of determination of COM via the ARIEL kinematic program (Ariel Dynamics Inc., Trabuco Canyon, CA, USA).

3. Results

The difference in body weight between competitors was only 4 kg. An even greater difference was in body height and was 10 cm in favor of Robles. Both measurements significantly differentiated hurdlers in terms of a measure of body fat (the ratio of the weight of the body in kilograms to the square of its height in meters), which was 1.21 in favor of Robles (Table 1). The time difference between those two world records is 0.04s. Jackson set his world record at the age of 26 and Robles at the age of 22. The age difference between competitors on the day of the experiment was approximately 10 years in favor of Jackson, and Robles obtained a better result by 0.47s in the 110 m performance.

Based on biomechanical analyses (Table 2), the following results were obtained: Robles's total stride length was 3.66 m, and the stride was completed in 0.33 s, while Jackson's stride length was 3.67 m, and it was slightly slower, lasting 0.36 s. During hurdle clearance, Dayron Robles reached the highest COM point at 1.38 m (0.32 m above the height of the hurdle), which corresponded to 72.2% of his body height. Colin Jackson reached the COM trajectory point at 1.52 m (0.45 m above the hurdle height), which was 83.4% of his height. The difference between the lowest COM point in the eccentric phase of the take-off was 1.11 m for Robles and 0.95 m for Jackson; and the highest COM point during the flight phase was 1.387 m for Robles and 1.517 m for Jackson. The height of the COM at the end of the concentric phase of take-off for Robles was 1.24 m and 1.08 m for Jackson.

Table 2. Biomechanical variables of the clearance of the fifth hurdle.

Variables	Colin Jackson	Dayron Robles	Difference	Δ (%)
Horizontal velocity 4 H–5 H (m/s)	9.14	9.18	0.04	0.43
	Take-off (braking phase)			
Horizontal velocity of COM (m/s	8.81	8.70	0.11	1.25
Vertical velocity of COM m/s	–0.43	–0.70	0.37	62.79
Velocity resultant of COM (m/s	8.82	8.73	0.09	1.03
Height of COM (m)	0.95	1.11	0.16	16.84
Foot to hurdle distance (m)	2.09	2.43	0.34	16.26
	Take-off (propulsion phase)			
Horizontal velocity of COM (m/s)	9.11	9.00	0.11	1.21
Vertical velocity of COM (m/s)	2.35	1.80	0.55	23.41
Velocity resultant of COM (m/s)	9.41	9.18	0.23	2.45
Height of COM (m)	1.08	1.24	0.16	14.81
Push-off angle (°)	72.9	78.7	5.80	7.95
Contact time (s)	0.10	0.10	0.0	0.0
	Flight			
Flight time (s)	0.36	0.33	0.03	8.34
Height of COM above the hurdle (m)	0.45	0.32	0.13	28.89
Maximal height COM (m)	1.44	1.52	0.08	5.55
	Landing (braking phase)			
Horizontal velocity of COM m/s	8.77	8.80	0.03	0.34
Vertical velocity of COM (m/s)	–1.02	–1.00	–0.02	1.97
Velocity resultant of COM (m/s)	8.84	8.86	0.02	0.22
Height of COM (m)	1.15	1.30	0.15	13.04
Foot to hurdle distance (m)	1.58	1.23	0.35	22.16
	Landing (propulsion phase)			
Horizontal velocity of COM (m/s)	8.41	9.35	1.06	11.17
Vertical velocity of COM (m/s)	–1.32	–1.00	–0.32	24.25
Velocity resultant of COM (m/s)	8.53	9.40	1.13	10.19
Height of COM (m)	1.06	1.23	0.17	16.03
Contact time (s)	0.08	0.07	0.01	12.50

4. Discussion

The entire process of hurdle clearance took 0.50 s for Robles; it took 0.10 s for take-off, 0.33 s for the flight phase, and 0.07 s for the landing phase. Meanwhile, Colin Jackson completed the hurdle clearance a little more slowly, as it took him 0.54 s. Jackson also spent 0.10 s for take-off, 0.36 s for the flight phase, and 0.08 s for the landing phase. For comparison, the measurement of Amara [23]—a medium level athlete (13.90 s at 110 m hurdles) showed differences in the abovementioned parameters of 0.60 s, 0.36 s, 0.21 s, and 0.12 s (respectively for each variable). Jackson's slower clearance of the hurdle is associated with a higher rise in his COM above the hurdle and a longer landing distance over the hurdle, extending both the flight phase and the shock absorption phase. A slower hurdler [30] had a similar problem; his excessive height of the vertical COM displacement together with a high take-off angle had a negative impact on the time to clear the hurdle. The difference in the flight parabola between the two athletes can be attributed mainly to the difference in their height and the difference in their functional abilities. Based on the kinematic parameters of the parabola, we can, therefore, conclude that Dayron Robles has a more rational hurdle clearance technique (Figure 1).

The take-off distance for Robles was 2.43 m, which was 66.4% of the total clearance length over the hurdle. For Jackson, the take-off distance was 2.09 m, which was 57.0% of the total length of clearance. Jackson's landing distance was 1.58 m (43.0% of his total stride length), while Robles's was 1.23 m (33.6% of his total stride length). It can be compared with some other studies [10,30], which indicate that the optimal ratio between take-off spot and landing place should be 40–60%, which is comparable with Amara's [17] findings (i.e., 58:42). This ratio was confirmed by previous researchers [8,18,24,28,31,32], which indicated that take-off distance should range from 2.04 cm to 2.31 cm. In turn, the landing distance was shorter. We can identify two different hurdle clearance strategies. Robles has a faster hurdle clearance; his take-off is elongated, and his landing is closer to the hurdle. The duration of Robles's flight phase is 0.33 s, and that of Jackson is 0.36 s. A technical model of When [33] indicated that the optimal over the hurdle time should range between 0.30 and 0.33 s for a world class hurdler. This confirms the importance of the take-off (the angle between the top of the foot and the hip) and landing distances in high hurdler races, as was previously mentioned by Coh and Iskra [31] and Lopez at el. [24].

In the concentric phase, Robles had a take-off angle of 78.7 °, and Jackson's was 72.9 °. The COM velocity resultant during the braking phase of the take-off was 8.73 m/s for Robles and 8.82 m/s for Jackson. This velocity resultant of COM is defined as the vector sum of the vertical COM velocity (0.70 m/s for Robles, –0.43 m/s for Jackson) and horizontal COM velocity (8.70 m/s for Robles and 8.81 m/s for Jackson). It changes until the last contact of the take-off when it measured 9.18 m/s for Robles and 9.41 m/s for Jackson. Robles's vertical COM velocity at that time was 1.80 m/s, and Jackson's was 2.35 m/s; their horizontal COM velocities were 9.00 m/s and 9.11 m/s, respectively. The COM horizontal velocity during take-off thus increased by 0.30 m/s for both Robles and Jackson. The relative increase in the horizontal velocity of COM for Robles was 3.30% and 3.29% for Jackson (Figure 2). For both athletes, the duration of their take-off was the same. Robles's COM height during take-off increased by 0.13 m, equal to Jackson's (Figure 1). It is comparable with data of Amara [17], Li and Fu [34], and Lopez at el. [24], who claimed that during take-off (propulsion phase), the average height of the COM should be around 1.12 m.

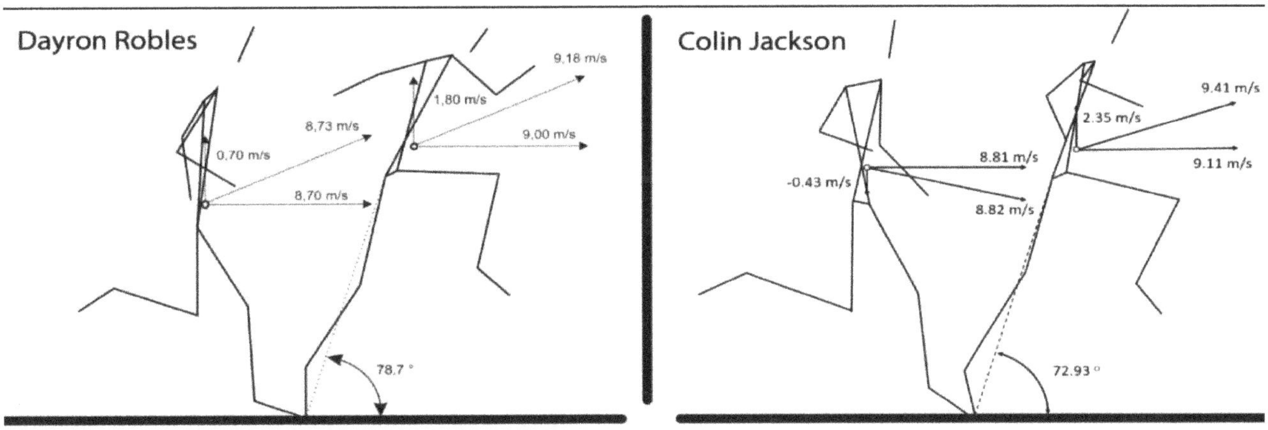

Figure 2. Comparison of the biomechanical parameters of take-off before the hurdle.

The transition between hurdle clearance and the sprint between hurdles is dependent on the landing phase. For Robles, the horizontal velocity at landing was 8.80 m/s, which means that the horizontal velocity decreased by 0.20 m/s (2.2%). For Jackson, the horizontal velocity decreased by 0.34 m/s (3.7%). During the landing phase, Robles's height of COM decreased by 0.07 m (5.4%) and 0.09 m (7.8%) for Jackson. The short duration of the landing phase (0.07 s for Robles and 0.08 s for Jackson) indicated a high level of reactive power [35] for both athletes (Figure 3), and an efficient transition to sprinting between hurdles [4,36].

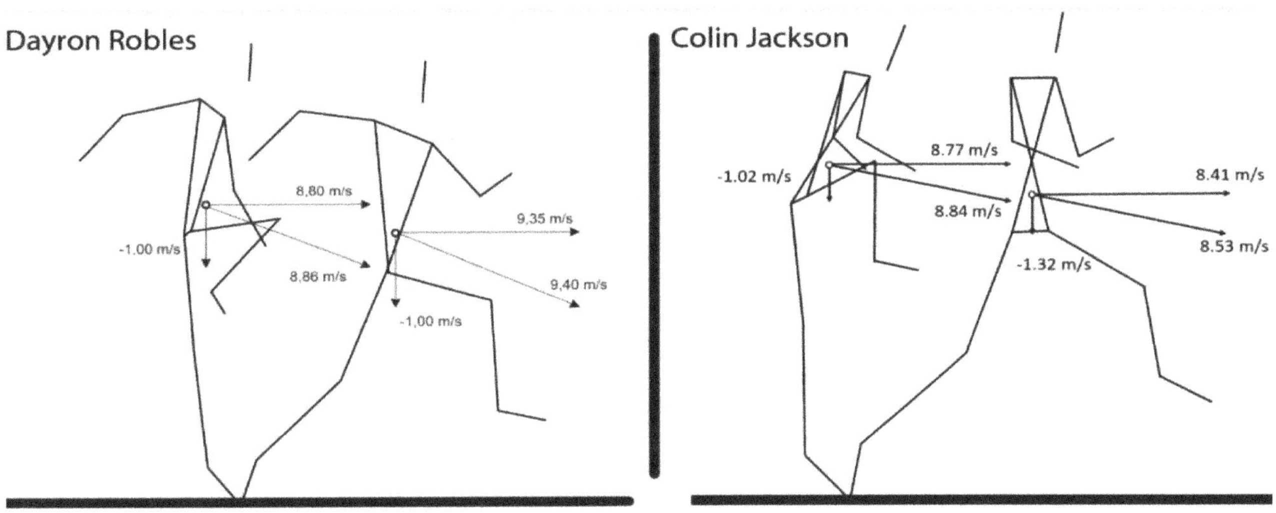

Figure 3. Comparison of the biomechanical parameters of the landing.

For Jackson, the reduction in the horizontal velocity of COM was greater than that of Robles, and the height of his center of mass (COM) was lower at landing, so it can be concluded that Robles has a slightly more biomechanically rational hurdle clearance technique. In addition, our results do not contradict the research of Amara [23], who claimed that the vertical component of COM velocity and the lead-leg/trail-leg at take-off and at flight phase constituted key factors of optimum hurdle clearance. According to Amara [17,23] and Shibayama et al. [37], in addition to the take-off angle, the knee and the hip angles are very important in high hurdles clearance, as also found in previous studies done by Coh [18,38], Xi et al. [22], Bubaj [21] and Sidhu [39]. Liu [40] just confirmed this statement and additionally indicated that the flight-phase duration is also defined by the takeoff angle, which should be lower.

5. Conclusions

In the present study, we analyzed the rationality of the 110 m hurdle clearance technique of Colin Jackson and Dayron Robles, using diagnostic technology for kinematic analysis. Both athletes have roughly the same personal record in the 110 m hurdle races (Jackson 12.91 s, Robles 12.87 s). The two hurdlers are quite different in morphological constitution, with Dayron Robles being 10 cm taller than Colin Jackson. Based on the results obtained, it can be concluded that Dayron Robles has a more effective hurdle clearance technique. It is characterized by a smaller loss of horizontal velocity of COM during clearance, a better COM flight parabola over the hurdle, and a smaller difference between the hurdle height and the height of the highest COM point, compared to Jackson's achievement. It proves that their hurdle clearance efficiencies differ but depend on the same kinematic parameters. Therefore, it can be considered that their individual technique of overcoming the hurdle their reached individual highest efficiency at this time. On this basis, we can also assume that the difference in overcoming one hurdle (the fifth) accumulated in the remaining hurdles until the end of the race, which reflects the final results of the races. Here Robles obtained a better running time in the 110 m hurdles.

6. Practical Application

From a practical point of view, based on some of the spatiotemporal parameters presented in the present analysis, there are some high hurdle common performance indicators. In order to optimize high hurdle performance with special regard to clearance hurdle movement performance, lower vertical displacement of COM, combined with right angle of take-off and short contact-time at the take-off and landing phases must be considered. These elements help improve a quick turn between horizontal and vertical velocity of forward propulsion and fast return of the trail leg at landing. To improve these indicators, appropriate training needs to be applied. It should consider high technical proficiency training and first of all activities which improve a higher rate of force development.

Author Contributions: Conceptualization, M.Č. and K.M.; Data curation, S.Š. and K.M.; Formal analysis, M.Č., N.B., S.Š. and K.M.; Investigation, M.Č., N.B. and S.Š.; Methodology, M.Č., N.B., S.Š. and K.M.; Resources, M.Č.; Software, N.B. and S.Š.; Supervision, M.Č. and K.M.; Validation, M.Č. and N.B.; Writing–original draft, M.Č., N.B. and K.M.; Writing–review & editing, M.Č. and K.M. All authors have read and agreed to the published version of the manuscript.

Acknowledgments: The authors would like to acknowledge the involvement of the participants for their contribution to this study.

References

1. Brüggemann, G.P.; Koszewski, D.; Müller, H. *Biomechanical Research Project*; Athens 1997, Final report; Meyer & Meyer Sport: Oxford, UK, 1999; pp. 12–41.
2. Bollschweiler, L. A biomechanical Analysis of Male and Female Intermediate Hurdles and Steeplechasers. Master's Thesis, Brigham Young University, Brigham, MA, USA, 2008.
3. Salo, A.I.; Scarborough, S. Athletics: Changes in technique within a sprint hurdle run. *Sport Biomech.* **2006**, *5*, 155–166. [CrossRef]
4. Iskra, J. The most effective technical training for the 110 metres hurdles. *New Stud. Athl.* **1995**, *10*, 51–55.
5. Schluter, W. Kinematic features of the 110-meter hurdle technique (Kinematische Merkmale der 110-m Hurdentechnik). *Leistungssport* **1981**, *2*, 118–127.
6. Mero, A.; Luhtanen, P. Biomechanical examination of the hurdle race during the World Championships in Helsinki. (Biomechanische Untersuchung des Hurdenlaufs während der Weltmeisterschaften in Helsinki. *Leistungssport* **1986**, *1*, 42–43. (In German)
7. La Fortune, M.A. Biomechanical analysis of 110 m hurdles. *Track Field News* **1988**, *105*, 3355–3365.

8. McDonald, C.; Dapena, J. Linear kinematics of the men's and woman's hurdles races. *Med Sci. Sports Exerc.* **1991**, *23*, 1382–1402. [CrossRef]
9. Dapena, J. Hurdle clearance technique. *Track Field Quart Rev.* **1991**, *116*, 710–712.
10. Mclean, B. The biomechanics of hurdling: Force plate analysis to assess hurdling technique. *New Stud. Athl.* **1994**, *4*, 55–58.
11. Kampmiller, T.; Slamka, M.; Vanderka, M. Comparative biomechanical analysis of 110 m hurdles of Igor Kovač and Peter Nedelicky. *Kinesiol. Slov.* **1991**, *1–2*, 26–30.
12. Lee, J. The Kinematic analysis of the hurdling of men's 110 m hurdle. *Korean J. Sport Biomech.* **2004**, *14*, 83–98. [CrossRef]
13. Iskra, J.; Coh, M. A review of biomechanical studies in hurdle races. *Kinesiol. Slov.* **2006**, *1*, 84–102.
14. Sidhu, A.; Singh, M. Kinematical analysis of hurdle clearance technique in 110 m hurdle race. *Int. J. Behav. Soc. Mov. Sci.* **2015**, *4*, 28–35.
15. Amritpals, S.; Shamsher, S. Relationship among the Technique of Hurdle Clearance Over the DifferentHurdles in 110 m Race. *Int. J. Sci. Res.* **2015**, *4*, 1591–1594.
16. Chin-Shan, H.; Chi-Yao, C.; Kuo-Chuan, L. The wearable devices application for evaluation of 110 meter high hurdle race. *J. Hum. Sport Exerc.* **2020**, *151*, 1–9.
17. Amara, S.; Mkaouer, B.; Chaabene, H.; Negra, Y.; Hammoudi-Riahi, S.; Ben- Salah, F. Key kinetic and kinematic factors of 110-m hurdles performance. *J. Phys. Educ. Sport.* **2019**, *19*, 658–668.
18. Coh, M.; Zvan, M.; Bubanj, S. *XXIIth International Symposium on Biomechanics in Sports*; Lamontagne, M., Gordon, D., Robertson, E., Sveistrup, H., Eds.; ISBS: Ottawa, ON, Canada, 2004; pp. 311–314.
19. Salo, A.; Grimshaw, P. 3–D biomechanical analysis of sprint hurdles at different competitive level. *Med. Sci. Sports Exerc.* **1997**, *29*, 231–237. [CrossRef]
20. Lee, J.; Park, Y.; Ryu, J.; Kim, J. The kinematic analysis of the third hurdling motion of the 110 m hurdles elite. *Korean J. Sport Biomech.* **2008**, *18*, 31–39.
21. Bubaj, R.; Stankovic, R.; Rakovic, A.; Bubanj, S.; Petrovic, P.; Mladenovic, D. Comparative biomechanical analysis of hurdle clearance techniques on 110 m running with hurdles of elite and non-elite athletes. *Serb. J. Sports Sci.* **2008**, *2*, 37–44.
22. Li, X.; Zhou, J.; Li, N.; Wang, J. Comparative biomechanics analysis of hurdle clearance techniques. *Port. J. Sport Sci.* **2011**, *11*, 307–309.
23. Amara, S.; Mkaouer, B.; Chaabene, H.; Negra, Y.; Hammoudi-Riahi, S.; Ben- Salah, F. Kinetic and kinematic analysis of hurdle clearance of an African and a world champion athlete: A comparative study. *S. Afr. J. Res. Sport PH* **2017**, *39*, 1–12.
24. López, J.; Padullés, J.M.; Olsson, H.J. Biomechanical analysis and functional assessment of D. Robles, world record holder and Olympic champion in 110 m hurdles. In Proceedings of the 29th International Conference on Biomechanics in Sports, Porto, Portugal, 20–23 June 2011; Vilas-Boas, J.P., Ed.; ISBS: Porto, Portugal, 2011; pp. 315–318.
25. Park, Y.J.; Ryu, J.K.; Ryu, J.S.; Kim, T.S.; Hwang, W.S.; Park, S.K.; Yoon, S. Kinematic analysis of hurdle clearance technique for 110-m men's hurdlers at IAAF World Championships, Daegue 2011. *Korean J. Sport Biomech.* **2011**, *21*, 529–540. [CrossRef]
26. Tsiokanos, A.; Tsaopoulos, D.E.; Tsarouchas, E.; Giavroglou, A. Race pattern of Men's 110-H hurdles: Time analysis of Olympic performance. *Biol. Exerc.* **2018**, *14*, 15–36. [CrossRef]
27. Graubner, R.; Nixdorf, E. Biomechanical analysis of the sprint and hurdles events at the 2009 IAAF World Championships in Athletics. *New Stud. Athl.* **2011**, *26*, 19–53.
28. Pollitt, L.; Walker, J.; Bissas, A.; Merlino, S. Biomechanical report for the IAAF world championships 2017: 110 m hurdles men's in 2017. In *IAAF World Championships Biomechanics Research Project*; International Association of Athletics Federations: London, UK, 2018.
29. Walker, J.; Pollitt, L.; Paradisis, G.P.; Bezodis, I.; Bissas, A.; Merlino, S. *Biomechanical Report for the IAAF World Indoor Championships 2018: 60 Metres Hurdles Men*; International Association of Athletics Federations: Birmingham, UK, 2019.
30. Dempster, W.T. *Space Requirements of the Seated Operator*; USAF, WADC, Tech. Rep.; Wright-Patterson Air Force Base: Greene County, OH, USA; pp. 55–159.
31. Coh, M.; Iskra, J. Biomechanical studies of 110 m hurdle clearance technique. *Sport Sci.* **2012**, *5*, 10–14.

32. González-Frutos, P.; Veiga, S.; Mallo, J.; Navarro, E. Spatiotemporal Comparisons between Elite and High-Level 60 m Hurdlers. *Front. Psychol.* **2019**, *10*, 1–9. [CrossRef]
33. Wen, C. *The High-Grade Tutorial of Track and Field*; People's Sports Press: Beijing, China, 2003; pp. 386–389.
34. Li, J.; Fu, D. The kinematic analysis on the transition technique between run and hurdle clearance of 110 m hurdles. In *XVIIIth International Symposium on Biomechanics in Sports*; Hong, Y., Johns, D.P., Sanders, R., Eds.; ISBS: Hong Kong, China, 2000; pp. 213–217.
35. Gollhofer, A.; Kyrolainen, H. Neuromuscular control of the human leg extensor muscles in jump exercises under various stretch-load conditions. *Int. J. Sports Med.* **1991**, *12*, 34–40. [CrossRef]
36. Lee, J. Kinematic analysis of hurdling of elite 110 m hurdlers. *Korean J. Sport Biomech.* **2009**, *19*, 761–770. [CrossRef]
37. Shibayama, K.; Fujii, N.; Shimizu, Y.; Ae, M. Analysis of angular momentum in hurdling by world and Japanese elite sprint hurdlers. In *XXXth International Symposium on Biomechanics in Sports*; Bradshaw, E.J., Burnett, A., Hume, P.A., Eds.; ISBS: Melbourne, Australia, 2012; pp. 54–57.
38. Coh, M. Biomechanical analysis of Colin Jackson's hurdle clearance technique. *New Stud. Athl.* **2003**, *18*, 37–45.
39. Sidhu, A.S. Three-dimensional kinematic analysis of hurdle clearance technique. *Global J. Res. Anal.* **2016**, *4*, 4–6.
40. Liiu, Y. A Kinesiological Analysis of the Hurdling Techniques of China's 110 m Hurdlers Liu Xiang and Shi Dongpeng. Master's Thesis, Shanxi University, Shanxi, China, 2008.

13

Analysis of the Effects of Dietary Pattern on the Oral Microbiome of Elite Endurance Athletes

Nida Murtaza [1], Louise M. Burke [2,3,*], Nicole Vlahovich [3,4], Bronwen Charlesson [3], Hayley M. O'Neill [4], Megan L. Ross [2,3], Katrina L. Campbell [4], Lutz Krause [1] and Mark Morrison [1,*]

1 Faculty of Medicine, Translational Research Institute, University of Queensland Diamantina Institute, Brisbane, QLD 4102, Australia; nida.murtaza@uqconnect.edu.au (N.M.); l.krause@uq.edu.au (L.K.)

2 Centre for Exercise & Nutrition, Mary MacKillop Institute for Health Research, Australian Catholic University, Melbourne, VIC 3000, Australia; meg.ross@ausport.gov.au

3 Australian Institute of Sport, Canberra, ACT 2617, Australia; Nicole.Vlahovich@ausport.gov.au (N.V.); bronwen.charlesson@outlook.com (B.C.)

4 Faculty of Health Sciences & Medicine, Bond University, Robina, QLD 4226, Australia; haoneill@bond.edu.au (H.M.O.); Katrina.Campbell@health.qld.gov.au (K.L.C.)

* Correspondence: Louise.Burke@ausport.gov.au (L.M.B.); m.morrison1@uq.edu.au (M.M.)

Abstract: Although the oral microbiota is known to play a crucial role in human health, there are few studies of diet x oral microbiota interactions, and none in elite athletes who may manipulate their intakes of macronutrients to achieve different metabolic adaptations in pursuit of optimal endurance performance. The aim of this study was to investigate the shifts in the oral microbiome of elite male endurance race walkers from Europe, Asia, the Americas and Australia, in response to one of three dietary patterns often used by athletes during a period of intensified training: a High Carbohydrate (HCHO; n = 9; with 60% energy intake from carbohydrates; ~8.5 g kg^{-1} day^{-1} carbohydrate, ~2.1 g kg^{-1} day^{-1} protein, 1.2 g kg^{-1} day^{-1} fat) diet, a Periodised Carbohydrate (PCHO; n = 10; same macronutrient composition as HCHO, but the intake of carbohydrates is different across the day and throughout the week to support training sessions with high or low carbohydrate availability) diet or a ketogenic Low Carbohydrate High Fat (LCHF; n = 10; 0.5 g kg^{-1} day^{-1} carbohydrate; 78% energy as fat; 2.1 g kg^{-1} day^{-1} protein) diet. Saliva samples were collected both before (Baseline; BL) and after the three-week period (Post treatment; PT) and the oral microbiota profiles for each athlete were produced by 16S rRNA gene amplicon sequencing. Principal coordinates analysis of the oral microbiota profiles based on the weighted UniFrac distance measure did not reveal any specific clustering with respect to diet or athlete ethnic origin, either at baseline (BL) or following the diet-training period. However, discriminant analyses of the oral microbiota profiles by Linear Discriminant Analysis (LDA) Effect Size (LEfSe) and sparse Partial Least Squares Discriminant Analysis (sPLS-DA) did reveal changes in the relative abundance of specific bacterial taxa, and, particularly, when comparing the microbiota profiles following consumption of the carbohydrate-based diets with the LCHF diet. These analyses showed that following consumption of the LCHF diet the relative abundances of *Haemophilus, Neisseria* and *Prevotella* spp. were decreased, and the relative abundance of *Streptococcus* spp. was increased. Such findings suggest that diet, and, in particular, the LCHF diet can induce changes in the oral microbiota of elite endurance walkers.

Keywords: oral microbiome; elite athletes; diet

1. Introduction

Recent technological advances have enabled a more holistic definition and characterisation of the microbes that colonise the human body, the "microbiomes". The human oral cavity serves as the habitat for a numerically large and diverse microbiome [1], which has been extensively characterised with respect to infectious and periodontal diseases, and caries, as well as for its contributions to the onset and progression of chronic conditions such as diabetes, cardiovascular disease and cancer [2]. However, the impacts of dietary pattern on the oral microbiome are not well defined, neither for the general population nor for cohorts who may follow specialised diets, such as elite athletes. In that context, recent studies have revealed a positive symbiotic association between the oral bacteria and host with respect to an enterosalivary nitrate-nitrite-nitric oxide pathway, which contributes to nitric oxide (NO) homeostasis [3,4]. Here, facultative anaerobic bacteria in the mouth reduce salivary gland concentrated nitrate to nitrite, which is then swallowed and absorbed into the bloodstream before further reduction to NO. The critical role of the oral microbiota in this effect has been demonstrated, where a seven-day period of antiseptic mouth wash treatment was shown to disrupt the oral microbiota of healthy non-athletes and, in the absence of any dietary modifications, was associated with reductions in plasma and oral nitrite levels and an increase in blood pressure [5]. These findings raise the spectre that diet may also invoke changes in the oral microbiota that manifest in alterations of this enterosalivary pathway and NO homeostasis but remains unexplored.

A recent investigation [6] of the effect of diet and training on exercise metabolism and performance in elite endurance athletes provided an opportunity for pilot work on this theme. The "Supernova 1" study investigated parameters around endurance capacity in a cohort of elite endurance race walkers who followed one of the three popular dietary approaches during a three-week period of intensified training: a ketogenic Low Carbohydrate High Fat diet (LCHF), or a diet high in carbohydrates consumed either ad libitum (HCHO) or at specific periods on a daily/weekly basis (PCHO). While the HCHO diet is focused on optimal muscle and brain carbohydrate (CHO) stores for each training session, the PCHO diet involves a strategic combination of sessions with such dietary support as well as other which are undertaken with low muscle glycogen availability to promote greater metabolic stress and cellular adaptation [7,8]. Finally, the LCHF diet involves severe CHO restriction to promote adaptations that increase muscle capacity for fat oxidation [7,8]. Details on the rationale for these radically different types of nutrition [6,8] and the actual protocols employed in this study can be found elsewhere [6,7]. In summary, the Supernova 1 study found that each group of athletes achieved a significant improvement in their aerobic capacity over the training block, which was undertaken during the base phase of the annual training plan. However, while this was associated with improved economy and real-world race performance in the two groups who trained while consuming the HCHO and PCHO diets, the LCHF group experienced an increase in the oxygen cost of exercise supported by high rates of fat oxidation, and thereby failed to improve their race performance despite the gain in aerobic capacity [6]. Based on these differential results, the overall aim of this study was to examine whether and how the oral microbiome of these athletes was affected by their diet during intensified training. This appears to be the first study that provides an in-depth investigation of diet x oral microbiome interactions in elite athletes.

2. Materials and Methods

2.1. Study Design

The group of world-class race walkers and the design of the "Supernova 1" study are described in detail by Burke et al. [6] and Mirtschin et al. [7]. In summary, these male race walkers (aged 20–35 years, BMI range 16–23 kg/m^2) were from Australia, Canada, Japan, Italy, Poland, Sweden, Chile and South Africa, and all met International Association of Athletics Federations (IAAF) standards for international competition, with more than 75% participating in the major championships during the year of the study (i.e., 2016 Rio Olympic Games and 2016 World Walking Cup). Twenty-nine study experiences were gained from 21 elite athletes who participated in either one (n = 13) or both (n = 8) of the Supernova 1 research camps conducted at the Australian Institute of Sport. Each camp involved three weeks of intensified training and rigorously supervised dietary interventions.

2.2. Allocation to Dietary Interventions

The athletes were involved over several months of planning and received education about the range of likely effects of the diets on various aspects of health and performance. Each had ample time to choose a diet(s) according to his beliefs of the performance benefits from the chosen diet. Although this type of assignment was non-random, given that all athletes choose freely to be in the study and to be fed their diet of choice, this approach both promoted adherence to the intervention and controlled for the random effects of such rigorous dietary control (e.g., feeling anxious about losing personal freedom of dietary choice). Therefore, any effects on the oral microbiome could be attributed to the diet, including any additional intrinsic biochemical, physiological or psychological overlay that belongs to the diet itself.

Three diets were compared: (i) a diet high in carbohydrate availability (HCHO; n = 9) comprised of 60% of energy intake from CHO (~8.5 g/kg body mass (BM)/day), 16% protein (~2.1 g/kg BM/day), 20% fat; (ii) a diet with periodised carbohydrate availability (PCHO; n = 10) of similar overall macronutrient composition as HCHO but consumed at different intervals across the day and throughout the week to support different training sessions with high or low CHO availability and (iii) a ketogenic low carbohydrate-high fat diet (LCHF; n = 10) comprised of 78% fat, 17% protein (~2.2 g/kg/day) and 0.50 g/kg/day carbohydrate (3.5% energy). All the meals were prepared taking into consideration the nutritional requirement within the allocated dietary intervention. Mirtschin et al. reported the detailed nutritional information and meal plans for the above three dietary interventions of this study [7].

2.3. Sample Collection, Genomic DNA Extraction and 16S rRNA Gene Amplicon Preparation

Saliva samples were collected from the athletes prior (baseline, BL) and after the three -week training-diet intervention using the OMNIgene saliva collection and preservative kit and according to the manufacturer's instruction (fasted collection, saliva collected by spitting into the tube). Total DNA was extracted from 0.25 mL aliquots of the preserved saliva samples using the repeated bead-beating procedure for cell lysis [9] and an automated column-based DNA purification procedure (Maxwell® 16MDx system, Promega Corporation, WI, USA) as described by Shanahan et al. [10]. Bar-coded PCR amplicon libraries of the V6-V8 hypervariable regions of 16S rRNA genes from Bacteria/Archaea were produced also following the protocols described by Shanahan et al. [10], and then sequenced via the Illumina MiSeq platform and workflows established by the Australian Centre for Ecogenomics at the University of Queensland.

2.4. Bioinformatics Analysis

The sequence data were analysed using the Quantitative Insights into Microbial Ecology (QIIME) software package on an Ubuntu Linux virtual machine. QIIME was used to demultiplex and perform quality control checking and filtering of the sequence data [11]. USEARCH 6.1 was used for the removal of candidate chimeric sequences [12]. The chimera checked filtered sequences were then clustered into Operational Taxonomic Units (OTUs) using the open reference OTU picking method. Threshold setting of 97% sequence identity was applied and Greengenes (version 13.8) database was used as the reference database [13]. Following the OTU picking step, OTUs that were not identified as Bacteria or Archaea, and/or OTUs that comprised $\leq$ 0.01% of the total sample sequence count, were discarded from further analysis. All of the samples with less than 1000 reads were also excluded from the OTU table. Single rarefaction was done by random sampling to the minimum read count (6861 reads) to generate a subsampled OTU table.

2.5. Statistical Analysis

The rarefied OTU table was used to generate the taxonomy plots from phylum to genus levels and used to calculate alpha- and beta-diversity metrics. Alpha diversity was measured by Shannon index as an estimator for richness and evenness of microbiota communities. Weighted and unweighted UniFrac distance matrices were constructed in QIIME and used for Principle Coordinate Analysis (PCoA) of beta (between sample) diversity analysis. Redundancy Analysis (RDA) and Analysis of Similarity (ANOSIM) measures were also performed on these data within the Calypso web server to identify any clustering with respect to BL or the specific dietary patterns. Linear Discriminant Analysis (LDA) Effect Size (LEfSe) and sparse Partial Least Squares Discriminant Analysis (sPLS-DA) analyses via the Mixomics mixMC package within Calypso were then used to identify whether any individual taxa are discriminatory for the different dietary patterns [14,15]. The multiple linear regression analysis available via Calypso was used to perform pairwise comparisons between the BL and post-diet training microbiome profiles. A p-value < 0.05 was considered significant for all the statistical analysis. Tukey's test was used to compare age and BMI data for the athletes assigned to each dietary group.

2.6. Ethics Approval, Trial Registration and Consent to Participate

The study was approved by the Ethics committee of the Australian Institute of Sports (AIS, no. 20150802) and UQ-HREC 2015001965. The clinical trial is registered by the Australian New Zealand Clinical Trials Registry (ANZCTR) and has been assigned the number ACTRN12618001529235. The raw sequence paired-end files are deposited in the European Nucleotide Archive with the primary accession number PRJEB29801. All the subjects were informed and consented to do this research.

3. Results

As mentioned previously, 21 elite race walkers were recruited in the study (with eight athletes recruited in both the camps). Table 1 provides the anthropometric details of the subjects enrolled in the study. According to Tukey's multiple comparisons test, there were no significant differences in the age ($p = 0.53$ for HCHO vs. PCHO; $p = 0.28$ for HCHO vs. LCHF and $p = 0.87$ for PCHO vs. LCHF) and the BMI scores ($p = 0.36$ for HCHO vs. PCHO; $p = 0.84$ for HCHO vs. LCHF and $p = 0.67$ for PCHO vs. LCHF) when athletes were grouped according to the dietary intervention they received.

Table 1. Athlete cohort characteristics.

	High Carbohydrate (HCHO) Diet	Periodised Carbohydrate (PCHO) Diet	Low Carbohydrate High Fat (LCHF) Diet
Sample size	$n = 9$	$n = 10$	$n = 10$
Age (years)	25.4 ± 4	27.4 ± 4.6	28.3 ± 3.5
BMI (kg/m^2)	20 ± 1.6	21 ± 1.3	20.4 ± 1.8
Country of origin	Australia, Canada, Japan, South Africa	Australia, Canada, Japan, Poland, Sweden, Italy	Australia, Canada, Japan, Poland, Sweden, Chile, South Africa
Gender	Male	Male	Male

Note: Data for Age and body mass index (BMI) are shown as mean ± standard deviation.

The Shannon alpha diversity was reduced following the diet-training interventions when compared to their subject-matched BL measures; however, these reductions were not statistically significant ($p = 0.1$ for BL vs. HCHO and BL vs PCHO; $p = 0.62$ for BL vs. LCHF). The PCoA analysis of the weighted UniFrac distances are shown in Figure 1 and did not reveal any distinct clustering of the saliva microbiome profiles, either with respect to the ethnic origin of the athletes or the dietary intervention. Similarly, the supervised analyses by RDA and ANOSIM did not identify any significant differences between the microbiota community composition at BL and following any of the three dietary interventions (data not shown). Taken together, these results suggest that the dietary interventions do not result in dramatic changes in the overall biodiversity of the oral microbiome, but rather more subtle changes in community composition. As mentioned previously in the Methods section, eight athletes were recruited in both the camps, and the two baseline profiles (B1 vs. B2) of these eight athletes were compared. No substantive differences between the two microbiota profiles were apparent, as assessed by Shannon alpha-diversity and ANOSIM beta-diversity analyses. These tests indicate that the time between the study camps was sufficiently long to ensure a "washout" between the two camps, and, thereby, no potential carryover effects from the previous diet on the subsequent results/profiles.

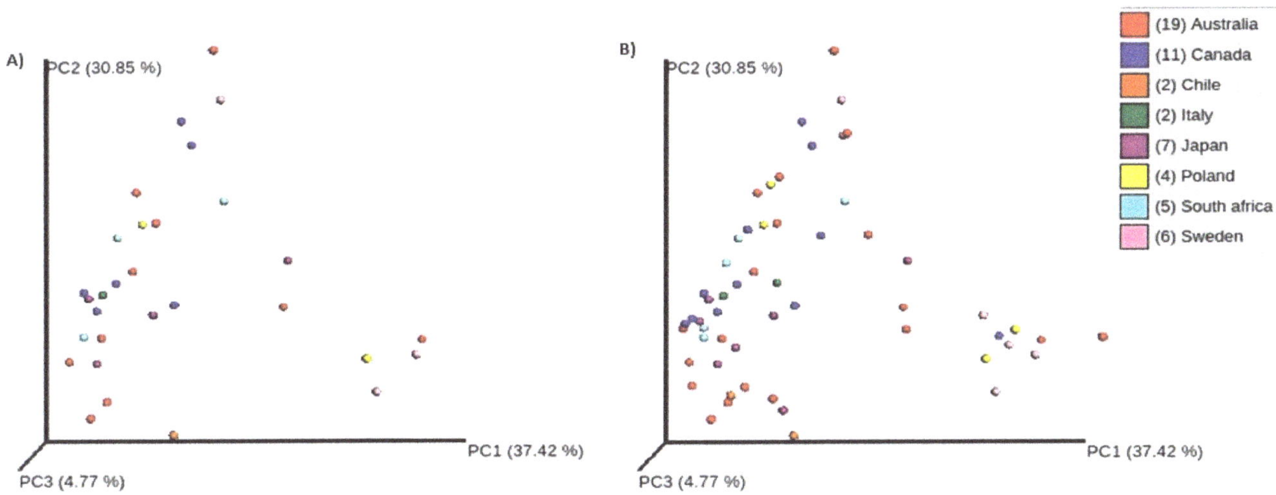

Figure 1. Principle component analysis of weighted UniFrac distances for the oral microbiomes of athletes at Baseline only (BL, **A**); and when combined with their profiles obtained after the diet-training intervention period (**B**). Samples are colored based on the athlete's country of origin and show no significant clustering indicative of a dietary and/or ethnic effect on the oral microbiomes.

3.1. Comparisons of Community Profiles of Saliva Samples between Baseline and Post Interventions

LefSe analyses was used to identify discriminating taxa between baseline (BL) and post diet-training interventions. OTU's affiliated to *Streptococcus, Peptostreptococcus, Actinomyces, Granulicatella, Atopobium, Veillonella* and *Prevotella* were found to be enriched following the consumption of HCHO diet, whereas *Parvimonas* was discriminatory and enriched for the BL samples from these same athletes (Supplementary Figure S1). Analysis by the sPLS-DA of the same athlete samples identified *Prevotella, Actinobacillus, Fusobacterium, Haemophilus* and *Gemella* to be associated and increased in BL samples (Figure 2). Pairwise comparisons (Supplementary Figure S2) of the oral microbiota profiles at BL and following HCHO diet training intervention was also examined using mixed effect linear regression, and the relative abundance of *Atopobium* was found to increase ($p = 0.015$), whereas *Capnocytophaga* ($p = 0.027$) and *Porphyromonas* ($p = 0.03$) were decreased after consumption of HCHO diet, when compared to the BL. However, no significant differences were observed once correction for multiple testing using false discovery rate was applied (FDR = 0.49).

LefSe analysis was then used to compare the microbiota profiles between BL and PCHO diet and revealed that the OTU's affiliated with *Leptotrichia, Neisseria, Moryella and Actinomyces* to be discriminatory and enriched for BL, whereas OTU's affiliated with *Streptococcus, Kingella,* unclassified members of *Neisseriaceae* and *Prevotella* were increased and discriminatory in the same athletes after consumption of the PCHO diet (Supplementary Figure S3). Analysis by sPLS-DA further showed that the relative abundances of *Haemophilus, Neisseria, Porphyromonas, Leptotrichia, Kingella, Prevotella, Unclassified Neisseriaceae, Rothia, Selenomonas and Tannerella* were increased following the consumption of the PCHO diet *whereas Unc. Aerococcaceae, Unc. CW040, Lautropia and Parvimonas* were distinct and increased in the BL samples of the same athletes who later received the PCHO dietary intervention (Figure 3). Repeated measures mixed effect linear regression analysis showed that the genus *Actinomyces* ($p = 0.04$), *Moryella* ($p = 0.05$), *Oribacterium* ($p = 0.04$), *Peptostreptococcus* ($p = 0.009$) and some unclassified *Erysipelotrichaceae* ($p = 0.04$) were reduced in response to the PCHO diet as compared to BL (Supplementary Figure S4). However, the statistical significance of all these differences was lost once correction for multiple testing using the false discovery rate was applied (FDR = 0.4) (Supplementary Figure S4).

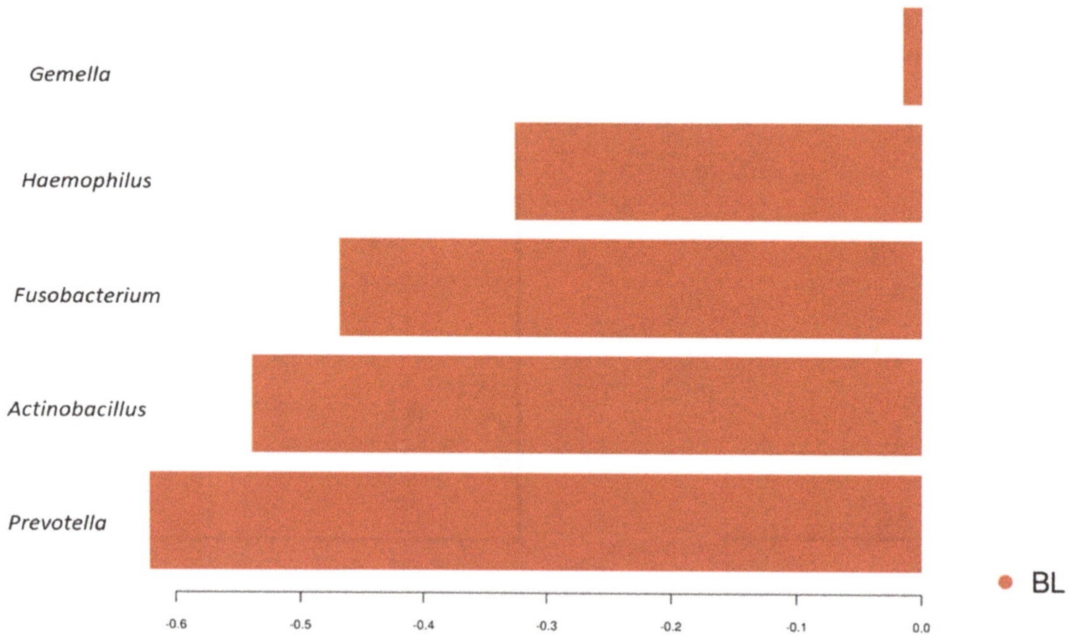

Figure 2. Genera differentiating between the oral microbiota profiles of athletes at baseline (BL, red) and after their consumption of the High Carbohydrate diet (HCHO) identified by sparse Partial Least Squares Discriminant Analysis (sPLS–DA).

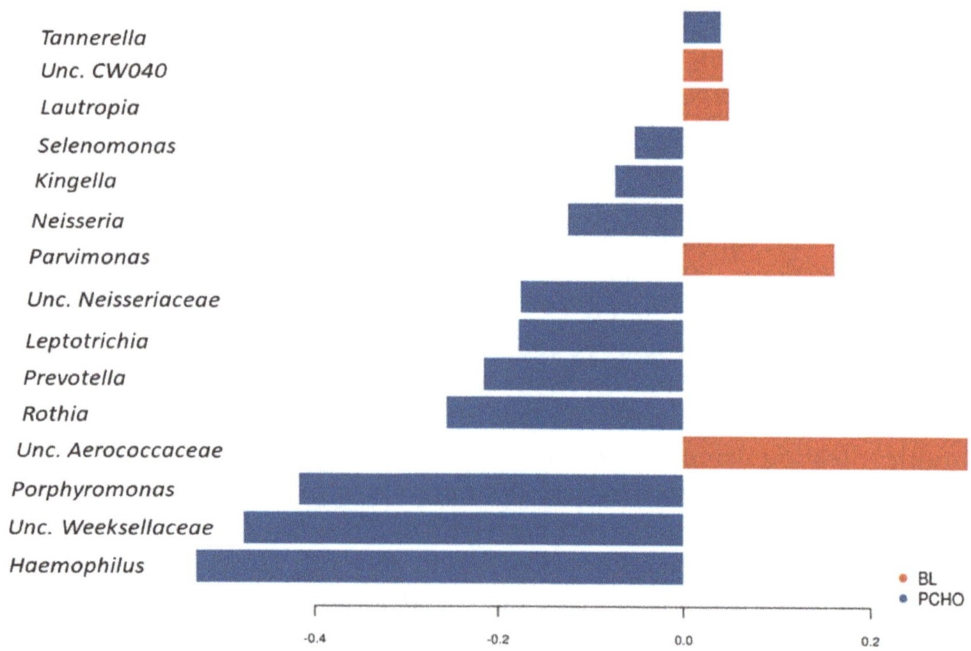

Figure 3. Genera differentiating between the oral microbiota profiles of athletes at baseline (BL, red) and after their consumption of the Periodised Carbohydrate diet (PCHO, blue) identified by sparse Partial Least Squares Discriminant Analysis (sPLS–DA).

Discriminating taxa for BL and for the same samples following the LCHF diet. Training intervention was also identified using LefSE and sPLS-DA. LefSe analysis revealed *Leptotrichia, Lachnospiraceae* and *TM-7* affiliated OTU's to be increased in the BL samples, whereas *Lactobacillales, Streptococcus, Neisseria* affiliated OTU's were discriminatory and increased in the LCHF group (Supplementary Figure S5). The sPLS-DA identified *Selenomonas, Unc. Planococcaceae, Unc. Enterobacteriaceae, Peptostreptococcus, Gemella, Granulicatella, Parvimonas Unc. Clostridiaceae* to increase following LCHF diet training intervention, whereas *Unc. F16, Unc. Neisseriaceae, Leptotrichia, Lactobacillus, Lautropia* and *Kingella* to be distinct and enriched in the BL samples of same athletes (Figure 4). According to repeated measures analysis using mixed effect linear regression, the genus *Fusobacterium* ($p = 0.02$), *Lautropia* ($p = 0.05$), *Aggregatibacter* ($p = 0.04$), *Leptotrichia* ($p = 0.040$) and some unclassified *F16* ($p = 0.04$) were reduced, whereas *Granulicatella* ($p = 0.03$), some unclassified Planococcaceae ($p = 0.03$) and *Streptococcus* ($p = 0.048$) were increased in response to LCHF diet when compared to microbiota profiles at their BL (Supplementary Figure S6). However, no significant differences were observed once correction for multiple testing using false discovery rate was applied (FDR = 0.4).

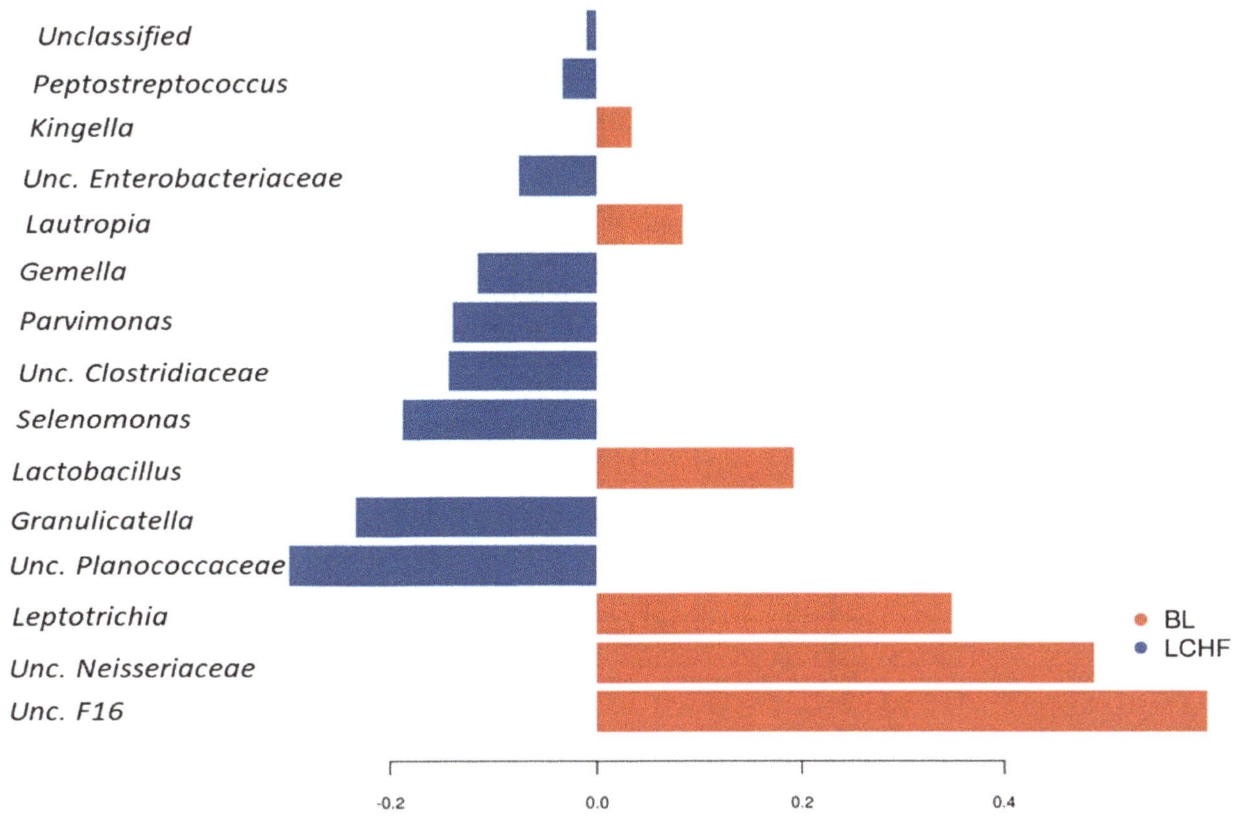

Figure 4. Genera differentiating between the oral microbiota profiles of athletes at baseline (BL, red) and after their consumption of the Low Carbohydrate High Fat diet (LCHF, blue) identified by sparse Partial Least Squares Discriminant Analysis (sPLS–DA).

3.2. Comparisons of Community Profiles of Saliva Samples at the Conclusion of Dietary Interventions

Figure 5 summarises the results of these analyses, showing the community profiles present in saliva samples at the conclusion of the dietary intervention periods, with annotations around some key genera and their inferred nitrate reductase capacity (Figure 5A). These profiles were compared with each other using sPLS-DA, which can be used to extract those taxa that most strongly discriminate the community structure between treatment groups (Figure 5B). Longitudinal comparison of the taxonomic profiles in the samples using sPLS-DA (Figure 5B) showed the strongest effect of the LCHF dietary intervention and in particular increase in the abundance of Gram-positive (Firmicutes) bacteria such as *Streptococcus*, *Peptostreptococcus*, and *Rothia*.

LefSe analyses was also used to examine the differences in oral microbiomes post intervention and these analyses showed that the discriminating and enriched taxa (at the OTU level) were *Streptococcus* affiliated OTUs for the LCHF diet intervention, whereas Gram-negative bacteria (e.g., *Haemophilus* and *Leptotrichia* spp.) were among the enriched and discriminating taxa for the HCHO/PCHO diets (Figure 6A,B).

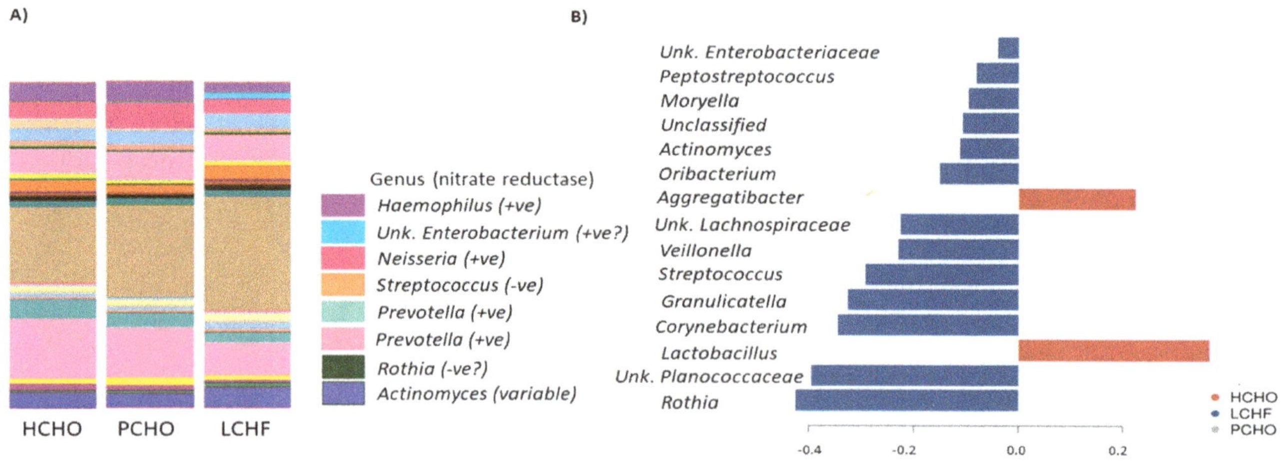

Figure 5. Oral microbiome profiles (genus-level) of athletes consuming either a high carbohydrate (HCHO), periodised carbohydrate (PCHO) or a low-carbohydrate high-fat diet (LCHF) after the diet-training intervention where bar plots represent: (**A**) relative abundance of genera in saliva samples after dietary interventions and their inferred nitrate reductase activity; (**B**) microbial families associated with different diets as identified by sparse Partial Least Squares Discriminant Analysis (sPLS-DA).

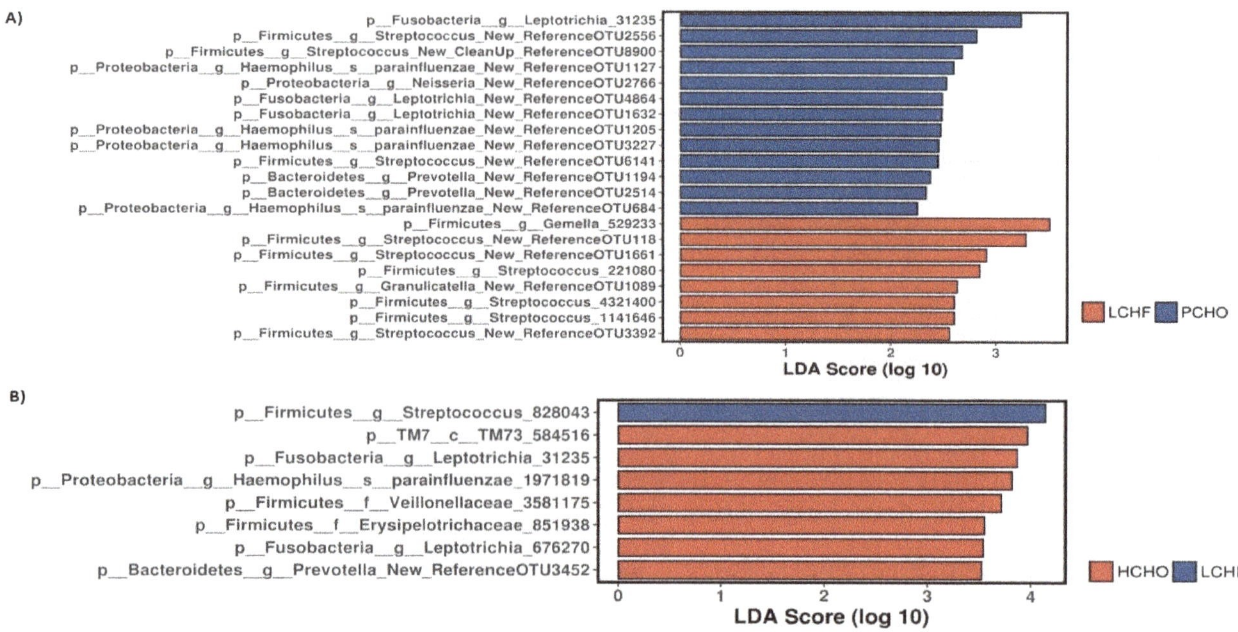

Figure 6. Linear Discriminant Analysis (LDA) Effect Size (LefSe) analysis at Operational Taxonomic Unit (OTU) level to compare the oral microbiome profiles of athletes post training diet interventions between Periodised Carbohydrate/Low Carbohydrate High Fat diet (PCHO/LCHF) (**A**) and High carbohydrate-Low Carbohydrate high-fat diet (HCHO/LCHF) (**B**), respectively.

4. Discussion

Despite the relatively small number of participants in this study, the dietary pattern consumed by these elite athletes during intensified training was shown to invoke remarkable effects on specific oral bacterial taxa—the bacterial communities in the mouth. The lack of a matching cohort of non-athletes (non-race walkers) and the lack of comprehensive data on the habitual dietary intake of athletes (i.e., BL samples) are acknowledged but were beyond the logistical and financial scope of the trial design. Furthermore, but understandably, the elite nature of the athletes ensured the group size is quite small, which also reduces the power needed for stringent statistical tests of significance, or the further subgrouping of the athletes according to ethnicity, etc. However, and despite these limitations, this is the first study of its type with elite endurance athletes, and one of the very few studies of the diet/nutrients × oral microbiota interactions affecting the physiology and/or metabolism of healthy human subjects. Furthermore, while fluctuations in the abundance and/or activities of nitrate-reducing bacteria in the oral microbiome are recognised to affect an individual's responsiveness to nitrate supplementation [16], this is the first study of the effects of dietary manipulation on this specific microbiome.

The bacterial taxa found in this study are similar to those represented in the Human Oral Microbiome Database (HOMD), as well as those typically reported in other studies of mainstream human subjects [17,18]. The beta-diversity UniFrac principal coordinates analysis showed no apparent clustering of the oral microbial communities based on the ethnicity of the athletes nor any distinct effects of the dietary interventions under investigation in this study. This is similar to the findings of other studies of healthy individuals in which no significant clustering and bacterial taxa changes in the oral cavity have been reported [17]. Nevertheless, more subtle changes within the bacterial communities in association with the diets were observed, with some of these representing potential alterations in community–host symbiosis. Here, the comparisons of the oral microbiome collected after three weeks of consuming one of three widely used diets by elite athletes during intensified training revealed that, unlike the CHO-rich diets, a ketogenic-LCHF diet appears to shift the balance of bacterial taxa that are widely considered to be key governors of the enterosalivary nitrate-nitrite-nitric oxide (NO) axis within the oral cavity. This is an important finding since previous studies have demonstrated functional effects on host health when alterations to the oral microbiome interfere with this pathway [19]. Facultative anaerobic bacteria in the mouth reduce salivary gland concentrated nitrate to nitrite, which is then swallowed and absorbed into the bloodstream, before further reduction to NO [3,4,20].

The critical role of the oral microbiome in this effect has been recently demonstrated in healthy non-athletes, where a seven-day period of antiseptic mouth wash treatment was shown to disrupt the oral microbiota and, in the absence of any dietary modifications, was associated with reductions in plasma and oral nitrite levels and an increase in blood pressure [20]. Taken together, the changes seen following consumption of the LCHF diet, with respect to reductions in the relative abundances of well-known Gram-negative nitrate/nitrite reducers such as *Haemophilus*, *Prevotella* and *Neisseria*; and an increase in *Streptococcus* spp., which are not recognised to be directly involved in nitrate/nitrite reduction; raises the spectre that consumption of the LCHF diet can impair the enterosalivary nitrate-nitrite-NO axis. Indeed, further indirect support for this hypothesis can be found in a recent brief report that a three-day LCHF diet was associated with an impaired plasma nitrate/nitrite conversion following supplementation with potassium nitrate, compared with the response observed when people consumed a HCHO diet [21]. This suggests that a LCHF diet might alter the baseline contribution of the nitrate-nitrite-NO pathway to NO-related health and performance benefits in athletes, as well as reduce their responsiveness to nitrate/beetroot juice supplementation as a performance aid [22]. Further supporting evidence comes from the major outcome of the Supernova 1 study, which is the primary study to the current project and from which these saliva samples were derived [6]. The study found a reduction in exercise economy (i.e., an increased oxygen cost of exercise) across a range of walking speeds in the LCHF group. It was originally hypothesised that this contributed to the failure of the LCHF group to improve their performance of a 10,000 m race walking event, despite the improvement in aerobic capacity that was seen across each of the study groups in response to the three week block of intensified training It is plausible to attribute this loss of economy to the substantial increase in the contribution of fat oxidation to exercise substrate needs in the LCHF group, noting the longstanding recognition that CHO oxidation is slightly more economical in generating ATP than fat oxidation per unit of oxygen utilization [23]. Additionally, the increase in exercise tolerance and performance following acute and/or chronic nitrate supplementation include improved oxygen delivery to the muscle via the vasodilatory effects of NO, as well as a direct effect on mitochondria to reduce proton leak [22]. However, these benefits are not universally observed across and within studies, and this variability is partially attributed to individual responsiveness, in addition to the more obvious contribution of unsuitable study protocols in relation to both the supplementation and exercise elements. However, based on the findings reported here, it is also plausible that part of the reduced exercise efficiency observed in the Supernova 1 study might be attributed to an altered oral microbiome, resulting in a reduction in nitrate/nitrite reducing activity and NO generation, with coordinate effects on circulation and mitochondrial function.

5. Conclusions

In conclusion, the results presented here are the first direct comparison of the oral microbiota profiles of elite athletes, and the effects of the dietary pattern consumed during intensified training for race-walking. The LCHF diet resulted in the most dramatic effects on the oral microbiota, with reductions in the relative abundance (*Haemophilus, Neisseria* and *Prevotella)*, and with a coincident increase in the relative abundance of *Streptococcus* spp. The athletes participating in this study following consumption of the LCHF diet also showed a loss of exercise economy (i.e., an increased oxygen cost of exercise) across a range of walking speeds compared to athletes consuming the carbohydrate rich diets [6]. The findings reported here therefore justify the need to examine how diet x oral microbiome interactions affect elite athlete performance; and, particularly, NO homeostasis, and any coordinate impacts on cardiovascular and circulatory physiology.

Supplementary Materials
Figure S1: Genera differentiating between the oral microbiota profiles of athletes at baseline (BL, red) and after their consumption of the High Carbohydrate diet (HCHO, blue) identified by LefSE; Figure S2: Mixed effect linear regression identified significant reductions in the relative abundances of *Capnocytophaga* (p = 0.027) and *Porphyromonas* (p = 0.032) whereas significant increase in the relative abundance of *Atopobium* (p = 0.015) after consumption of the High carbohydrate (HCHO) diet. Relative abundance was compared by mixed effect linear regression, including sampling time point as fixed effect and athlete as random effect. BL: baseline. Samples collected from the same individual are connected by lines; Figure S3: Genera differentiating between the oral microbiota profiles of athletes at baseline (BL, red) and after their consumption of the Periodised Carbohydrate diet (PCHO, blue) identified by LefSE; Figure S4: Mixed effect linear regression identified significant reductions in the relative abundances of *Actinomyces* (p = 0.043), *Moryella* (p = 0.053), *Oribacterium* (p = 0.042), *Peptostreptococcus* (p = 0.009) and *Unc. Erysipelotrichaceae* (p = 0.042) after consumption of the Periodised carbohydrate (PCHO) diet. Relative abundance was compared by mixed effect linear regression, including sampling time point as fixed effect and athlete as random effect. BL: baseline. Samples collected from the same individual are connected by lines; Figure S5: Genera differentiating between the oral microbiota profiles of athletes at baseline (BL, red) and after their consumption of the Low Carbohydrate High Fat diet (LCHF, blue) identified by LefSE; Figure S6: Mixed effect linear regression identified significant reductions in the relative abundances of *Fusobacterium* (p = 0.020), *Lautropia* (p = 0.048), *Leptotrichia* (p = 0.040), *Aggregatibacter* (p = 0.044) and *Unc. F16* (p = 0.040) whereas significant increase in the relative abundances of *Granulicatella* (p = 0.038), *Streptococcus* (p = 0.048) and *Planococcaceae* (p = 0.038) after consumption of the low carbohydrate high fat (LCHF) diet. Relative abundance was compared by mixed effect linear regression, including sampling time point as fixed effect and athlete as random effect. BL: baseline. Samples collected from the same individual are connected by lines.

Author Contributions: Conceptualization, L.M.B. and M.M.; methodology, L.M.B., M.M., and L.K.; formal analysis, N.M.; investigation, N.M.; resources, L.M.B. and M.M.; original draft preparation, N.M.; manuscript review and editing, L.M.B., M.M., L.K., N.V., B.C., H.M.O., M.L.R., and K.L.C.; visualization, N.M.; supervision, M.M.; project administration, L.M.B. and M.M.; funding acquisition, L.M.B. and M.M.

Acknowledgments: The authors thank all the subjects for their participation in this study and N.M. especially acknowledges the support and guidance from Alicia Kang, Erin Shanahan, Naoki Fukuma and Luisa Gomez Arango.

References

1. Dewhirst, F.E.; Chen, T.; Izard, J.; Paster, B.J.; Tanner, A.C.; Yu, W.H.; Lakshmanan, A.; Wade, W.G. The Human Oral Microbiome. *J. Bacteriol.* **2010**, *192*, 5002–5017. [CrossRef]
2. He, J.; Li, Y.; Cao, Y.; Xue, J.; Zhou, X. The oral microbiome diversity and its relation to human diseases. *Folia Microbiol.* **2015**, *60*, 69–80. [CrossRef]
3. Lundberg, J.O.; Weitzberg, E.; Cole, J.A.; Benjamin, N. Nitrate, bacteria and human health. *Nat. Rev. Microbiol.* **2004**, *2*, 593. [CrossRef] [PubMed]
4. Lundberg, J.O.; Weitzberg, E.; Gladwin, M.T. The nitrate-nitrite-nitric oxide pathway in physiology and therapeutics. *Nat. Rev. Drug Discov.* **2008**, *7*, 156–167. [CrossRef] [PubMed]
5. Petersson, J.; Carlström, M.; Schreiber, O.; Phillipson, M.; Christoffersson, G.; Jägare, A.; Roos, S.; Jansson, E.A.; Persson, A.E.; Lundberg, J.O.; et al. Gastroprotective and blood pressure lowering effects of dietary nitrate are abolished by an antiseptic mouthwash. *Free Radic. Biol. Med.* **2009**, *46*, 1068–1075. [CrossRef] [PubMed]
6. Burke, L.M.; Ross, M.L.; Garvican-Lewis, L.A.; Welvaert, M.; Heikura, I.A.; Forbes, S.G.; Mirtschin, J.G.; Cato, L.E.; Strobel, N.; Sharma, A.P.; et al. Low carbohydrate, high fat diet impairs exercise economy and negates the performance benefit from intensified training in elite race walkers. *J. Physiol.* **2017**, *595*, 2785–2807. [CrossRef]
7. Mirtschin, J.G.; Forbes, S.F.; Cato, L.E.; Heikura, I.A.; Strobel, N.; Hall, R.; Burke, L.M. Organization of Dietary Control for Nutrition-Training Intervention Involving Periodized Carbohydrate Availability and Ketogenic Low-Carbohydrate High-Fat Diet. *Int. J. Sport Nutr. Exerc. Metab.* **2018**, 1–10. [CrossRef] [PubMed]
8. Burke, L.M.; Hawley, J.A.; Jeukendrup, A.; Morton, J.P.; Stellingwerff, T.; Maughan, R.J. Toward a Common Understanding of Diet-Exercise Strategies to Manipulate Fuel Availability for Training and Competition Preparation in Endurance Sport. *Int. J. Sport Nutr. Exerc. Metab.* **2018**, *28*, 451–463. [CrossRef] [PubMed]
9. Ó Cuív, P.; Aguirre de Cárcer, D.; Jones, M.; Klaassens, E.S.; Worthley, D.L.; Whitehall, V.L.; Kang, S.; McSweeney, C.S.; Leggett, B.A.; Morrison, M. The effects from DNA extraction methods on the evaluation of microbial diversity associated with human colonic tissue. *Microb. Ecol.* **2011**, *61*, 353–362. [CrossRef]
10. Shanahan, E.R.; Zhong, L.; Talley, N.J.; Morrison, M.; Holtmann, G. Characterisation of the gastrointestinal mucosa-associated microbiota: A novel technique to prevent cross-contamination during endoscopic procedures. *Aliment. Pharmacol. Ther.* **2016**, *43*, 1186–1196. [CrossRef]
11. Caporaso, J.G.; Kuczynski, J.; Stombaugh, J.; Bittinger, K.; Bushman, F.D.; Costello, E.K.; Fierer, N.; Peña, A.G.; Goodrich, J.K.; Gordon, J.I.; et al. QIIME allows analysis of high-throughput community sequencing data. *Nat. Methods* **2010**, *7*, 335–336. [CrossRef] [PubMed]
12. Haas, B.J.; Gevers, D.; Earl, A.M.; Feldgarden, M.; Ward, D.V.; Giannoukos, G.; Ciulla, D.; Tabbaa, D.; Highlander, S.K.; Sodergren, E.; et al. Chimeric 16S rRNA sequence formation and detection in Sanger and 454-pyrosequenced PCR amplicons. *Genome Res.* **2011**, *21*, 494–504. [CrossRef]
13. DeSantis, T.Z.; Hugenholtz, P.; Larsen, N.; Rojas, M.; Brodie, E.L.; Keller, K.; Huber, T.; Dalevi, D.; Hu, P.; Andersen, G.L. Greengenes, a chimera-checked 16S rRNA gene database and workbench compatible with ARB. *Appl. Environ. Microbiol.* **2006**, *72*, 5069–5072. [CrossRef] [PubMed]
14. Cao, K.-A.L.; Costello, M.-E.; Lakis, V.A.; Bartolo, F.; Chua, X.-Y.; Brazeilles, R.; Rondeau, P. MixMC: A Multivariate Statistical Framework to Gain Insight into Microbial Communities. *PLoS ONE* **2016**, *11*, e0160169. [CrossRef]
15. Zakrzewski, M.; Proietti, C.; Ellis, J.J.; Hasan, S.; Brion, M.-J.; Berger, B.; Krause, L. Calypso: A user-friendly web-server for mining and visualizing microbiome–environment interactions. *Bioinformatics* **2017**, *33*, 782–783. [CrossRef] [PubMed]
16. Burleigh, M.C.; Liddle, L.; Monaghan, C.; Muggeridge, D.J.; Sculthorpe, N.; Butcher, J.P.; Henriquez, F.L.; Allen, J.D.; Easton, C. Salivary nitrite production is elevated in individuals with a higher abundance of oral nitrate-reducing bacteria. *Free Radic. Biol. Med.* **2018**, *120*, 80–88. [CrossRef] [PubMed]

17. Bik, E.M.; Long, C.D.; Armitage, G.C.; Loomer, P.; Emerson, J.; Mongodin, E.F.; Nelson, K.E.; Gill, S.R.; Fraser-Liggett, C.M.; Relman, D.A. Bacterial diversity in the oral cavity of 10 healthy individuals. *ISME J.* **2010**, *4*, 962. [CrossRef]
18. Aas, J.A.; Paster, B.J.; Stokes, L.N.; Olsen, I.; Dewhirst, F.E. Defining the normal bacterial flora of the oral cavity. *J. Clin. Microbiol.* **2005**, *43*, 5721–5732. [CrossRef] [PubMed]
19. Vanhatalo, A.; Blackwell, J.R.; L'Heureux, J.E.; Williams, D.W.; Smith, A.; van der Giezen, M.; Winyard, P.G.; Kelly, J.; Jones, A.M. Nitrate-responsive oral microbiome modulates nitric oxide homeostasis and blood pressure in humans. *Free Radic. Biol. Med.* **2018**, *124*, 21–30. [CrossRef]
20. Qu, X.M.; Wu, Z.F.; Pang, B.X.; Jin, L.Y.; Qin, L.Z.; Wang, S.L. From Nitrate to Nitric Oxide: The Role of Salivary Glands and Oral Bacteria. *J. Dent. Res.* **2016**, *95*, 1452–1456. [CrossRef]
21. Piatrikova, E. The Impact of High-Carbohydrate and High-Fat Diets in Combination with Nitrate on O_2 Uptake Kinetics and Performance during High-Intensity Exercise. Published Online First: 16 March 2017. Available online: https://ore.exeter.ac.uk/repository/handle/10871/28215 (accessed on 16 December 2017).
22. Jones, A.M. Influence of dietary nitrate on the physiological determinants of exercise performance: A critical review. *Appl. Physiol. Nutr. Metab. Physiol. Appl. Nutr. Metab.* **2014**, *39*, 1019–1028. [CrossRef] [PubMed]
23. Krogh, A.; Lindhard, J. The Relative Value of Fat and Carbohydrate as Sources of Muscular Energy. *Biochem. J.* **1920**, *14*, 290–363. [CrossRef] [PubMed]

14

Lower Back Complaints in Adolescent Competitive Alpine Skiers

Attilio Carraro [1,*], Martina Gnech [2], Fabio Sarto [3,*], Diego Sarto [2], Jörg Spörri [4,5] and Stefano Masiero [6]

1 Faculty of Education, Free University of Bolzano, 39042 Bressanone (Bolzano), Italy
2 School of Human Movement Sciences, University of Padova, 35122 Padova, Italy; gnechmartina@gmail.com (M.G.); centrostudi@diegosarto.it (D.S.)
3 Department of Biomedical Sciences, University of Padova, 35131 Padova, Italy
4 Sports Medical Research Group, Department of Orthopaedics, Balgrist University Hospital, University of Zurich, 8006 Zurich, Switzerland; joerg.spoerri@balgrist.ch
5 University Centre for Prevention and Sports Medicine, Department of Orthopaedics, Balgrist University Hospital, University of Zurich, 8006 Zurich, Switzerland
6 Department of Neurosciences, Section of Rehabilitation, University of Padova, 35128 Padova, Italy; stef.masiero@unipd.it
* Correspondence: attilio.carraro@unibz.it (A.C.); fabio.sarto.2@phd.unipd.it (F.S.)

Abstract: Background: Little is known about lower back complaints in adolescent competitive alpine skiers. This study assessed their prevalence and severity (i.e., intensity and disability) with respect to sex, category, discipline preference, and training attributes. Methods: 188 competitive skiers aged 15 to 18 years volunteered in this study. Data collection included (i) questions on participants' demographics, sports exposure, discipline preferences, and other sports-related practices; (ii) the Nordic Musculoskeletal Questionnaire on lower back complaints; and (iii) the Graded Chronic Pain Scale. Results: As many as 80.3% and 50.0% of all skiers suffered from lower back complaints during the last 12 months and 7 days, respectively. A total of 50.7% reported their complaints to be attributable to slalom skiing, and 26% to giant slalom. The majority of complaints were classified as low intensity/low disability (Grade I, 57.4%) and high intensity/low disability complaints (Grade II, 21.8%). The Characteristic Pain Intensity was found to be significantly related to the skiers' years of sports participation, number of competitions/season, and number of skiing days/season. Conclusion: This study further supports the relatively high magnitudes of lower back-related pain in adolescent competitive alpine skiers, with a considerable amount of high intensity (but low disability) complaints, and training attributes being a key driver.

Keywords: alpine skiing; athletes' health; epidemiology; spine; musculoskeletal injuries

---

1. Introduction

Competitive alpine skiing is a popular yet high-risk sport. At all competition levels, health problems are frequent [1–7]. In particular, lower back has been reported to be one of the most affected body regions for overuse complaints [8]. Adolescent competitive alpine skiers are also known to suffer from relatively high rates of radiographic abnormalities in the thoracolumbar spine [9]. Specifically, degenerative disc changes were observed to be more prevalent in adolescent competitive alpine skiers than in age-matched controls [10]. Moreover, a recent study found such disc degenerations (particularly disc dehydration and disc protrusion) to be significantly more prevalent in symptomatic than in asymptomatic athletes [11]. However, little is known about the prevalence of lower back complaints in adolescent skiers with respect to severity (i.e., intensity and disability). Additionally, the role of discipline preference is widely unexplored as of yet.

The link between lower back pain and physical activity has been described as a U-shaped relationship, whereas increased risk was found for both sedentary subjects and those practicing strenuous physical activities [12]. According to this association, athletes may be considered a high-risk population, mainly due to the training and competition loads they are subjected to. Moreover, as a result of their musculoskeletal and spinal immaturity and excessive height growth, adolescent athletes are especially vulnerable [11,13].

From a biomechanical perspective, the following factors may contribute to overloading of the lower back structures in alpine ski racing [14]: (a) repetitive and heavy mechanical loads, particularly when accompanied by insufficient recovery between the training sessions [15]; (b) unphysiological postures (i.e., frontal bending, lateral bending, and torsion), associated with high ground reaction forces (up to 2.89 times the body weight) [16]; and (c) excessive exposure to low-frequency whole-body vibrations [17–20]. Since all of these factors are typical characteristics of alpine skiing-specific sports exposure, studying the relations between training attributes and lower back complaints is of superior importance.

Therefore, the aims of this study were: (1) to describe the demographics, sports exposure, and other sports- or warm-up-related practices of adolescent competitive alpine skiers; (2) to assess the prevalence of lower back complaints in this specific cohort with respect to sex, category, and discipline preference; (3) to explore their lower back complaints severity (i.e., intensity and disability); and (4) to investigate the potential relations with training attributes.

2. Materials and Methods

2.1. Study Design and Setting

This study was designed as a cross-sectional observation and was based on a structured and customized questionnaire package. Data were collected in the participants' sport clubs facilities at the end of the competition season. Questionnaires were spread physically. A member of the research team introduced the questionnaires to the participants, explaining all the questionnaire items and scales. Subsequently, the participants filled the questionnaires independently and individually.

2.2. Participants and Recruitment

Participants were included if they were members of ski clubs associated with the FISI (Italian Winter Sports Federation) Veneto region section and competed in the categories under 16 (U-16) and under 18 (U-18) years old. There were no study exclusions. All the ski clubs associated with the FISI Veneto region were contacted and invited to take part in the study. Finally, 188 adolescent competitive alpine skiers (110 males and 78 females) volunteered for the purpose of the current study; 128 belonged to the category U-16 and 60 to the U-18. The entire study sample represented about 70% of all U-16 and U-18 competitive alpine skiers affiliated to the FISI clubs in that region. The Ethics Committee of the Department of Biomedical Sciences of the University of Padua approved the study (HEC-DSB/02-19). Prior to the study, all the participants and their parents or legal representatives provided written informed consent. The participants did not receive any reward for their participation in the study.

2.3. Assessment Methods and Parameters

The questionnaire package comprised four parts: (1) questions on participants' demographics, sports exposure (years of sports participation, number of competitions/season, number of skiing days/season, number of athletic preparation days/season) and other sports- or warm-up-related practices; (2) the Nordic Musculoskeletal Questionnaire (NMQ), Italian version [21,22]; (3) specific questions on how their skiing discipline (e.g., Slalom—SL; Giant Slalom—GS; Super-G—SG;

or Downhill (DH)) was related to the occurrence of lower back complaints; (4) the Graded Chronic Pain Scale (GCPS), Italian version [23,24].

The NMQ aimed on investigating the time prevalence of musculoskeletal complaints in the lower back during the last 12 months and 7 days, respectively, as well as on whether these complaints resulted in any restrictions while carrying out normal activities or whether they required medical attention or not. Questionnaire completion was supported by a body map displaying the pain area. The GCPS was used to grade the severity of the lower back complaints. The underlying methodology consists of seven questions related to pain intensity items and disability items with respect to the 6 months preceding the questionnaire. Answers were provided on a scale from 0 (e.g., "no pain" or "no interference/change") to 10 (e.g., "pain as bad it could be" or "unable to carry on any activity/extreme change") [23]. Based on these scale points, as well as on a specific scoring system, the Characteristic Pain Intensity (0–100), Disability Score (0–100), and Disability Points (0–3) were calculated and, subsequently, were assigned to five severity grades, as described in Von Korff et al. [23]: Grade 0 (pain-free); Grade I (low disability—low intensity); Grade II (low disability, high intensity); Grade III (high disability, moderately limiting); and Grade IV (high disability—severely limiting).

2.4. Statistical Analysis

Participant demographics, sports exposure, and training/competition/other sports practices were expressed as the mean ± SD and percentage proportions, respectively. NMQ-related measures and GCPS-based classifications were expressed as the absolute number and percentage of participants affected. The GCPS scores were described as the mean ± SD. All the measures were presented for the entire sample and the subgroups based on sex (female and male) and competition category (U-16 and U-18). Prevalence was additionally described with respect to the discipline to which they were perceived as being attributable. Pearson's Chi-squared tests were used to assess the potential sex and category differences in measures with percentage proportions at $p < 0.05$. Independent sample t-tests were used to evaluate the sex and category differences in interval scaled measures at $p < 0.05$. Pearson's correlation analysis was performed on GCPS items and scores, as well as on the relationship between GCPS scores, years of sports participation, number of competitions/season, number of skiing days/season, and number of athletic preparation days/season. For any correlation analysis, statistical significance was set at $p \leq 0.05$.

3. Results

3.1. Participant Demographics, Sports Exposure and Training/Competition/Other Sports Practices

Male participants were characterized as follows: age: 16.1 ± 1.1 y; weight: 65 ± 10 kg; height: 1.74 ± 0.08 m; BMI: 21.5 ± 2.3 kg/m^2; years of sports participation: 8.1 ± 2.4 y. The group of female participants had the following characteristics: age: 16 ± 1 years; weight: 56.2 ± 6.4 kg; height: 1.65 ± 0.05 m; BMI: 20.7 ± 1.9 kg/m^2; years of sports participation: 7.1 ± 2.9 y. Over the past competition (i.e., winter) season, the participants reported a mean of 85.4 ± 47.2 days (3.5 ± 1.3 days/week) of ski training and participated in 17.2 ± 12.0 competitions on average. Independent sample t-tests revealed no significant differences between the sexes. However, there were significant differences in the number of skiing days/season ($t(186) = 2.18$, $p = 0.029$) and the number of competitions in the last season ($t(186) = 7.22$, $p < 0.001$) between the U-16 and U-18 categories, with athletes in the U-18 category who performed more skiing days and competitions. Most participants (62.8%) declared that they practiced one or more sports other than alpine skiing, 83.5% reported that they participated in specific athletic preparation programs, and 78.3% declared that they regularly warm-up before skiing. The Chi-squared tests revealed, however, no significant sex or category differences in these variables at $p < 0.05$.

3.2. Prevalence of Lower Back Complaints

An overview of the NMQ-related results is presented in Table 1. A total of 80.3% of all participants reported having suffered from lower back complaints during the last 12 months, and 50.0% during the last 7 days. As many as 28.2% reported that they have been restricted in normal activities (e.g., job and leisure activities) during the last 12 months, and 27.7% indicated that their lower back complaints required medical attention during the last 12 months. Except for lower back complaints during the last 7 seven days, which were more frequent in females, there were found no sex or category differences. Interestingly, 50.7% of the participants reported their lower back complaints being attributed to performing SL, 26.0% to GS, and 7.3% to SG; meanwhile, no participants attributed their lower back complaints to DH skiing. A remarkable season period-related difference in the frequency patterns of lower back complaints was found between the competition period and the off-season period. During the off-season period, only 3.3% reported their lower back complaints to last longer than two weeks, while during the competition period this percentage proportion was more than six times higher (21.3%).

Table 1. Overview of the Nordic Musculoskeletal Questionnaire (NMQ)-based results and differences between sexes and categories.

NMQ Measure	Overall $n = 188$	Male $n = 110$	Female $n = 78$	χ^2(df), p	U-16 $n = 128$	U-18 $n = 60$	χ^2(df), p
Lower back complaints during the last 12 months	(151) 80.3%	(89) 80.9%	(62) 79.5%	n.s.	(103) 80.5%	(48) 80%	n.s.
Lower back complaints during the last 7 days	(94) 50%	(42) 42.7%	(47) 60.3%	5.61(1) 0.018	(65) 50.8%	(29) 48.3%	n.s.
Restricted in normal activities during the last 12 months	(53) 28.2%	(31) 28.2%	(22) 28.2%	n.s.	(36) 28.1%	(17) 28.3%	n.s.
Required medical attention during the last 12 months	(52) 27.7%	(33) 30%	(19) 24.4%	n.s.	(35) 27.3%	(17) 28.3%	n.s.

All NMQ-related measures are expressed as absolute numbers and the percentage proportion on the overall group/subgroups (number of affected skiers/number of skiers per group × 100). Levels of significance for sex and category differences are based on Pearson chi-square tests. n.s.: not significant at $p < 0.05$; U-16: under 16 years; U-18: under 18 years.

3.3. Severity of Lower Back Complaints

The GCPS-related results are summarized in Table 2. The mean value of Characteristic Pain Intensity was 37.53 ± 18.0 and the Disability Score was 13.27 ± 14.59 on average. There were no significant sex or category differences at $p < 0.05$. Most participants (57.4%) suffered from low intensity—low disability complaints (Grade I), and 21.8% from high intensity—low disability complaints (Grade II). Again, there were no significant differences between males and females, or between U-16 and U-18 skiers.

Table 2. Overview of the Graded Chronic Pain Scale (GCPS) scores and differences between sexes and categories.

GCPS Score	Overall $n = 188$	Male $n = 110$	Female $n = 78$	t(df), p	U-16 $n = 128$	U-18 $n = 60$	t(df), p
Characteristic Pain Intensity	37.53 ± 18.0	28.30 ± 21.98	32.26 ± 22.11	n.s.	30.62 ± 22.71	28.50 ± 20.70	n.s.
Disability Score	13.27 ±14.59	11.29 ±15.22	9.61 ±12.32	n.s	11.51 ±15.06	8.64 ±11.59	n.s
GCPS Classification				$\chi 2$			$\chi 2$
Grade 0 Pain free	(39) 20.7%	(23) 20.9%	(16) 20.5%	n.s.	(27) 21.1%	(12) 20%	n.s.
Grade I Low intensity-Low disability	(108) 57.4%	(64) 58.2%	(44) 56.4%	n.s.	(70) 54.7%	(38) 63.3%	n.s.
Grade II High intensity-Low disability	(41) 21.8%	(23) 20.9%	(18) 23.1%	n.s.	(31) 24.2%	(10) 16.7%	n.s
Grade III High Disability-Moderately Limiting	—	—	—	—	—	—	—
Grade IV High Disability-Severely Limiting	—	—	—	—	—	—	—

GCPS scores are expressed as mean ± SD. GCPS classifications are expressed as absolute numbers and the percentage proportion of the overall group/subgroups (number of affected skiers/number of skiers per group × 100). Levels of significance for sex and category differences are based on independent sample *t*-tests and Pearson chi-square tests, respectively. n.s.: not significant at $p < 0.05$; U-16: under 16 years; U-18: under 18 years.

3.4. Relationship between Different Severity Measures, as well as between Severity and Training Attributes

We found a medium-correlation Characteristic Pain Intensity and Disability Score (r = 0.62, $p < 0.01$). Moreover, the average lower back complaint intensity, as well as the intensity at the time of filling out the questionnaire, positively correlated with the worst pain intensity experienced within the last 6 months (r = 0.63, $p < 0.01$; r = 0.47, $p < 0.01$, respectively).

The results of the correlation analysis between the GCPS scores and different training attributes are highlighted in Table 3. There were small yet significant correlations between the Characteristic Pain Intensity and the training attributes "years of sports participation", "number of competitions/season", and "number of skiing days/season". Moreover, an additional independent *t*-test showed a significant difference (t (186) = 2.12, p = 0.035, d = 0.31) in the lower back complaint severity (i.e., GCPS—Characteristic Pain Intensity) between skiers who exclusively practiced alpine skiing and those who also practiced other sports, with the first group reporting higher intensities.

Table 3. Correlation between the Grading Chronic Pain Scale scores and questions on sports exposure.

	Characteristic Pain Intensity	Disability Score
Years of sports participation	0.28 **	0.15 *
Number of competitions/season	0.21 **	−0.02
Number of skiing days/season	0.27 **	0.12
Number of athletic preparation days/season	0.03	−0.09

Level of significance based on Pearson correlation analysis: * $p < 0.05$, ** $p < 0.01$.

4. Discussion

The main findings of this study were: (1) as many as 80.3% of all participating adolescent skiers suffered from lower back complaints during the last 12 months (50.0% during the last 7 days; 28.2% with restrictions in normal activities; and 27.7% requiring medical attention); (2) 50.7% of the participants reported their lower back complaints being attributable to SL, and 26.0% to GS; (3) despite the fact that the majority of the participants experienced lower back complaints of a low intensity/low disability (Grade I, 57.4%), a considerable portion suffered from a high intensity/low disability complaints (Grade II, 21.8%); (4) there were small yet significant correlations between the Characteristic Pain Intensity and the training attributes "years of sports participation", "number of competitions/season", and "number of skiing days/season".

4.1. Prevalence of Lower Back Complaints with Respect to Sex, Category and Discipline Preference

The current study found relatively high rates of lower back complaints in adolescent competitive alpine skiers. Indeed, 50.0% and 80.3% of the participants displayed lower back complaints in the last 7 days and 12 months, respectively. These values are considerably higher than those was previously reported for other populations. For example, a 12 months lower back pain prevalence of between 49.8% and 65.0% was observed in previous studies in elite athletes of different sports [25–27]. A 7 days lower back pain prevalence between 19.4% and 25.3% was reported for endurance athletes [25]. Previous works found a 12 months lower back complaints prevalence ranging from 20.5% to 57.0% in non-athletic adolescents [25,28,29], while a 7 days lower back complaints prevalence of about 20.0% was reported for young non-athletes [25].

The higher prevalence of lower back complaints observed in the present study compared to other athletic (and non-athletic) adolescents suggests that competitive alpine skiers are especially prone for lower back complaints. Indeed, in the sport of alpine ski racing, repetitive and heavy mechanical loads, high ground reaction forces, and the exposure to low-frequency whole-body vibrations have been shown to adversely affect the spinal structures while skiing [14,16,17]. Moreover, in young skiers, the immaturity of the musculoskeletal system may exacerbate the damage experienced by the spine during the practice of this sport [13].

Despite these plausible sports-related adverse loading patterns, only a few studies, however, have investigated the occurrence of lower back complaints in competitive alpine skiers. Moreover, due to focusing on a different age group and reporting other time prevalence measures or absolute injury rates, most of them are not directly comparable to the results of the current study [3,4,6,8,11]. The only study directly comparable to our investigation reported similar magnitudes of current low back pain (67.0%) in ski high school athletes aged 15–19 years [30].

Noteworthy, in our study, a higher 7 days lower back complaints prevalence was observed in females with respect to males (60.3% vs. 42.7%). These results are in agreement with previous works and, on the one hand, may be explained by a different pain threshold and symptom perception between males and females [31,32]. On the other hand, this sex difference may also be explained by the different anatomical characteristics of the female body (e.g., greater spine flexibility), as well as the different pubertal growth and hormonal states [33,34].

Furthermore, our study revealed that, during the 12 months prior to data collection, 28.2% of the participants were restricted in carrying out normal daily life activities, while 27.2% needed to see a physician. This latter percentage is similar to the magnitudes found in previous studies (range between 24.0 and 33.0%) including large cohorts of children and adolescents [35,36].

Interestingly, we found different skiing disciplines to have different perceived impacts on lower back complaints. Indeed, 50.7% attributed their lower back complaints to SL, while 26.0% reported to have suffered them in connection with GS and 7.3% with SG. None of the participants attributed their lower back complaints to DH. A possible explanation is that, in SL, there are more pronounced and larger ground reaction force peaks (approximately plus 20.0%) after gate passage than in GS [37].

Regarding the prevalence of lower back complaints according to the annual programming period, we found that the prevalence of lower back complaints lasting less than 7 days was 86.0% in the off-season and 33.3% in the competition season. Conversely, the frequency of lower back complaints lasting more than two weeks changed from 3.3% in the off-season to 21.3% in the period of the competition season. This fact may suggest that more severe lower back complaints emerge from skiing rather than from off-snow training [3].

4.2. Severity of Lower Back Complaints with Respect to Intensity and Disability

Another aim of this work was to study the severity (i.e., pain intensity and disability) of lower back complaints in adolescent competitive alpine skiers. Despite the fact that most of the participants (57.4%) reported low intensity—low disability complaints (Grade I of the GCPS), 21.8% showed high intensity—low disability complaints (Grade II). These findings showed that a considerable part of the participants suffered from a relatively high severity of lower back complaints already at a relatively young age (15–18 y). However, the pain resulted in being of low disability, which is in agreement with previous studies in adolescent athletes [25,38]. One potential explanation for this finding may be the consideration that the cohort of the current study consisted of relatively young athletes, who may not have suffered from an extensive accumulation of adverse loadings over time yet.

4.3. Relationship between Lower Back Complaints Severity and Training Attributes

The current study revealed small yet significant correlations between Characteristic Pain Intensity and the training attributes "years of sports participation", "number of competitions/season", and "number of skiing days/season". These findings further support our current understanding of the development of lower back overuse injuries, according to which an accumulation of adverse loadings on the athletes' spine is a key driver for inducing pain [16]. However, the present sample was homogeneous with respect to training attributes, since the participants of our study belonged to ski clubs of the same region. Therefore, the results of this study may be specific to our cohort and should be interpreted with caution.

4.4. Methodological Considerations

Despite providing valuable new insights into the prevalence and severity of lower back complaints in adolescent competitive alpine skiers, this study has some limitations that one should be aware of. First, the retrospective nature of the NMQ and GCPS methodologies may cause them to suffer from a recall bias. Recent and more severe complaints are more likely to be remembered than older and less severe ones. Second, the background and experience of the participants filling out the questionnaires may influence the outcomes. Third, other potential cofounders for lower back complaints, such as smoking, hours of sleep per night, and psychosocial factors (depression, stress, poor academic performance, poor competitive results, etc.), were not evaluated in this study.

5. Conclusions

This study provides a new set of data regarding the prevalence and severity of lower back complaints in a sample of adolescent competitive alpine racers. It further supports the relatively high magnitudes of lower back-related pain, with a considerable amount of high intensity but low disability complaints. Interestingly, more low back complains were reported during SL and GS than other skiing disciplines. Moreover, this study further highlights an accumulation of adverse loadings on the athletes' spine being a key driver for developing pain conditions. Accordingly, adolescent competitive alpine skiers should be particularly protected by rigorous prevention strategies already before reaching adolescence.

Author Contributions: Conceptualization, A.C., D.S., and S.M.; investigation, M.G.; resources, D.S. and M.G.; data curation, A.C., F.S., and M.G.; writing—original draft preparation, F.S., M.G. and J.S.; writing—review and editing A.C., J.S., and S.M. All authors have read and agreed to the published version of the manuscript.

Acknowledgments: The authors would like to thank the participants for their kind participation and their coaches, ski clubs, and the FISI Veneto Committee for supporting and facilitating the completion of this study.

References

1. Flørenes, T.W.; Bere, T.; Nordsletten, L.; Heir, S.; Bahr, R. Injuries among male and female World Cup alpine skiers. *Br. J. Sports Med.* **2009**, *43*, 973–978. [CrossRef] [PubMed]
2. Bere, T.; Flørenes, T.W.; Nordsletten, L.; Bahr, R. Sex differences in the risk of injury in World Cup alpine skiers: A 6-year cohort study. *Br. J. Sports Med.* **2014**, *48*, 36–40. [CrossRef] [PubMed]
3. Schoeb, T.; Peterhans, L.; Fröhlich, S.; Frey, W.O.; Gerber, C.; Spörri, J. Health problems in youth competitive alpine skiing: A 12-month observation of 155 athletes around the growth spurt. *Scand. J. Med. Sci. Sports* **2020**. [CrossRef] [PubMed]
4. Fröhlich, S.; Helbling, M.; Fucentese, S.F.; Karlen, W.; Frey, W.O.; Spörri, J. Injury risks among elite competitive alpine skiers are underestimated if not registered prospectively, over the entire season and regardless of whether requiring medical attention. *Knee Surgery Sport. Traumatol. Arthrosc.* **2020**. [CrossRef]
5. Müller, L.; Hildebrandt, C.; Müller, E.; Oberhoffer, R.; Raschner, C. Injuries and illnesses in a cohort of elite youth alpine ski racers and the influence of biological maturity and relative age: A two-season prospective study. *Open Access J. Sport. Med.* **2017**, *8*, 113–122. [CrossRef]
6. Alhammoud, M.; Racinais, S.; Rousseaux-Blanchi, M.P.; Bouscaren, N. Recording injuries only during winter competitive season underestimates injury incidence in elite alpine skiers. *Scand. J. Med. Sci. Sport.* **2020**, *30*, 1177–1187. [CrossRef]
7. Westin, M.; Alricsson, M.; Werner, S. Injury profile of competitive alpine skiers: A five-year cohort study. *Knee Surgery Sport. Traumatol. Arthrosc.* **2012**, *20*, 1175–1181. [CrossRef] [PubMed]

8. Hildebrandt, M.C.; Raschner, A.C. Traumatic and overuse injuries among elite adolescent alpine skiers: A two-year retrospective analysis. *Int. Sport. J.* **2013**, *14*, 245–255.
9. Rachbauer, F.; Sterzinger, W.; Eibl, G. Radiographic Abnormalities in the Thoracolumbar Spine of Young Elite Skiers. *Am. J. Sports Med.* **2001**, *29*, 446–449. [CrossRef]
10. Witwit, W.A.; Kovac, P.; Sward, A.; Agnvall, C.; Todd, C.; Thoreson, O.; Hebelka, H.; Baranto, A. Disc degeneration on MRI is more prevalent in young elite skiers compared to controls. *Knee Surg. Sport. Traumatol. Arthrosc.* **2018**, *26*, 325–332. [CrossRef]
11. Peterhans, L.; Fröhlich, S.; Stern, C.; Frey, W.O.; Farshad, M.; Sutter, R.; Spörri, J. High Rates of Overuse-Related Structural Abnormalities in the Lumbar Spine of Youth Competitive Alpine Skiers: A Cross-sectional MRI Study in 108 Athletes. *Orthop. J. Sport. Med.* **2020**, *8*, 1–10. [CrossRef]
12. Heneweer, H.; Vanhees, L.; Picavet, H.S.J. Physical activity and low back pain: A U-shaped relation? *Pain* **2009**, *143*, 21–25. [CrossRef]
13. Meyer, M.; Laurent, C.; Higgins, R.; Skelly, W. Downhill ski injuries in children and adolescents. *Sport. Med.* **2007**, *37*, 485–499. [CrossRef]
14. Spörri, J.; Kröll, J.; Supej, M.; Müller, E. Reducing the back overuse-related risks in alpine ski racing: Let's put research into sports practice. *Br. J. Sports Med.* **2019**, *53*, 2–3. [CrossRef]
15. Soligard, T.; Schwellnus, M.; Alonso, J.M.; Bahr, R.; Clarsen, B.; Dijkstra, H.P.; Gabbett, T.; Gleeson, M.; Hägglund, M.; Hutchinson, M.R.; et al. How much is too much? (Part 1) International Olympic Committee consensus statement on load in sport and risk of injury. *Br. J. Sports Med.* **2016**, *50*, 1030–1041. [CrossRef]
16. Spörri, J.; Kroll, J.C.H.; Fasel, B.; Muller, E. Potential Mechanisms Leading to Overuse Injuries of the Back in Alpine Ski Racing A Descriptive Biomechanical Study. *Am. J. Sports Med.* **2015**, *43*, 2042–2048. [CrossRef]
17. Spörri, J.; Kröll, J.; Fasel, B.; Aminian, K.; Müller, E. The Use of Body Worn Sensors for Detecting the Vibrations Acting on the Lower Back in Alpine Ski Racing. *Front. Phyisiol.* **2017**, *8*, 522. [CrossRef]
18. Supej, M.; Ogrin, J.; Holmberg, H. Whole-Body Vibrations Associated With Alpine Skiing: A Risk Factor for Low Back Pain? *Front. Phyisiol.* **2018**, *9*, 204. [CrossRef]
19. Supej, M.; Ogrin, J. Transmissibility of whole-body vibrations and injury risk in alpine skiing. *J. Sci. Med. Sport* **2019**, *22*, S71–S77. [CrossRef]
20. Tarabini, M.; Saggin, B.; Scaccabarozzi, D. Whole-body vibration exposure in sport: Four relevant cases. *Ergonomics* **2015**, *58*, 1143–1150. [CrossRef]
21. Kuorinka, I.; Jonsson, B.; Kilbom, A.; Vinterberg, H.; Biering-Sørensen, F.; Andersson, G.; Jørgensen, K. Standardised Nordic questionnaires for the analysis of musculoskeletal symptoms. *Appl. Ergon.* **1987**, *18*, 233–237. [CrossRef]
22. Gobba, F.; Ghersi, R.; Martinelli, S.; Richeldi, A.; Clerici, P.; Grazioli, P. Traduzione in lingua italiana e validazione del questionario standardizzato Nordic IRSST per la rilevazione di disturbi muscoloscheletrici. *Med. del Lav.* **2008**, *99*, 424–443.
23. Von Korff, M.; Ormel, J.; Keefe, F.J.; Dworkin, S.F. Clinical Section Grading the severity of chronic pain. *Pain* **1992**, *50*, 133–149. [CrossRef]
24. Salaffi, F.; Stancati, A.; Grassi, W. Reliability and validity of the Italian version of the Chronic Pain Grade questionnaire in patients with musculoskeletal disorders. *Clin. Rheumatol.* **2006**, *25*, 619–631. [CrossRef] [PubMed]
25. Bahr, R.; Andersen, S.O.; Løken, S.; Fossan, B. Low Back Pain Among Endurance Athletes With and Without Specific Back Loading—A Cross-Sectional Survey of Cross-Country Skiers, Rowers, Orienteerers, and Nonathletic Controls. *Spine* **2004**, *29*, 449–454. [CrossRef]
26. Schulz, S.S.; Lenz, K.; Büttner-Janz, K. Severe back pain in elite athletes: A cross-sectional study on 929 top athletes of Germany. *Eur. Spine J.* **2016**, *25*, 1204–1210. [CrossRef]
27. Fett, D.; Trompeter, K.; Platen, P. Back pain in elite sports: A cross-sectional study on 1114 athletes. *PLoS ONE* **2017**, *12*, e0180130. [CrossRef]
28. Masiero, S.; Carraro, E.; Celia, A.; Sarto, D.; Ermani, M. Prevalence of nonspecific low back pain in schoolchildren aged between 13 and 15 years. *Acta Pædiatrica* **2008**, *97*, 212–216. [CrossRef]
29. Kędra, A.; Czaprowski, D. Epidemiology of back pain in children and youth aged 10–19 from the area of the southeast of Poland. *Biomed Res. Int.* **2013**, *2013*. [CrossRef]
30. Bergstrøm, K.A.; Brandseth, K.; Fretheim, S.; Tvilde, K.; Ekeland, A. Back injuries and pain in adolescents attending a ski high school. *Knee Surgery Sport. Traumatol. Arthrosc.* **2004**, *12*, 80–85. [CrossRef]

31. Keogh, E.; Eccleston, C. Sex Differences in Adolescent Chronic Pain and Pain-Related Coping. *Pain* **2006**, *12*, 275–284. [CrossRef] [PubMed]
32. Mingheli, B.; Raul, O.; Nunes, C. Non-specific Low Back Pain in Adolescents From the South of Portugal: Prevalence and Associated Factors. *J. Orthop. Sci.* **2014**, *19*, 883–892. [CrossRef]
33. Shehab, D.K.; Al-Jarallah, K.F. Nonspecific low-back pain in Kuwaiti children and adolescents: Associated factors. *J. Adolesc. Heal.* **2005**, *36*, 32–35. [CrossRef]
34. Balanguè, F.; Damidot, P.; Nordin, M.; Parnianpour, M.; Waldburger, M. Cross-sectional Study of the Isokinetic Muscle Trunk Strength Among School Children. *Spine* **1993**, *18*, 1199–1205. [CrossRef] [PubMed]
35. Masiero, S.; Carraro, E.; Sarto, D.; Bonaldo, L.; Ferraro, C. Healthcare service use in adolescents with non-specific musculoskeletal pain. *Acta Paediatr.* **2010**, *99*, 1224–1228. [CrossRef]
36. Watson, K.D.; Papageorgiou, A.C.; Jones, G.T.; Taylor, S.; Symmons, D.P.M.; Silman, A.J.; Macfarlane, G.J. Low back pain in schoolchildren: Occurrence and characteristics. *Pain* **2002**, *97*, 87–92. [CrossRef]
37. Spörri, J.; Kröll, J.; Fasel, B.; Aminian, K.; Müller, E. Course Setting as a Prevention Measure for Overuse Injuries of the Back in Alpine Ski Racing. *Orthop. J. Sport. Med.* **2016**, *4*, 1–8. [CrossRef]
38. Müller, J.; Müller, S.; Stoll, J.; Fröhlich, K.; Otto, C.; Mayer, F. Back pain prevalence in adolescent athletes. *Scand. J. Med. Sci. Sports* **2017**, *27*, 448–454. [CrossRef]

15

The Effect of Branched-Chain Amino Acids, Citrulline and Arginine on High-Intensity Interval Performance in Young Swimmers

Chun-Fang Hsueh [1], Huey-June Wu [2], Tzu-Shiou Tsai [3], Ching-Lin Wu [4] and Chen-Kang Chang [5,*]

1 Graduate Institute of Sport Coaching Science, Chinese Culture University, Taipei 114, Taiwan; swim_speedo@hotmail.com
2 Department of Combat Sports and Martial Arts, Chinese Culture University, Taipei 114, Taiwan; wuhc0123@gmail.com
3 Taipei Municipal Nan Gang High School, Taipei 115, Taiwan; Tsai481026@gmail.com
4 Graduate Institute of Sports and Health Management, National Chung Hsing University, Taichung 402, Taiwan; psclw@dragon.nchu.edu.tw
5 Department of Sport Performance, National Taiwan University of Sport, 16, Section 1, Shaun-Shih Road, Taichung 404, Taiwan
* Correspondence: wspahn@seed.net.tw

Abstract: High-intensity interval training has drawn significant interest for its ability to elicit similar training responses with less training volume compared to traditional moderate-intensity protocols. The purpose of this study was to examine the effect of co-ingestion of branched-chain amino acids (BCAA), arginine, and citrulline on 8×50 m high-intensity interval swim performance in trained young swimmers. This study used a randomized cross-over design. Eight male (age 15.6 ± 1.3 years) and eight female (age 15.6 ± 0.9 years) swimmers completed both amino acids (AA) and placebo (PL) trials. The participants ingested 0.085 g/kg body weight BCAA, 0.05 g/kg body weight arginine and 0.05 g/kg body weight citrulline before the swim test in the AA trial. The average 50 m time was significantly shorter in the AA trial than that in the PL trial. The AA trial was faster than the PL trial in the first, second, and the seventh laps. The AA trial showed significantly higher plasma BCAA concentrations and lower tryptophan/BCAA ratio. The other biochemical parameters and ratings of perceived exertion were similar between the two trials. The results showed that BCAA, arginine, and citrulline, allowed the participants to swim faster in a high-intensity interval protocol in young swimmers.

Keywords: central fatigue; tryptophan; ammonia; nitric oxide; stroke rate; stroke count

1. Introduction

High-intensity interval training (HIIT) has drawn significant interest from athletes of various sports, as well as general or less-fit populations [1,2]. The high-intensity nature of this protocol recruits both type-I and -II muscle fibers [3], resulting in significant improvement in cardiopulmonary and anaerobic capabilities [1,2,4,5]. Several studies have shown that HIIT can elicit similar training responses in competitive swimmers with less training volume compared to traditional moderate-intensity protocols [6,7]. One of the important factors for the success in HIIT is the ability to maintain the training intensity, especially at the later stages. However, the accumulation of peripheral and/or central fatigue, resulting from repeated high-intensity bouts, leads to declines in exercise intensity at the later stages of HIIT, and potentially reduce the training effect [1,2].

The peripheral factors for fatigue in HIIT include limitations in anaerobic and aerobic energy supply, and intramuscular accumulation of metabolic by-products such as H^+ and inorganic phosphate [8,9]. Moreover, the central nervous system may also be involved, as the capacity of the motor cortex to drive the knee extensors after high-intensity intermittent cycling was significantly decreased [10]. One of the mechanisms that contributes to central fatigue is the increase in cerebral concentration of the neurotransmitter serotonin (5-hydroxytryptamine) during exercise. The increased cerebral serotonin could lead to the feeling of fatigue and the loss of central drive and motivation [11]. An increase in serotonin concentration in presynaptic neutrons would lead to increased serotonin release and serotonin binding to postsynaptic receptors during nerve stimulation [12]. In addition, cerebral serotonin concentration was inversely correlated to running time to fatigue in rodents [13,14]. The rate of cerebral serotonin synthesis is regulated by the transport of free tryptophan, the precursor to serotonin, across the blood brain barrier [15]. Branched-chain amino acids (BCAA) have been hypothesized to alleviate central fatigue by competing with tryptophan in crossing the blood brain barrier through the L-system transporter [16]. Indeed, the decreased plasma free tryptophan/BCAA ratio would reduce the uptake of tryptophan, and subsequently, serotonin synthesis in the brain [14].

Nitric oxide (NO), a signaling molecule with a wide range of physiological functions, has been suggested to improve exercise performance by enhancing exercise-induced vasodilation [17], increasing the oxygenation status in the working muscles, and improving VO_2 kinetics [18]. Supplementations of arginine or citrulline, both of which are precursors to NO, have been suggested to improve performance in high-intensity exercise [19,20].

Previously, we revealed that supplementation of BCAA and arginine could improve repeated sprint performance in handball players [21]. We later added citrulline to the supplementation regimen [22,23] because the combined ingestion of citrulline and arginine may be more effective in increasing plasma arginine concentration than consuming either amino acid individually [24]. Although the nutritional strategies to support HIIT have been proposed, most results were obtained from land-based exercise [25]. In addition, the combination of BCAA, arginine, and citrulline on high-intensity interval swimming performance has not been investigated. With the increasing application of HIIT in swimming training, the aim of this study was to examine the effect of co-ingestion of BCAA, arginine, and citrulline on 8×50 m swim performance in trained young swimmers. The biochemical and stroke parameters were analyzed to investigate the potential mechanism of the supplementation.

2. Materials and Methods

2.1. Participants

Eight male (age: 15.6 ± 1.3 years; height: 1.74 ± 0.05 m; weight: 64.4 ± 7.6 kg) and eight female (age: 15.6 ± 0.9 years; height: 1.58 ± 0.06 m; weight: 54.0 ± 8.4 kg) swimmers were recruited from a high school in northern Taiwan. All participants have been participating in swimming training for at least 7 years and have competed at the national or international level. The characteristics and personal best performance of the participants are presented in Table 1. The exclusion criteria included cardiovascular disease risks, musculoskeletal injuries, smoking, or consumption of protein supplements in the past three months. After the experimental procedure and potential risks were explained, all participants and their legal guardians gave their written informed consent. The study protocol was approved by the Research Ethics Committee of China Medical University Hospital (CRREC-105-003).

Table 1. Basic characteristics of participants.

Gender *	Age (Year)	Height (m)	Weight (kg)	Body Mass Index	Best Style	Personal Best † 50 m (s)	Personal Best † 100 m (s)
M	15	1.78	67.1	21.18	Backstroke	29.8	62.2
M	17	1.78	71.1	22.44	Breaststroke	31.2	69.1
M	17	1.77	70.2	22.41	Front crawl	25.7	54.9
M	17	1.78	70.5	22.25	Front crawl	25.6	52.7
M	15	1.69	53.6	18.77	Front crawl	27.3	56.2
M	14	1.68	52.6	18.64	Butterfly	28.9	57.3
M	16	1.69	68.8	24.09	Butterfly	26.8	57.3
M	14	1.71	61.1	20.90	Front crawl	26.2	54.8
Mean ‡	15.6	1.74	64.4	21.33			
SD ‡	1.3	0.05	7.6	1.89			
F	16	1.46	46.3	21.72	Front crawl	29.7	65.2
F	15	1.59	45.4	17.96	Front crawl	29.8	66.1
F	17	1.60	51.4	20.08	Front crawl	28.2	59.9
F	16	1.64	60.9	22.64	Front crawl	28.0	61.2
F	15	1.53	44.1	18.84	Front crawl	29.5	61.1
F	16	1.58	56.5	22.63	Butterfly	31.3	69.2
F	16	1.65	60.9	22.37	Butterfly	33.5	71.8
F	14	1.60	66.6	26.02	Butterfly	31.7	68.9
Mean §	15.6	1.58	54.0	21.53			
SD §	0.9	0.06	8.4	2.55			

* M: male; F: female; † personal best record in their respective best style; ‡ mean and standard deviation of male participants; § mean and standard deviation of female participants.

2.2. *Study Design*

This study used a double-blind, placebo-controlled, randomized cross-over design. The study protocol is outlined in Figure 1. Each participant completed two trials, amino acids (AA) and placebo (PL), in a random order, separated by a wash-out period of at least seven days. The regular training schedule and dietary habits were maintained during the study period. The participants refrained from all training activity on the day prior to the trial. The study was conducted in January, 2017.

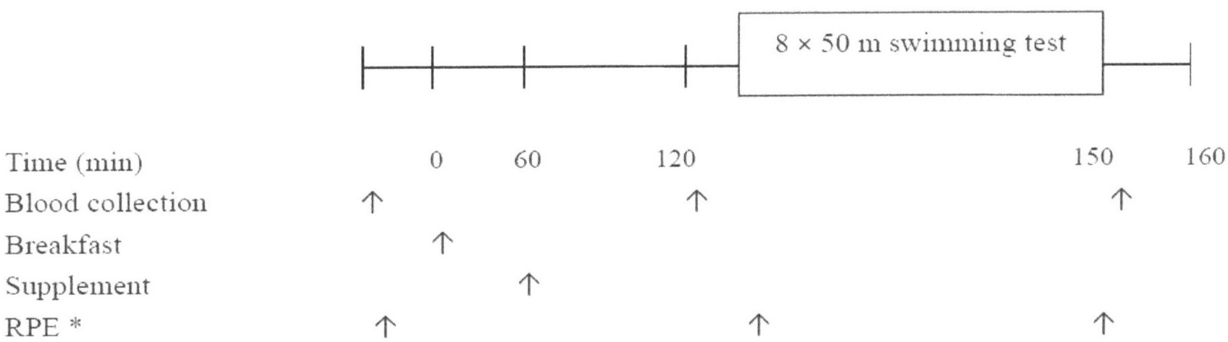

Figure 1. Study protocol. * RPE: ratings of perceived exertion. The symbols (↑) pointed out the actions at the specific time point.

2.3. *Dietary Control*

During the two days prior to each trial, the participants were provided with the same three meals per day, purchased from local convenience stores. The meals provided approximately

1624 kcal/day with 55% energy from carbohydrate, 25% from fat, and 18% from protein, according to the manufacturer's label. A standardized breakfast was given on the days of trials, including white bread 0.5 g/kg body weight, jam 0.1 g/kg body weight, butter 0.1 g/kg body weight, and soybean milk 5 mL/kg body weight (6.2 kcal/kg body weight, containing carbohydrate 1.0 g/kg body weight, protein 0.24 g/kg body weight, and fat 0.14 g/kg body weight).

2.4. Supplementation

On the days of the trials, the participants reported to a 25 m swimming pool in the morning after an overnight fast. After collecting blood samples from the antecubital vein, the participants consumed the standard breakfast, followed by one of the two interventions. In the AA trial, the participants ingested 0.085 g/kg body weight BCAA (leucine: isoleucine: valine = 10:7:3, containing vitamin E 6.67 IU/g BCAA, capsule, General Nutrition Corporation, Pittsburgh, PA, USA), 0.05 g/kg body weight arginine, and 0.05 g/kg body weight citrulline (arginine: citrulline = 1:1, tablet, General Nutrition Corporation). In the placebo (PL) trial, the participants consumed the identical number of empty capsules and tablets containing starch (Chung-Yu Biotech Co LTD, Taichung, Taiwan) and one capsule of vitamin E (100 IU, General Nutrition Corporation). All capsules and tablets were taken with water within 15 min.

2.5. High-Intensity Interval Swimming Test

Thirty min after consuming the amino acids or placebo, the participants began a controlled 1000 m warm-up. The warm-up included 8 × 50 m easy swim focusing on individual skills, 200 m mixed style, and 4 × 100 m free style. The warm-up lasted approximately 20 min. The 8 × 50 m high-intensity interval swimming test started 60 min after consuming the amino acids or placebo, following the international rules with push starts. There was a 3-min active recovery period between each sprint. The approximate work to rest ratio of 1:6 is chosen to allow the better recovery of acid/base balance and creatine phosphate resynthesis [2]. The participants were asked to swim with their best style with the best effort in each sprint. Four male and five female participants swam front crawl, two male and three female participants swam butterfly, one male participant swam breaststroke and another male participant swam backstroke. Participants from both trials were grouped into 3 or 4 according to their best record, and competed at the same time to encourage the best performance. No food or fluid was provided during the test. The ratings of perceived exertion (RPE) were recorded immediately before and after the test using Borg's 20-point scale [26].

2.6. Stroke Characteristics

The stroke characteristics were analyzed by an experienced swimmer/coach by reviewing the video files of the entire trials. The time to finish three consecutive strokes, measured by a stop watch, was recorded during approximately 35–40 m in each lap. The stroke rate was determined by dividing the time by three. For front crawl and backstroke, the timing started when the right hand entered the water, and ended immediately before the right hand entered the water for the second time. For breaststroke, the timing started when the arms started the outsweep, and ended when the arms completed the forward extension for the third time. For butterfly, the timing started when the arms entered the water, and ended immediately before the arms entered the water for the third time. The stroke count was measured during the entire lap, excluding the sculling or flipper movement after the start or turn.

2.7. Measurement of Blood Biochemical Parameters

The time point of blood sampling is shown in Figure 1. Venous blood samples were collected into tubes containing EDTA. After centrifugation at 1500× g for 15 min at 4 °C, the plasma samples were aliquoted and stored at −70 °C until further analysis. Plasma BCAA concentrations were measured enzymatically (Biovision, Milpitas, CA, USA) with a microplate spectrophotometer (Benchmark Plus, Bio-Rad, Hercules, CA, USA). Plasma tryptophan concentrations were analyzed with a fluorescence assay (Bridge-It, Mediomics, St. Louis, MO, USA). The fluorescence at excitation 485 nm and emission

665 nm was read by a microplate fluorescence reader (Plate Chameleon, Hidex, Turku, Finland). Plasma NO_x concentrations were determined using Griess reagent [27]. Plasma concentrations of urea, glucose, lactate, NH_3, glycerol, and non-esterified fatty acids (NEFA) were measured enzymatically with an automatic analyzer (Hitachi 7020, Tokyo, Japan) using commercial kits (Randox, Antrim, UK). Hemoglobin concentration and hematocrit in whole blood were measured by a blood cell analyzer (Sysmex Kx-21, Diamond Diagnostics, Holliston, MA, USA) to correct potential changes in plasma volume during the study periods [28].

2.8. Statistical Analysis

The results were initially analyzed by three-way (gender × trial × time) analysis of variance with repeated measurements. However, gender effect was insignificant in all performance, biochemical and stroke parameters. Therefore, the data from both genders were pulled together and analyzed by two-way (trial × time) analysis of variance with repeated measurements. If the interaction effect was to be found significant, the differences between the two trials were identified by Ryan-Holm-Bonferroni post hoc analysis [29]. If the time or lap effect was to be found significant, the differences within the same trial were identified with Bonferroni post hoc analysis. A $p < 0.05$ is considered statistically significant. With the power of 0.80 and sample size of 16, the minimal detectable difference is 1.06 standard deviation (SD). The data are presented as mean ± SD.

3. Results

The average 50 m time of the eight laps in the high-intensity interval swimming test was significantly shorter in the AA trial than that in the PL trial (AA: 30.50 ± 2.87 s vs. PL: 30.94 ± 3.02 s, $p < 0.001$, Figure 2a). Thirteen participants (6 male and 7 female) out of total 16 had faster average lap time in the AA trial (Figure 2a). When each lap was considered separately, there were significant trial, lap, and interaction effects (all $p < 0.001$, $\eta^2 = 0.795$, 0.452, 0.236, respectively). The post-hoc analysis showed that AA trial was faster than the PL trial in the first (AA: 30.47 ± 0.44 s vs. PL: 31.34 ± 0.57 s, $p < 0.001$), second (AA: 32.76 ± 2.54 s vs. PL: 33.58 ± 2.48 s, $p < 0.001$), and the seventh laps (AA: 31.64 ± 4.30 s vs. PL: 32.50 ± 4.60 s, $p < 0.001$) (Figure 2b).

The AA trial showed significantly higher plasma BCAA concentrations before and after the 8 × 50 m test (Figure 3a). Plasma tryptophan concentrations were decreased after the interval swim in both trials at the similar magnitude (Figure 3b). Nevertheless, the elevated plasma BCAA concentrations lead to significantly lower tryptophan/BCAA ratios before and after the interval swim in the AA trial (Figure 3c). Plasma NO_x levels showed a significant time effect ($p < 0.001$), but the post hoc analysis did not find significant difference among the three time points in either trials (Table 2). Plasma concentrations of NH_3, urea, lactate, glycerol, and NEFA were similar in both trials (Table 2). The participants also reported similar RPE before and after the 8 × 50 m test in both trials (Table 2).

(A)

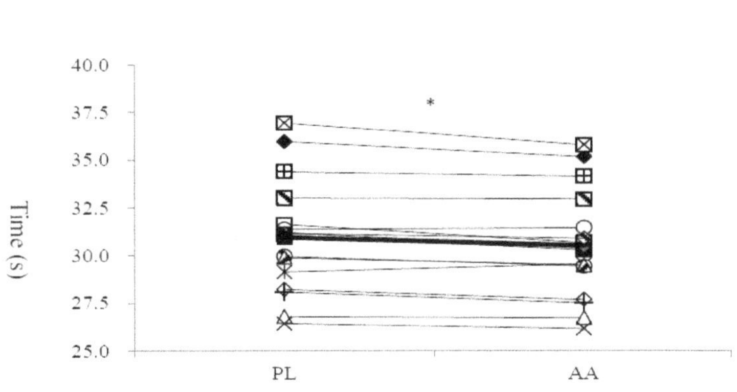

Figure 2. *Cont.*

(B)

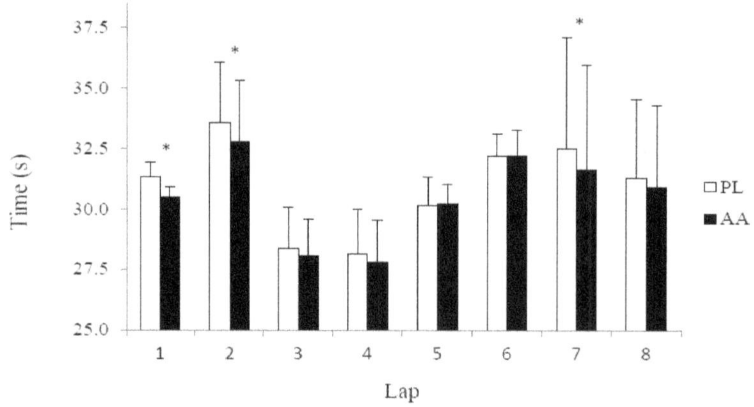

Figure 2. The performance of the 8 × 50 m high-intensity interval swimming test in the AA (amino acids supplemented) and PL (placebo) trials. (**A**) the average lap time of each participant.* Significant difference between the AA and PL trials, $p < 0.05$; (**B**) the average time in each lap. Trial effect: $p < 0.001$; lap effect: $p < 0.001$; interaction effect: $p < 0.001$; * Significant difference between the AA and PL trials, $p < 0.05$.

(A)

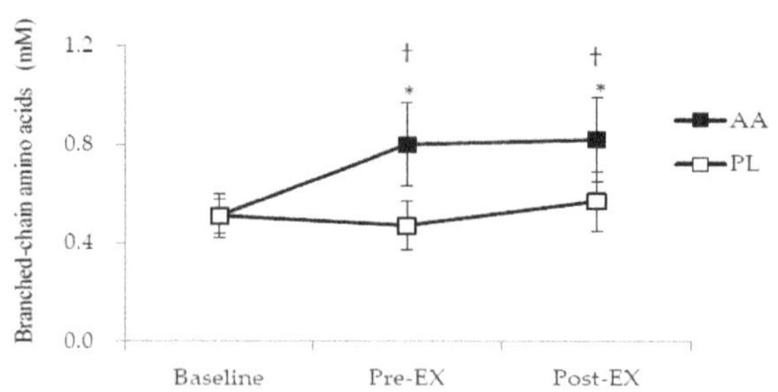

(B)

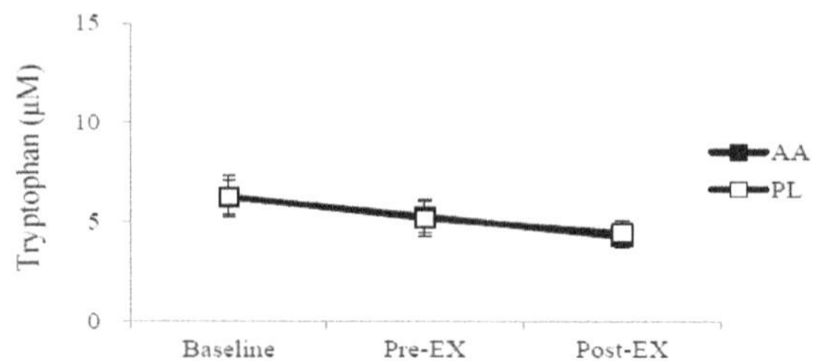

(C)

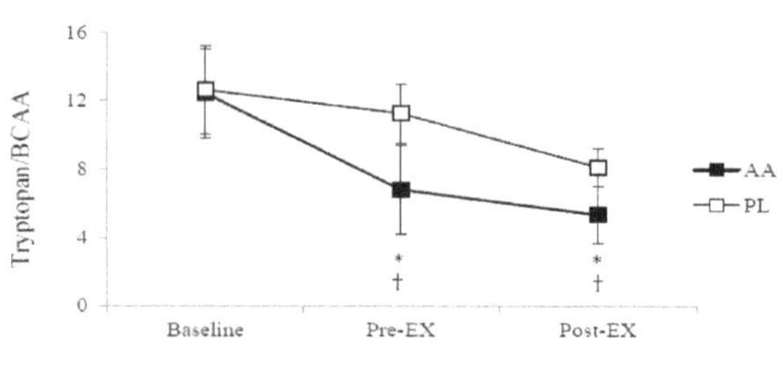

Figure 3. Plasma amino acid concentrations at baseline, before, and after the 8 × 50 m high-intensity interval swimming test in the AA (amino acids supplemented) and PL (placebo) trials. (**A**) Branched-chain amino acids, trial effect: $p < 0.001$; time effect: $p < 0.001$; interaction effect: $p < 0.001$. (**B**) Tryptophan, trial effect: $p = 0.821$; time effect: $p < 0.001$; interaction effect: $p = 0.383$. (**C**) Tryptophan/branched-chain amino acids ratio, trial effect: $p < 0.001$; time effect: $p < 0.0001$; interaction effect: $p < 0.001$; * Significantly different from the baseline in the same trial, $p < 0.05$; † AA trial vs. PL trial at the same time point, $p < 0.05$. Pre-Ex: before 8 × 50 m swim test; Post-Ex: immediately after 8 × 50 m swim test.

Table 2. Biochemical parameters and ratings of perceived exertion at the baseline, before, and after 8 × 50 m test in the in the AA (amino acids supplemented) and PL (placebo) trials.

	Trial	Baseline	Pre-Ex	Post-Ex
NO_x (μM)	AA	11.61 ± 4.94	31.65 ± 29.56	23.06 ± 15.28
	PL	12.68 ± 7.42	25.84 ± 29.39	18.36 ± 11.71
NH_3 (μM)	AA	115.20 ± 103.49	123.72 ± 66.29	123.86 ± 65.35
	PL	116.59 ± 40.69	109.02 ± 50.89	114.81 ± 50.31
Urea (mM)	AA	4.64 ± 0.77	5.38 ± 0.90	5.11 ± 0.91
	PL	4.77 ± 0.65	5.01 ± 0.87	4.63 ± 0.73
Lactate (mM)	AA	1.36 ± 0.56	1.91 ± 0.59	14.75 ± 4.43 *,†
	PL	1.43 ± 0.34	1.71 ± 0.38	14.12 ± 2.79 *,†
Glycerol (μM)	AA	46.00 ± 21.00	81.89 ± 28.83 *	240.89 ± 96.61 *,†
	PL	44.63 ± 25.27	71.35 ± 26.45	227.44 ± 58.36 *,†
NEFA (mM) [1]	AA	0.49 ± 0.27	0.42 ± 0.16	0.22 ± 0.09 †
	PL	0.44 ± 0.25	0.38 ± 0.10	0.20 ± 0.08 †
RPE [2]	AA	9.1 ± 2.4	15.0 ± 1.8 *	17.2 ± 2.3 *
	PL	9.7 ± 2.4	14.8 ± 2.2 *	17.3 ± 1.8 *

[1] NEFA. non-esterified fatty acids; [2] RPE: ratings of perceived exertion; * Significantly different from the baseline in the same trial, $p < 0.001$; † Significantly different from Pre-Ex in the same trial, $p < 0.05$. Pre-Ex: before 8 × 50 m swim test; Post-Ex: immediately after 8 × 50 m swim test.

The data of stroke rate and stroke count are shown in Table 3. None of the main effects was significant in stroke rate. However, the participants in the AA trial showed a trend of faster stroke rate in the first (p = 0.011) and second lap (p = 0.011 and 0.002, respectively, according to paired t-test), compared to those in the PL trial. The last lap showed the highest stroke count in both trials. In the AA trial, the participants swam the last lap with significantly higher stroke count than in the third lap (p = 0.015), while in the PL trial, the stroke count in the last lap was significantly higher than in the third (p = 0.038) and fourth lap (p = 0.041).

Table 3. Stroke rate and stroke count in the 8 × 50 m high-intensity interval swimming test in the AA and PL trials.

Trial		Lap								
		1	2	3	4	5	6	7	8	Mean
Stroke rate [1] (count/min)	PL	70.6 ± 19.5	71.2 ± 19.3	72.3 ± 19.0	71.4 ± 20.2	70.2 ± 18.7	69.2 ± 18.5	69.4 ± 18.2	69.4 ± 18.3	70.5 ± 19.0
	AA	74.5 ± 18.5	76.0 ± 18.3	72.7 ± 19.5	72.4 ± 18.4	70.7 ± 16.5	71.4 ± 18.0	70.1± 17.4	71.9 ± 18.2	72.7 ± 18.1
Stroke count [2] (count/lap)	PL	30.7 ± 9.0 [a,b]	30.6 ± 9.5 [a,b]	30.8 ± 9.1 [a]	30.8 ± 9.2 [a,b]	31.1 ± 9.4 [a,b]	31.7 ± 9.5 [a,b]	31.6 ± 9.4 [a,b]	31.9 ± 9.0 [b]	31.1 ± 9.3
	AA	31.1 ± 8.5 [a,b]	30.6 ± 8.2 [a,b]	30.6 ± 8.2 [a]	31.1 ± 8.6 [a]	31.2 ± 8.3 [a,b]	31.3 ± 8.1 [a,b]	31.5 ± 8.4 [a,b]	32.1 ± 8.4 [b]	31.2 ± 8.3

[1] Trial effect $p = 0.102$, lap effect $p = 0.489$, interaction effect $p = 0.513$; [2] Trial effect $p = 0.910$, lap effect $p < 0.001$, interaction effect $p = 0.643$; The values with different superscripts (a, b) were significantly different within the same trial.

4. Discussion

The results of this study suggested that the combined supplementation of BCAA, arginine, and citrulline significantly improved performance in 8 × 50 m high-intensity interval swims in well-trained young swimmers. The participants in the AA trial showed significantly lower plasma tryptophan/BCAA ratio before and after the interval swims. In addition, the participants were able to swim faster under a similar degree of perceived effort, indicating the possibility of alleviated central fatigue.

The participants in the AA trial showed significantly higher plasma BCAA concentrations and lower tryptophan/BCAA ratio after the interval swims, compared to the PL trial. This is in agreement with our previous studies using the same supplements [22,23]. It has been revealed that central nervous system plays a role in the development of fatigue in repeated high-intensity exercise [9]. Several studies using functional magnetic resonance imaging have found increased activations in sensory processing and motor-related brain regions such as primary motor cortex, supplementary motor area and pre-motor cortex while performing fatiguing exercise tasks [30]. These activations suggest a greater perception of effort under fatigue and the need for higher motor output to sustain the same physical workload [31]. The decreased plasma tryptophan/BCAA ratio in the AA trial would reduce the cerebral uptake of tryptophan, leading to lower cerebral serotonin synthesis [14].

Although previous studies have reported that oral supplementation of BCAA could reduce RPE and mental fatigue in maximal exercise in untrained participants [32], our results suggest that the participants in the AA trial had better performance under the same level of RPE. This contradiction may result from the different protocols to measure physical performance. Blomstrand et al. used a fixed-rate protocol, followed by a 20-min maximal exercise on a bicycle treadmill [32]. On the other hand, the time-trial style of the present protocol required the participants to swim at their best effort in each lap. Therefore, the participants in both trials reached similar RPE, which is in agreement with our previous study [33].

A recent study revealed that a short-term citrulline supplementation could increase peak power output by 9% and total power output by 7% in 60-s all-out sprint that followed the 6-min bout of severe-intensity exercise [20]. In addition, a single dose of citrulline malate could improve performance in repeated high-intensity anaerobic resistance exercises [34]. Acute beetroot juice supplementation, which is rich in citrulline, also improved peak and mean power output, while reducing the time required to reach peak power output in the Wingate test [35]. A recent review summarized that acute beetroot juice could improve the performance in repeated high-intensity exercise by increasing phosphocreatine resynthesis and muscle shortening velocity [36]. These ergogenic effects could be mediated by the increased tissue oxygenation and improved O_2 kinetics. In the first and second lap during which central fatigue may not have been accumulated, it is possible that ergogenic effect was partially the result of the role of citrulline in improving short-term anaerobic performance. At the later stage of repeated high-intensity exercise, the aerobic system becomes an important energy source despite the all-out effort [9]. For example, the contribution of aerobic energy increased from 25% in the first sprint to approximately 50% in the second to forth sprints in 30 s × 4 swimming with 30 s rest in between [37]. Our participants also showed significantly elevated plasma glycerol concentrations after 8 × 50 m swim (Table 2), indicating greater lipolysis. The increased phosphocreatine resynthesis and muscle work efficiency, combining with delayed central fatigue, may lead to the better performance in the later stage of the high-intensity interval swim.

Our results showed that plasma ammonia and urea were similar between the two trials. In addition, ammonia concentrations remained unchanged after exercise in both trials, indicating that BCAA oxidation was not significantly increased in the AA trial. It is possible that the breakfast and the appropriate warm up before 8 × 50 m swim had already increased plasma ammonia levels. This is in agreement with Peyrebrune et al., who reported that plasma ammonia concentration was decreased after 8 × 50 yards sprint swimming [38]. These results agree with the notion that the major source of ATP turnover comes from aerobic metabolism, rather than adenosine monophosphate (AMP) deamination, towards the end of the repeated swims.

In previous studies we have shown that 0.17 g/kg body weight BCAA, twice of the dosage in the present study, could delay the development of central fatigue and prevent the decline in perceptual-motor functions [22,23]. Although the dosage can be tolerated, the large number of capsules may discourage some athletes from following this supplement regime. The lower dosage of 0.085 g/kg body weight in this study still resulted in an average plasma BCAA concentration of 0.8 mM prior to exercise, which was similar or slightly lower to the previous results [21–23]. The combined dosage of citrulline and arginine is 0.1 g/kg body weight, which is in line with previous studies using acute citrulline supplementations [22,23,39].

We specifically use the acute supplementation protocol for the purpose of creating higher plasma BCAA concentration during exercise to compete with free tryptophan in cross blood brain barrier. The longer-term of BCAA supplementation would not lead to significantly higher plasma concentrations compared to the acute regimen. In addition, it has been shown that acute supplements of citrulline-malate or other nitrate sources 40 min to 2.5 h prior to exercise could improve performance and lead to lower steady-state VO_2 at the same intensity [40–42], while several days of beetroot juice supplementation did not elicit greater improvements [40]. Therefore, the acute supplementation regime used in this study would be sufficient for the ergogenic effect.

HIIT has been reported to elicit similar, or even better effects on performance compared to high-volume lower-intensity training in competitive swimmers [6,43]. The shorter duration and lower training volume make HIIT ideal for most athletes and general populations who are living on a tight schedule. Most HIIT in swimming includes repeated sprints of 10 to 30 s duration with resting intervals of 2 to 5 min [44]. Our study adopted this protocol so that the results can be applied to practical training situations. It appears that our participants can maintain speed throughout the present protocol with 3-min recovery between each lap, whereas those with shorter (60 s) recovery periods resulted in significant decrements in performance toward the end [45]. Plasma lactate values in the present study are in line with others using similar protocols in swimmers [37,46], and similar to that after a 100 m swimming competition [47].

Swimming velocity is the product of stroke rate, the number of stroke cycle per min, and stroke length, the distance travelled with each stroke cycle [48]. Elite swimmers usually increase stroke rate, while ignoring stroke length, in order to increase or maintain speed when fatigue is accumulating [49]. In the present study, the participants in the AA trial swam significantly faster in the first and second lap with a trend of higher stroke rate. It is possible that the supplements provided higher central drive in the early stages of 8×50 m swim. In the seventh lap, the stroke rate is similar between the two trials. Therefore, the faster speed may result from the longer stroke length, indicating higher muscle strength or technical efficiency in the AA trial during the lap. In the third and fourth laps, the participants swam the fastest, while using the lowest stroke count. This suggests that the participants swam with the highest efficiency in the middle of the 8×50 m test.

One of the limitations to this study is the low energy provided in the standard meals during the two days prior to the trial. The meal boxes provided were similar to the participants' usual diet, both in terms of energy content and food choice. The participants may have had relatively low muscle glycogen levels on the morning of the trials. However, the breakfast before the trial, containing 1.0 g/kg body weight carbohydrate, would ensure the euglycemic state throughout the test. Another limitation is the relatively short exercise time. Whether the ergogenic effect shown in this study can be extended to the entire training period requires further investigation. The lack of data in oxygen consumption and phosphocreatine concentration in the muscle also prevented us from gaining further understanding of the mechanisms.

5. Conclusions

The present results showed that BCAA, arginine, and citrulline allowed young participants to swim faster in a 8 × 50 m high-intensity interval protocol while feeling the same level of effort. Future research may focus on the modifications in training load to utilize the enhanced physiological and psychological mechanisms associated with these supplements.

Author Contributions: Conceptualization, C.-K.C. and C.-L.W.; Methodology, C.-K.C., H.-J.W. and C.-F.H.; Data acquisition and analysis, C.-F.H. and T.-S.T.; Interpretation of data, C.-K.C., T.-S.T. and C.-F.H.; Funding acquisition, C.-K.C.; Manuscript preparation: C.-K.C. and C.-L.W.

Acknowledgments: The authors thank Yu-Fang Huang for her technical assistance.

References

1. Buchheit, M.; Laursen, P.B. High-intensity interval training, solutions to the programming puzzle: Part I: Cardiopulmonary emphasis. *Sports Med.* **2013**, *43*, 313–338. [CrossRef] [PubMed]
2. Buchheit, M.; Laursen, P.B. High-intensity interval training, solutions to the programming puzzle. Part II: Anaerobic energy, neuromuscular load and practical applications. *Sports Med.* **2013**, *43*, 927–954. [CrossRef] [PubMed]
3. Altenburg, T.M.; Degens, H.; van Mechelen, W.; Sargeant, A.J.; de Haan, A. Recruitment of single muscle fibers during submaximal cycling exercise. *J. Appl. Physiol. (1985)* **2007**, *103*, 1752–1756. [CrossRef] [PubMed]
4. Garcia-Hermoso, A.; Cerrillo-Urbina, A.J.; Herrera-Valenzuela, T.; Cristi-Montero, C.; Saavedra, J.M.; Martinez-Vizcaino, V. Is high-intensity interval training more effective on improving cardiometabolic risk and aerobic capacity than other forms of exercise in overweight and obese youth? A meta-analysis. *Obes. Rev.* **2016**, *17*, 531–540. [CrossRef]
5. Midgley, A.W.; McNaughton, L.R.; Carroll, S. Reproducibility of time at or near VO2max during intermittent treadmill running. *Int. J. Sports Med.* **2007**, *28*, 40–47. [CrossRef] [PubMed]
6. Faude, O.; Meyer, T.; Scharhag, J.; Weins, F.; Urhausen, A.; Kindermann, W. Volume vs. intensity in the training of competitive swimmers. *Int. J. Sports Med.* **2008**, *29*, 906–912. [CrossRef] [PubMed]
7. Sperlich, B.; Zinner, C.; Heilemann, I.; Kjendlie, P.L.; Holmberg, H.C.; Mester, J. High-intensity interval training improves VO(2peak), maximal lactate accumulation, time trial and competition performance in 9-11-year-old swimmers. *Eur. J. Appl. Physiol.* **2010**, *110*, 1029–1036. [CrossRef] [PubMed]
8. Spencer, M.; Bishop, D.; Dawson, B.; Goodman, C. Physiological and metabolic responses of repeated-sprint activities:specific to field-based team sports. *Sports Med.* **2005**, *35*, 1025–1044. [CrossRef] [PubMed]
9. Girard, O.; Mendez-Villanueva, A.; Bishop, D. Repeated-sprint ability—Part I: Factors contributing to fatigue. *Sports Med.* **2011**, *41*, 673–694. [CrossRef]
10. Sidhu, S.K.; Bentley, D.J.; Carroll, T.J. Locomotor exercise induces long-lasting impairments in the capacity of the human motor cortex to voluntarily activate knee extensor muscles. *J. Appl. Physiol. (1985)* **2009**, *106*, 556–565. [CrossRef]
11. Davis, J.M.; Bailey, S.P. Possible mechanisms of central nervous system fatigue during exercise. *Med. Sci. Sports Exerc.* **1997**, *29*, 45–57. [CrossRef] [PubMed]
12. Newsholme, E.A.; Blomstrand, E. Branched-chain amino acids and central fatigue. *J. Nutr.* **2006**, *136*, 274S–276S. [CrossRef] [PubMed]
13. Soares, D.D.; Coimbra, C.C.; Marubayashi, U. Tryptophan-induced central fatigue in exercising rats is related to serotonin content in preoptic area. *Neurosci. Lett.* **2007**, *415*, 274–278. [CrossRef] [PubMed]
14. Yamamoto, T.; Azechi, H.; Board, M. Essential role of excessive tryptophan and its neurometabolites in fatigue. *Can. J. Neurol. Sci.* **2012**, *39*, 40–47. [CrossRef] [PubMed]
15. Pardridge, W.M. Blood-brain barrier carrier-mediated transport and brain metabolism of amino acids. *Neurochem. Res.* **1998**, *23*, 635–644. [CrossRef] [PubMed]
16. Fernstrom, J.D. Branched-chain amino acids and brain function. *J. Nutr.* **2005**, *135*, 1539S–1546S. [CrossRef] [PubMed]

17. Brown, M.D.; Srinivasan, M.; Hogikyan, R.V.; Dengel, D.R.; Glickman, S.G.; Galecki, A.; Supiano, M.A. Nitric oxide biomarkers increase during exercise-induced vasodilation in the forearm. *Int. J. Sports Med.* **2000**, *21*, 83–89. [CrossRef] [PubMed]
18. Bailey, S.J.; Vanhatalo, A.; Winyard, P.G.; Jones, A.M. The nitrate-nitrite-nitric oxide pathway: Its role in human exercise physiology. *Eur. J. Sport Sci.* **2012**, *12*, 309–320. [CrossRef]
19. Yavuz, H.U.; Turnagol, H.; Demirel, A.H. Pre-exercise arginine supplementation increases time to exhaustion in elite male wrestlers. *Biol. Sport* **2014**, *31*, 187–191. [CrossRef] [PubMed]
20. Bailey, S.J.; Blackwell, J.R.; Lord, T.; Vanhatalo, A.; Winyard, P.G.; Jones, A.M. l-Citrulline supplementation improves O2 uptake kinetics and high-intensity exercise performance in humans. *J. Appl. Physiol. (1985)* **2015**, *119*, 385–395. [CrossRef]
21. Chang, C.K.; Chang Chien, K.M.; Chang, J.H.; Huang, M.H.; Liang, Y.C.; Liu, T.H. Branched-chain amino acids and arginine improve performance in two consecutive days of simulated handball games in male and female athletes: A randomized trial. *PLoS ONE* **2015**, *10*, e0121866. [CrossRef] [PubMed]
22. Yang, C.C.; Wu, C.L.; Chen, I.F.; Chang, C.K. Prevention of perceptual-motor decline by branched-chain amino acids, arginine, citrulline after tennis match. *Scand. J. Med. Sci. Sports* **2017**, *29*, 935–944. [CrossRef] [PubMed]
23. Chen, I.F.; Wu, H.J.; Chen, C.Y.; Chou, K.M.; Chang, C.K. Branched-chain amino acids, arginine, citrulline alleviate central fatigue after 3 simulated matches in taekwondo athletes: A randomized controlled trial. *J. Int. Soc. Sports Nutr.* **2016**, *13*, 28. [CrossRef] [PubMed]
24. Suzuki, T.; Morita, M.; Hayashi, T.; Kamimura, A. The effects on plasma L-arginine levels of combined oral L-citrulline and L-arginine supplementation in healthy males. *Biosci. Biotechnol. Biochem.* **2016**, 1–4. [CrossRef] [PubMed]
25. Naderi, A.; Earnest, C.P.; Lowery, R.P.; Wilson, J.M.; Willems, M.E. Co-ingestion of Nutritional Ergogenic Aids and High-Intensity Exercise Performance. *Sports Med.* **2016**, *46*, 1407–1418. [CrossRef] [PubMed]
26. Borg, G.A. Psychophysical bases of perceived exertion. *Med. Sci. Sports Exerc.* **1982**, *14*, 377–381. [CrossRef] [PubMed]
27. Green, L.C.; Wagner, D.A.; Glogowski, J.; Skipper, P.L.; Wishnok, J.S.; Tannenbaum, S.R. Analysis of nitrate, nitrite, and [15N] nitrate in biological fluids. *Anal. Biochem.* **1982**, *126*, 131–138. [CrossRef]
28. Costill, D.L.; Fink, W.J. Plasma volume changes following exercise and thermal dehydration. *J. Appl. Physiol.* **1974**, *37*, 521–525. [CrossRef]
29. Atkinson, G. Analysis of repeated measurements in physical therapy research: Multiple comparisons amongst level means and multi-factorial designs. *Phys. Ther. Sport* **2002**, *3*, 191–203. [CrossRef]
30. Tan, X.R.; Low, I.C.C.; Stephenson, M.C.; Soong, T.W.; Lee, J.K.W. Neural Basis of Exertional Fatigue in the Heat: A Review of Magnetic Resonance Imaging Methods. *Scand. J. Med. Sci. Sports* 2017. [CrossRef]
31. Benwell, N.M.; Mastaglia, F.L.; Thickbroom, G.W. Changes in the functional MR signal in motor and non-motor areas during intermittent fatiguing hand exercise. *Exp. Brain Res.* **2007**, *182*, 93–97. [CrossRef] [PubMed]
32. Blomstrand, E.; Hassmen, P.; Ek, S.; Ekblom, B.; Newsholme, E.A. Influence of ingesting a solution of branched-chain amino acids on perceived exertion during exercise. *Acta Physiol. Scand.* **1997**, *159*, 41–49. [CrossRef]
33. Cheng, I.S.; Wang, Y.W.; Chen, I.F.; Hsu, G.S.; Hsueh, C.F.; Chang, C.K. The supplementation of branched-chain amino acids, arginine, and citrulline improves endurance exercise performance in two consecutive days. *J. Sports Sci. Med.* **2016**, *15*, 509–515. [PubMed]
34. Perez-Guisado, J.; Jakeman, P.M. Citrulline malate enhances athletic anaerobic performance and relieves muscle soreness. *J. Strength Cond. Res.* **2010**, *24*, 1215–1222. [CrossRef] [PubMed]
35. Cuenca, E.; Jodra, P.; Perez-Lopez, A.; Gonzalez-Rodriguez, L.G.; Fernandes da Silva, S.; Veiga-Herreros, P.; Dominguez, R. Effects of Beetroot Juice Supplementation on Performance and Fatigue in a 30-s All-Out Sprint Exercise: A Randomized, Double-Blind Cross-Over Study. *Nutrients* **2018**, *10*. [CrossRef]
36. Dominguez, R.; Mate-Munoz, J.L.; Cuenca, E.; Garcia-Fernandez, P.; Mata-Ordonez, F.; Lozano-Estevan, M.C.; Veiga-Herreros, P.; da Silva, S.F.; Garnacho-Castano, M.V. Effects of beetroot juice supplementation on intermittent high-intensity exercise efforts. *J. Int. Soc. Sports Nutr.* **2018**, *15*, 2. [CrossRef]
37. Peyrebrune, M.C.; Toubekis, A.G.; Lakomy, H.K.; Nevill, M.E. Estimating the energy contribution during single and repeated sprint swimming. *Scand. J. Med. Sci. Sports* **2014**, *24*, 369–376. [CrossRef]

16

Effects of Upper-Limb, Lower-Limb and Full-Body Compression Garments on Full Body Kinematics and Free-Throw Accuracy in Basketball Players

Duo Wai-Chi Wong [1,2], Wing-Kai Lam [3,4,5,*], Tony Lin-Wei Chen [1], Qitao Tan [1], Yan Wang [1,2] and Ming Zhang [1,2,*]

1 Department of Biomedical Engineering, Faculty of Engineering, The Hong Kong Polytechnic University, Hong Kong 999077, China; duo.wong@polyu.edu.hk (D.W.-C.W.); tony.l.chen@connect.polyu.hk (T.L.-W.C.); matthew.tan@connect.polyu.hk (Q.T.); annie.y.wang@polyu.edu.hk (Y.W.)
2 The Hong Kong Polytechnic University Shenzhen Research Institute, Shenzhen 518057, China
3 Guangdong Provincial Engineering Technology Research Center for Sports Assistive Devices, Guangzhou Sport University, Guangzhou 510000, China
4 Department of Kinesiology, Shenyang Sport University, Shenyang 110102, China
5 Li Ning Sports Science Research Center, Li Ning (China) Sports Goods Company, Beijing 101111, China
* Correspondence: gilbertlam@li-ning.com.cn (W.-K.L.); ming.zhang@polyu.edu.hk (M.Z.)

Abstract: Compression garments can enhance performance and promote recovery in athletes. Different body coverage with compression garments may impose distinct effects on kinematic movement mechanics and thus basketball free-throw accuracy. The objective of this study was to examine basketball free-throw shooting accuracy, consistency and the range of motion of body joints while wearing upper-, lower- and full-body compression garments. Twenty male basketball players performed five blocks of 20 basketball free-throw shooting trials in each of the following five compression garment conditions: control-pre, top, bottom, full (top + bottom) and control-post. All conditions were randomized except pre- and post-control (the first and last conditions). Range of motion of was acquired by multiple inertial measurement units. Free-throw accuracy and the coefficient of variation were also analyzed. Players wearing upper-body or full-body compression garments had significantly improved accuracy by 4.2% and 5.9%, respectively ($p < 0.05$), but this difference was not observed with shooting consistency. Smaller range of motion of head flexion and trunk lateral bending ($p < 0.05$) was found in the upper- and full-body conditions compared to the control-pre condition. These findings suggest that an improvement in shooting accuracy could be achieved by constraining the range of motion through the use of upper-body and full-body compression garments.

Keywords: range of motion; basketball shooting; proprioception

---

1. Introduction

Basketball is one of the most popular sports; at least 450 million people play basketball worldwide, ranging from registered elite players to amateurs [1]. Basketball skills can be categorized into offensive skills, including shooting, passing and dribbling and defensive skills, including blocking and stealing [2]. While shooting is the mean to score in the game, free-throws (or foul shots) are considered as one of the easiest movements, yet they can significantly influence the outcome of a game [3,4]. Movement mechanics and coordination are key to free-throwing performance [5,6] and may be regulated by wearing compression garments [7].

Compression garment can enhance performance and recovery in various sports [7,8]. Specifically, compression garments improve joint awareness, reduce muscle soreness and encourage blood circulation and thus, promote recovery [9]. Conversely, some studies have argued that upper-body compression garment may impose negative effects in hot environments and the claimed benefits may only be confined to perception of comfort [10,11]. Different movement tasks, selection of indicators, and the physical status of the athletes may also contribute to the variability and effectiveness of using compression garments during exercise, whereas garment design, such as type, coverage and tightness, may affect the functions of the garment [9]. The tightness of the compression garment has been hypothesized to change the interfacial pressure of the body [12]; however, there is a lack of studies exploring the influence of body coverage with different compression garments.

The benefits of compression garments could be attributed to the enhancement of proprioception to improve movement mechanics [13]. Hooper et al. [14] demonstrated the relationship between throwing velocity and accuracy, and improved proprioceptive signals in upper-body compression garments for baseball athletes. The compression on the cutaneous receptors or muscle spindle receptors not only enhanced the sensory information, but also filtered irrelevant mechanoreceptor information [15]. Depending on the task, the nervous system integrated these signals or information at multiple levels to mediate cutaneous and muscle afferent feedback, which is imperative for smooth coordination of movements [15–17].

There is insufficient evidence to support the use of compression garments (upper-body or lower-body) to enhance basketball performance. Atkins et al. [7] showed that wearing lower-body compression garments overnight produced negligible effects on the countermovement jump, repeated sprint and agility test performances, despite improvements in perceived fatigue and muscle soreness. Other evidence indicated that lower-leg compression garments were found to significantly reduce the range of abduction motion of the hip joint during a drop vertical jump, but produced minimal effects on the kinematics/kinetics of other lower extremity joints [13].

Furthermore, lower-body compression was shown to improve lower limb balance and stability in active females during a single-leg balance task [18]. Poor stability results in higher motion variability and may potentially weaken shooting accuracy [6,19,20]. How these findings affect other functional performances (e.g., basketball shooting) requires further investigation. Since compression garments produce mechanical restraints on body segments and joints, range of motion (ROM) has been one of the key parameters for the evaluation of kinematic effects during exercise in previous basketball studies [13,21].

Considering the relationship between compression garment coverage (upper-body, lower-body and combined) on the kinematics and shooting performance of basketball specific maneuvers is currently questionable, coaches and athletes are eager to understand what type of compression garment coverage could help them improve performance and consistency of performance. The objective of this study was to examine the effect of upper- and lower-body compression garment coverage (top, bottom and full) on the full body range of motion (ROM) and shooting accuracy of basketball free-throws. It was hypothesized that a certain compression garment condition would improve free-throw performance and consistency compared to the no-compression garment control group.

2. Materials and Methods

2.1. Participants

Twenty (n = 20) male basketball players were recruited from local universities. Their average age, height and body mass were 22.6 ± 1.1 years, 179.4 ± 3.4 cm and 72.7 ± 8.2 kg, respectively. All participants had at least 4 years of experiences in playing basketball and were right hand dominant single-handed shooters. The average basketball training experience and training time were 8.5 ± 2.4 years and 5.2 ± 1.6 h per week, respectively. All participants were physically fit and healthy and reported no injuries over the previous 6 months. Ethical approval (IRB-2017-BM-006) was granted from the institutional ethics committee. Written informed consent was obtained from all participants.

2.2. Experimental Conditions and Procedure

All free-throw shooting conditions were performed in our biomechanical laboratory. The free-throw distance and the height of the basketball rim were set according to the International Basketball Federation standards [19]. The participants performed single-handed free-throws under five different garment conditions, control-pre: no garment pre-control, Top: upper-body compression garment (Li Ning, Powershell, AULM043-I, Beijing, China), Bottom: lower-body compression garment bottom (Li Ning, Powershell, AUDL101-1, Beijing, China), full: both upper-body and lower-body compression garment and control-post: no garment post-control, as shown in Figure 1. Control-pre and control-post were the first and the last test conditions. The remaining three compression garment conditions (top, bottom and full) were randomly assigned as the second to the fourth conditions across participants. As the experimental protocol compared the first and last conditions, we were able to evaluate the fatigue effect [22]. For each free-throw condition, 20 free-throw shooting trials were performed. Testing of the next condition started immediately after the participant changed their garments.

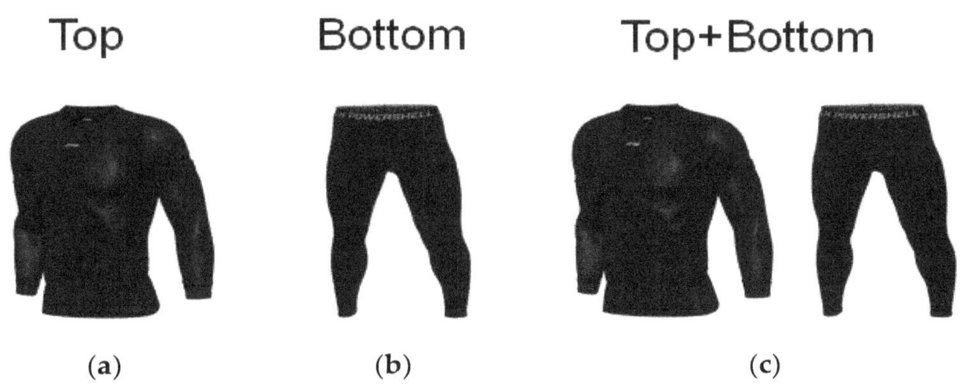

Figure 1. Compression garment conditions: (**a**) top; (**b**) bottom; (**c**) full (top + bottom).

The control conditions (control-pre and control-post) were self-selected comfortable sportswear that were not compression garments. The experimenters measured the height, waist and chest circumference of the participants to determine the appropriate garment [23]. The appropriate compression garment size was pre-determined by the manufacturer's sizing guidelines and was based on the body height and mass of each participant. Next, we assigned participants compression garments one size smaller than the pre-determined appropriate size in order to increase the interfacial pressure, as recommended by the experimental protocol detailed by Williams and colleagues [12].

A motion capturing system with multiple inertial measurement units (MyoMOTION, Noraxon, Inc., Scottsdale, AZ, USA) was used to measure full-body kinematics during the free-throw shooting trials. The inertial measurement units (IMU) were attached and strapped to each body segment according to the instrument guidelines. During each free-throw trial, the participants performed shooting from the same position behind the free-throw line. The sampling frequency of the IMU was 200 Hz. The kinematic data during the free-throw motion were post-processed using Matlab software (MathWorks, Inc., Natick, MA, USA) using a 6 Hz cutoff 4th order Butterworth low-pass filter.

2.3. Outcome Measures

Outcome measures including performance score (accuracy) and joint ROM variables were investigated. The performance score was gauged using an ordinal six-point (0 to 5 point) scoring system. Five, four and three points denoted a clean score, that the ball hit the rim and went in, and that the ball hit the backboard and went in, respectively. Two, one and zero points denoted that the ball hit the rim and missed, hit the backboard and missed and missed complete, respectively, as illustrated in Table 1 [19,24]. The consistency of the score was also assessed by the coefficient of variation (i.e., the ratio of the standard deviation to the mean of the trials).

Table 1. The six-point basketball shooting performance score system.

Performance	Scored			Missed		
	Clean (Swish)	Rim & In	Backboard & In	Rim & Out	Backboard & Out	Complete Miss
Score	5	4	3	2	1	0

ROM of the head, trunk, elbow, shoulder, wrist, hip, knee and ankle joints in the sagittal, coronal and frontal planes were calculated. Data were averaged across trials for each participant in each condition which served as the targeted average profile for subsequent statistical analysis [25]. We did not view the within-participant effect (trial) of ROM as an independent observation or random factor to be analyzed.

2.4. Data Analysis

All statistical analysis was performed in SPSS 21 (IBM, New York, NY, USA). Prior to statistical analysis, the Shapiro–Wilk test was performed to check for the normality of the kinematic data, and it was satisfied. The Wilcoxon signed-rank test was performed to compare free-throw performance scores between the control-pre- and control-post-control conditions to ensure that there was no learning or fatigue effect (i.e., Control pre- and post-control were not significantly different). Furthermore, one-way repeated measures analysis of variance (ANOVA) was performed to examine any significant difference for joint ROM variables between the control-pre, top, bottom and full conditions, followed by the post hoc pairwise comparison of Least Significant Difference (LSD) if a significant main effect was found. We chose the LSD approach as our research hypothesis was more focused on planned comparisons. As such, we regarded the ANOVA as an additional constraint [26]. Similarly, the comparison for the performance score and the coefficient of variation was performed using a nonparametric test (Friedman test), with the post hoc pairwise Wilcoxon signed-rank test, as the performance score was gauged in an ordinal scale. Level of significance was set at $p = 0.05$. The indices of effect size for the ANOVA and post hoc pairwise comparison were partial η^2 and Cohen's d, respectively.

3. Results

3.1. Control-Pre and Control-Post Conditions

There was no significant difference in performance score between the control-pre (Median = 2.975) and control-post (Median = 3.075) conditions ($Z = -1.430$, $p = 0.153$). Similarly, there was no significant difference in the coefficient of variation of performance score between the control-pre and control-post conditions ($Z = -1.382$, $p = 0.167$). We assumed that there was no pronounced carry-over or fatigue effect that significantly affected performance over the course of the experiment.

3.2. Free-Throw Accuracy

There were no significant differences in free-throw performance score ($\chi^2(4) = 6.510$, $p = 0.089$) or the coefficient of variation of the performance score ($\chi^2(4) = 5.629$, $p = 0.131$) between the conditions (control-pre, top, bottom or full). However, post hoc pairwise comparison showed that the free-throw performance scores of the top (Median = 3.1, $Z = -2.357$, $p = 0.018$) and full (Median = 3.15, $Z = -2.112$, $p = 0.035$) conditions were significantly larger than that of the control-pre condition (Median = 2.975), as shown in Tables 2 and 3.

Table 2. Descriptive statistics of the averaged and coefficient of variation of the free-throw performance score.

Condition	Performance Score		Coefficient of Variation (%)
	Median	Mean (Standard Deviation)	Mean (Standard Deviation)
Control-Pre	2.975	2.975 (0.419)	38.04 (6.67)
Top	3.100 *	3.168 (0.382)	36.78 (7.05)
Bottom	3.050	3.035 (0.411)	37.06 (7.07)
Full	3.150 *	3.175 (0.385)	36.19 (7.58)
Control-Post	3.075	3.123 (0.476)	35.88 (8.61)

* significant difference ($p < 0.05$) compared to the control-pre condition by post hoc Wilcoxon signed-rank test.

Table 3. Probability values (p-value) of the average (upper right triangle) and coefficient of variation (lower left triangle) of the free-throw performance score.

Coefficient of Variation	Performance Score			
	Control-Pre	Top	Bottom	Full
Control-Pre		0.018 *	0.230	0.035 *
Top	0.296		0.152	0.888
Bottom	0.227	0.654		0.159
Full	0.107	0.794	0.344	

* significant difference ($p < 0.05$) by post hoc Wilcoxon signed-rank test.

3.3. Full-Body Joint Range of Motion (RoM)

One-way ANOVA repeated measures showed that the variation in compression garments imposed significant effects on the ROM of head flexion ($p = 0.014$, partial $\eta^2 = 0.169$), trunk lateral bending ($p = 0.024$, partial $\eta^2 = 0.152$), left shoulder flexion ($p = 0.041$, partial $\eta^2 = 0.152$), right shoulder rotation ($p = 0.048$, partial $\eta^2 = 0.128$) and left knee flexion ($p = 0.003$, partial $\eta^2 = 0.212$). Post hoc pairwise comparison showed that the top condition significantly reduced the head flexion ($p = 0.037$; d = 0.503; 1.346, 95% CI 0.376 to 2.315) and trunk lateral bending ($p = 0.042$; d = 0.487; 1.039, 95% CI 0.041 to 2.036) ROM compared with the control-pre condition (Table 4). Similarly, the full condition significantly reduced head flexion ($p = 0.009$; d = 0.650; 1.346, 95% CI 0.376 to 2.315) and trunk lateral bending ($p = 0.028$; d = 0.532; 1.446, 95% CI 0.173 to 2.718) ROM compared to the control-pre condition.

Table 4. Descriptive statistics and one-way ANOVA repeated measures outcome of the range of motion of head and trunk in different compression garment conditions.

	Range of Motion, Mean (Standard Deviation)				ANOVA Repeated Measure	
	Control-Pre	Top	Bottom	Full	Effect Size	p-Value
Head FL/EX	10.57 (3.81)	9.53 (3.1) [a]	9.75 (3.37)	9.22 (3.07) [A]	0.169	0.014 *
Head lateral bending	6.14 (2.83)	5.80 (2.69)	6.05 (2.99)	5.87 (2.62)	0.019 [g]	0.694
Head axial rotation	13.17 (8.04)	17.11 (12.74)	15.02 (10.49)	14.42 (8.63)	0.053	0.368
Trunk FL/EX	19.20 (6.24)	17.15 (5.96)	18.43 (5.85)	18.15 (6.42)	0.11	0.082
Trunk lateral bending	10.21 (4.24)	9.17 (4.38) [a]	9.88 (3.63)	8.77 (4.01) [a]	0.152	0.024 *
Trunk axial rotation	11.05 (4.56)	11.46 (5.04)	10.99 (4.36)	11.39 (4.37)	0.018 [g]	0.687

FL/EX: flexion/extension; * significant difference ($p < 0.05$) using one-way ANOVA repeated measures; [g] Greenhouse–Geisser correction to adjust the lack of sphericity; [a] and [A] denote $p < 0.05$ and $p < 0.0125$ than the control-pre condition.

Compared to that of the bottom condition, both the top ($p = 0.01$; d = 0.642; 3.422, 95% CI 0.929 to 5.915) and full ($p = 0.003$; d = 0.778; 3.530, 95% CI 1.405 to 5.655) conditions significantly reduced the ROM of the left shoulder flexion, while the top condition had significantly larger right shoulder rotation compared with the control-pre ($p = 0.013$; d = 0.611; 38.316, 95% CI −8.98 to 67.65) and bottom ($p = 0.041$; d = 0.491; 23.028, 95% CI 1.08 to 44.976) conditions (Table 5). The control-pre condition had significantly larger left knee flexion ROM than the bottom (p = 0.026; d = 0.539; 2.605, 95% CI 0.345 to 4.864) and full (p = 0.002; d = 0.804; 2.908, 95% CI 1.214 to 4.602) conditions. Similarly, the top condition had a significantly larger left knee flexion ROM than the bottom (p = 0.044; d = 0.482; 2.047, 95% CI 0.059 to 4.035) and full (p = 0.018; d = 0.585; 2.351, 95% CI, 0.469 to 4.232) conditions (Table 6).

Table 5. Descriptive statistics and one-way ANOVA repeated measures outcome of the range of motion of the upper limb in different compression garment conditions.

	Range of Motion, Mean (Standard Deviation)				ANOVA Repeated Measure	
	Control-Pre	Top	Bottom	Full	Effect Size	p-Value
L elbow FL/EX	49.35 (23.12)	51.38 (23.28)	50.95 (22.82)	51.24 (24.05)	0.048	0.417
R elbow FL/EX	93.30 (13.27)	89.43 (12.46)	89.14 (13.79)	89.82 (14.38)	0.098	0.116
L shoulder FL/EX	30.06 (12.77)	26.98 (11.58)	30.40 (12.66) [B]	26.87 (10.48) [C]	0.152 [g]	0.041 *
R shoulder FL/EX	44.11 (18.88)	40.48 (16.96)	44.01 (19.11)	41.47 (17.2)	0.148 [g]	0.148
L shoulder AB/AD	124.84 (113.81)	125.37 (132.49)	133.85 (120.05)	132.36 (124.17)	0.022 [g]	0.66
R shoulder AB/AD	72.93 (51)	75.01 (55.07)	76.05 (48.47)	78.02 (71.69)	0.012 [g]	0.821
L shoulder rotation	50.50 (40.81)	58.41 (51.4)	67.74 (83.18)	59.95 (61.04)	0.089 [g]	0.176
R shoulder rotation	90.38 (45.46)	128.70 (81.71) [a]	105.67 (67.28) [b]	118.07 (73.94)	0.128	0.048 *
L wrist RA/UL	35.80 (26.08)	34.93 (27)	35.12 (28.48)	38.26 (32.93)	0.036	0.552
R wrist RA/UL	70.79 (27.55)	79.36 (29.02)	71.34 (33.37)	77.37 (31.8)	0.071 [g]	0.249
L wrist FL/EX	39.21 (33.56)	39.37 (41.11)	42.20 (43.93)	42.90 (45.34)	0.011 [g]	0.885
R wrist FL/EX	105.39 (34.39)	109.35 (36.59)	110.83 (35.36)	106.85 (35.66)	0.026	0.675
L palm rotation	49.54 (47.21)	51.35 (48.84)	60.70 (72.13)	52.23 (55.49)	0.067 [g]	0.269
R palm rotation	93.97 (46)	126.74 (77.75)	113.01 (81.54)	110.93 (66.53)	0.117	0.066

FL/EX: flexion/extension; AB/AD: abduction/adduction; RA/UL: Radial/Ulnar deviation; * significant difference ($p < 0.05$) using one-way ANOVA repeated measures; [g] Greenhouse–Geisser correction to adjust the lack of sphericity; [a] denotes $p < 0.05$ than the control-pre condition; [b] and [B] denote $p < 0.05$ and $p < 0.0125$ than the top condition; [C] denotes $p < 0.0125$ than the bottom condition.

Table 6. Descriptive statistics and one-way ANOVA repeated measures outcome of the range of motion of the lower limb in different compression garment conditions.

	Range of Motion, Mean (Standard Deviation)				ANOVA Repeated Measure	
	Control-Pre	Top	Bottom	Full	Effect Size	p-Value
L hip FL/EX	23.56 (6.8)	22.58 (6.65)	22.34 (7.8)	21.81 (7.19)	0.076 [g]	0.22
R hip FL/EX	26.47 (4.49)	25.14 (6.02)	26.19 (6.26)	25.93 (5.85)	0.065	0.274
L hip AB/AD	5.69 (1.73)	6.46 (2.38)	5.57 (1.64)	6.28 (2.36)	0.069	0.251
R hip AB/AD	6.95 (2.6)	7.22 (2.72)	6.31 (2.42)	6.97 (2.62)	0.069	0.248
L hip rotation	9.99 (3.57)	10.03 (3.52)	9.31 (3.04)	9.45 (2.53)	0.043 [g]	0.445
R hip rotation	12.62 (3.89)	12.83 (4.19)	12.43 (4.17)	12.30 (4.61)	0.013	0.861
L knee FL/EX	51.86 (8.63)	51.30 (8.15)	49.25 (10.08) [a, b]	48.95 (9.37) [A, b]	0.212	0.003 *
R knee FL/EX	53.77 (7.33)	52.90 (7.88)	53.61 (6.61)	52.94 (6.67)	0.036	0.549
L knee rotation	10.64 (4.39)	11.35 (5.59)	10.26 (3.99)	10.35 (4.21)	0.051 [g]	0.37
R knee rotation	14.96 (4.52)	14.72 (6.12)	15.68 (5.86)	15.43 (5.01)	0.031	0.61
L knee AB/AD	7.15 (4.52)	7.92 (4.46)	6.81 (2.89)	7.00 (3.28)	0.029 [g]	0.587
R knee AB/AD	8.32 (3.72)	7.67 (3.84)	9.10 (4.32)	8.48 (3.58)	0.048	0.418
L ankle PL/DO	61.22 (16.82)	64.36 (8.64)	61.71 (8.01)	61.83 (9.08)	0.049 [g]	0.362
R ankle PL/DO	60.93 (11.16)	61.97 (6.1)	60.76 (7.49)	61.82 (8.21)	0.019 [g]	0.682
L ankle EV/IV	25.31 (14.66)	22.84 (13.08)	24.29 (11.37)	23.38 (12.54)	0.041	0.49
R ankle EV/IV	26.49 (13.19)	23.04 (11.28)	22.95 (8.38)	21.27 (10.34)	0.123	0.056
L ankle AB/AD	15.28 (4.08)	15.47 (4.5)	15.52 (4.76)	16.12 (5.18)	0.016 [g]	0.732
R ankle AB/AD	13.98 (3.73)	14.69 (4.46)	15.17 (4.9)	14.43 (4.14)	0.077	0.204

FL/EX: flexion/extension; AB/AD: abduction/adduction; EV/IV: eversion/inversion; PL/DO: plantarflexion/dorsiflexion; * significant difference ($p < 0.05$) using one-way ANOVA repeated measures; [g] Greenhouse–Geisser correction to adjust the lack of sphericity; [a] and [A] denote $p < 0.05$ and $p < 0.0125$ than the control-pre condition; [b] denotes $p < 0.05$ than the top condition.

4. Discussion

This study examined the effect of upper and lower-body compression garments on the body kinematics and shooting accuracy of basketball free-throws. Our study found that upper-body (top) or full-body (top + bottom) compression garments significantly improved the performance of basketball free-throws; however, there was no significant improvement in the consistency of performance. Overall, mechanically, compression garments had a significant influence on the ROM of the head flexion, trunk lateral bending, left (non-dominant side) shoulder flexion, right (dominant side) shoulder rotation and left knee flexion as indicated by the ANOVA findings. Post hoc comparisons showed that wearing either upper- or full-body garments constrained the ROM of head flexion and trunk lateral bending which could be associated with improved trunk stability and thus, improved performance [27]. The relationship between the condition of the head movement and stability and free-throw accuracy was advocated previously, but not well understood [28]. On the other hand, garment coverage of the lower body (bottom or full-body gear) significantly reduced the ROM of the left (non-dominant) side knee joint in the sagittal plane, but not the right (dominant) side, because experienced players tended to adjust the knee joint of the dominant side to greater extent for better performance [29]. Theoretically, compression of the knee joint enhanced proprioception and thus performance [30,31] notwithstanding that our study did not demonstrate an improved shooting score for lower-body (bottom) garments. In addition, the reduced head flexion and trunk lateral bending ROM could implicate successful shooting performance.

Elbow and wrist movements are determinants of free-throw performance and player skill levels [20]. Skilled players coordinate the shooting arm by constantly compromising between elbow and wrist movements to adapt to subtle changes in release parameters of the ball (e.g., release height, angle of ball projection, velocity at ball release) [20]. In addition, more highly skilled players tend to maximize the ROM of the wrist joint [20]. top compression garments help to constrain the ROM of the elbow, and thus players can focus on optimizing distal joint (wrist) motion only [20]. In our study, although there were no significant main effects on the ROM of the elbow and wrist joints, pairwise comparisons showed that upper-body (top) garments significantly reduced the ROM of the right (dominant) side elbow, but increased that of the wrist radial/ulnar deviation and palmar rotation compared to that of the control-pre condition. This was likely due to the fact that the uncovered wrist joint compensated the reduced motion of the elbow [20]. In fact, some statisticians argued that conducting and interpreting post hoc analyses could still be valid even though the main effect was not significant [32,33].

The enhanced proprioception by compression garments may also facilitate the organization of compensatory behavior between joints for better performance. This was supported by existing studies that the proprioception (joint position sense) of the elbow and wrist joints was correlated with the success rate of the free-throw tasks [34]. More highly skilled players managed to optimize their performance based on the perceptual consequence of their actions [35].

A previous study suggested that the shoulder joint plays an important role in the action of basketball free-throws. Kaya et al. [36] found that free-throw performance was significantly correlated with the peak torque of the shoulder joint muscles and the shoulder joint position sense at 160° in the dominant side. While we anticipated that compression garments would amplify the proprioception [30], enhance stability and reduce the ROM of the shooting limb (right side), our study found that the ROM of the upper-body was significantly smaller when wearing top compression garments than when wearing bottom garments. Although there were no significant differences compared to that of the control-pre condition, we believe that the increased trend of the joint ROM may indicate that wearing lower-body (bottom) garments alone had a negative effect on the shoulder joint. From the kinetic chain perspective, intervention at the lower limb level may alter energy generation which can be transferred to the upper limbs and thus considerably influences upper limb movement tasks (e.g., racket and ball speed in racket sports) [19,37]. The influence of lower limb garments on the upper limbs may also be the reason that the full-body garments did not have an effect on the elbow and wrist joints, despite upper-body garments having an effect.

There were some limitations in this study. First, although we demonstrated no carry-over effect as revealed by the fact that there was no significant difference between the performance score of the control-pre and control-post conditions, there was an improvement trend on both the performance score and consistency. We believed that the randomized order assigned on the garment condition could minimize the carry-over effect. Second, our short adaptation time for each compression garment condition may not be adequate enough, despite that there is no consensus on the duration of adaptation in the past studies. Future studies may consider tests with longer adaptation in different days or weeks or considering the variation of kinematic variables [38]. Third, we presented only joint ROM in this study. More comprehensive analysis with discrete variables (peak angle, angular velocity), joint power, muscle force, proprioception as well as stability should be considered to evaluate their influence and underlying mechanism on the free-throw shooting performance. Asymmetry sport activity (e.g., single-handed shooting) may produce unique sequential coordination of the upper and lower limb with coherent patterns of muscle activation [39]. Forth, our study confined to non-professional basketball players. Playing level and sex effects may contribute to variations in movement strategy, skeletal alignment and muscle strength and could also be investigated. Lastly, the compression garments may impose different levels of pressure on the participants depending on their body built. Future study shall consider measuring the compression level in each condition.

5. Conclusions

Players wearing upper-body or full-body compression garment significantly improved basketball free-throw accuracy by 4.2% and 5.9%, respectively, but not on the intertrial consistency. full body kinematics data suggested that the improved performance could be attributed to the reduced ROM of head flexion and lateral bending of the trunk. Future studies investigating the relationship between shooting performance in basketball, reduced ROM and enhanced proprioception or stability are required.

Author Contributions: Conceptualization, D.W.-C.W. and W.-K.L.; data curation, D.W.-C.W. and T.L.-W.C.; formal analysis, D.W.-C.W. and T.L.-W.C.; funding acquisition, M.Z.; investigation, T.L.-W.C., Q.T. and Y.W.; methodology, D.W.-C.W., T.L.-W.C. and Q.T.; supervision, W.-K.L. and M.Z.; writing—original draft, D.W.-C.W.; writing—review & editing, W.-K.L. All authors have read and agreed to the published version of the manuscript.

References

1. Drinkwater, E.J.; Pyne, D.B.; McKenna, M.J. Design and interpretation of anthropometric and fitness testing of basketball players. *Sports Med.* **2008**, *38*, 565–578. [CrossRef] [PubMed]
2. Krause, J.V.; Nelson, C. *Basketball Skills & Drills*; Human Kinetics: Champaign, IL, USA, 2018.
3. Sampaio, J.; Janeira, M. Statistical analyses of basketball team performance: Understanding teams' wins and losses according to a different index of ball possessions. *Int. J. Perform. Anal. Sport* **2003**, *3*, 40–49. [CrossRef]
4. Csataljay, G.; O'Donoghue, P.; Hughes, M.; Dancs, H. Performance indicators that distinguish winning and losing teams in basketball. *Int. J. Perform. Anal. Sport* **2009**, *9*, 60–66. [CrossRef]
5. Okazaki, V.H.; Rodacki, A.L.; Satern, M.N. A review on the basketball jump shot. *Sports Biomech.* **2015**, *14*, 190–205. [CrossRef] [PubMed]
6. Verhoeven, F.M.; Newell, K.M. Coordination and control of posture and ball release in basketball free-throw shooting. *Hum. Mov. Sci.* **2016**, *49*, 216–224. [CrossRef] [PubMed]
7. Atkins, R.; Lam, W.-K.; Scanlan, A.T.; Beaven, C.M.; Driller, M. Lower-body compression garments worn following exercise improves perceived recovery but not subsequent performance in basketball athletes. *J. Sports Sci.* **2020**, *38*, 1–9. [CrossRef]
8. Marqués-Jiménez, D.; Calleja-González, J.; Arratibel, I.; Delextrat, A.; Terrados, N. Are compression garments effective for the recovery of exercise-induced muscle damage? A systematic review with meta-analysis. *Physiol. Behav.* **2016**, *153*, 133–148. [CrossRef]
9. MacRae, B.A.; Cotter, J.D.; Laing, R.M. Compression garments and exercise: Garment considerations, physiology and performance. *Sports Med.* **2011**, *41*, 815–843. [CrossRef]

10. Leoz-Abaurrea, I.; Aguado-Jiménez, R. Upper Body Compression Garment: Physiological Effects While Cycling in a Hot Environment. *Wilderness Environ. Med.* **2017**, *28*, 94–100. [CrossRef]
11. Ali, A.; Creasy, R.H.; Edge, J.A. Physiological effects of wearing graduated compression stockings during running. *Eur. J. Appl. Physiol.* **2010**, *109*, 1017–1025. [CrossRef]
12. Brophy-Williams, N.; Driller, M.W.; Shing, C.M.; Fell, J.W.; Halson, S.L. Confounding compression: The effects of posture, sizing and garment type on measured interface pressure in sports compression clothing. *J. Sports Sci.* **2015**, *33*, 1403–1410. [CrossRef] [PubMed]
13. Zamporri, J.; Aguinaldo, A. The Effects of a Compression Garment on Lower Body Kinematics and Kinetics During a Drop Vertical Jump in Female Collegiate Athletes. *Orthop. J. Sports Med.* **2018**, *6*, 2325967118789955. [CrossRef] [PubMed]
14. Hooper, D.R.; Dulkis, L.L.; Secola, P.J.; Holtzum, G.; Harper, S.P.; Kalkowski, R.J.; Comstock, B.A.; Szivak, T.K.; Flanagan, S.D.; Looney, D.P. Roles of an upper-body compression garment on athletic performances. *J. Strength Cond. Res.* **2015**, *29*, 2655–2660. [CrossRef] [PubMed]
15. Barss, T.S.; Pearcey, G.E.; Munro, B.; Bishop, J.L.; Zehr, E.P. Effects of a compression garment on sensory feedback transmission in the human upper limb. *J. Neurophysiol.* **2018**, *120*, 186–195. [CrossRef]
16. Zehr, P.E.; Collins, D.F.; Chua, R. Human interlimb reflexes evoked by electrical stimulation of cutaneous nerves innervating the hand and foot. *Exp. Brain Res.* **2001**, *140*, 495–504. [CrossRef]
17. Zehr, E.P.; Collins, D.F.; Frigon, A.; Hoogenboom, N. Neural control of rhythmic human arm movement: Phase dependence and task modulation of Hoffmann reflexes in forearm muscles. *J. Neurophysiol.* **2003**, *89*, 12–21. [CrossRef]
18. Michael, J.S.; Dogramaci, S.N.; Steel, K.A.; Graham, K.S. What is the effect of compression garments on a balance task in female athletes? *Gait Posture* **2014**, *39*, 804–809. [CrossRef]
19. Lam, W.-K.; Lee, W.C.-C.; Ng, S.-O.; Zheng, Y. Effects of foot orthoses on dynamic balance and basketball free-throw accuracy before and after physical fatigue. *J. Biomech.* **2019**, *96*, 109338. [CrossRef]
20. Button, C.; Macleod, M.; Sanders, R.; Coleman, S. Examining movement variability in the basketball free-throw action at different skill levels. *Res. Q. Exerc. Sport* **2003**, *74*, 257–269. [CrossRef]
21. Montgomery, P.G.; Pyne, D.B.; Hopkins, W.G.; Dorman, J.C.; Cook, K.; Minahan, C.L. The effect of recovery strategies on physical performance and cumulative fatigue in competitive basketball. *J. Sports Sci.* **2008**, *26*, 1135–1145. [CrossRef]
22. Thomas, J.R.; Nelson, J.K.; Silverman, S.J. *Research Methods in Physical Activity*; Human Kinetics: Champaign, IL, USA, 2015.
23. Watkins, W.B. Compression garment sizing: Challenges, issues, and a solution. *Plast. Surg. Nurs.* **2010**, *30*, 85–87. [CrossRef] [PubMed]
24. Martin, L. *Sports Performance Measurement and Analytics: The Science of Assessing Performance, Predicting Future Outcomes, Interpreting Statistical Models, and Evaluating the Market Value of Athletes*; FT Press: Upper Saddle River, NJ, USA, 2016.
25. Newell, J.; Aitchison, T.; Grant, S. *Statistics for Sports and Exercise Science: A Practical Approach*; Routledge: Abingdon, UK, 2014.
26. Holm, S. A simple sequentially rejective multiple test procedure. *Scand. J. Stat.* **1979**, *6*, 65–70.
27. Doan, B.; Kwon, Y.-H.; Newton, R.; Shim, J.; Popper, E.; Rogers, R.; Bolt, L.; Robertson, M.; Kraemer, W. Evaluation of a lower-body compression garment. *J. Sports Sci.* **2003**, *21*, 601–610. [CrossRef] [PubMed]
28. Humphries, K.M.; Ward, J.; Coats, J.; Nobert, J.; Amonette, W.; Dyess, S. Immediate effects of lower cervical spine manipulation on handgrip strength and free-throw accuracy of asymptomatic basketball players: A pilot study. *J. Chiropr. Med.* **2013**, *12*, 153–159. [CrossRef]
29. Ammar, A.; Chtourou, H.; Abdelkarim, O.; Parish, A.; Hoekelmann, A. Free throw shot in basketball: Kinematic analysis of scored and missed shots during the learning process. *Sport Sci. Health* **2016**, *12*, 27–33. [CrossRef]
30. Ghai, S.; Driller, M.; Ghai, I. Effects of joint stabilizers on proprioception and stability: A systematic review and meta-analysis. *Phys. Ther. Sport* **2017**, *25*, 65–75. [CrossRef]
31. Ghai, S.; Driller, M.W.; Masters, R.S.J.G. The influence of below-knee compression garments on knee-joint proprioception. *Gait Posture* **2018**, *60*, 258–261. [CrossRef]
32. Hsu, J. *Multiple Comparisons: Theory and Methods*; CRC Press: Boca Raton, FL, USA, 1996.

33. Maxwell, S.E.; Delaney, H.D.; Kelley, K. *Designing Experiments and Analyzing Data: A Model Comparison Perspective*; Routledge: Abingdon, UK, 2017.
34. Sevrez, V.; Bourdin, C. On the role of proprioception in making free throws in basketball. *Res. Q. Exerc. Sport* **2015**, *86*, 274–280. [CrossRef]
35. Handford, C.; Davids, K.; Bennett, S.; Button, C. Skill acquisition in sport: Some applications of an evolving practice ecology. *J. Sports Sci.* **1997**, *15*, 621–640. [CrossRef]
36. Kaya, D.; Callaghan, M.J.; Donmez, G.; Doral, M.N. Shoulder joint position sense is negatively correlated with free-throw percentage in professional basketball players. *Isokinet. Exerc. Sci.* **2012**, *20*, 189–196. [CrossRef]
37. Reid, M.; Elliott, B.; Alderson, J. Lower-limb coordination and shoulder joint mechanics in the tennis serve. *Med. Sci. Sports Exerc.* **2008**, *40*, 308. [CrossRef] [PubMed]
38. Lam, W.; Maxwell, J.; Masters, R. Analogy versus explicit learning of a modified basketball shooting task: Performance and kinematic outcomes. *J. Sports Sci.* **2009**, *27*, 179–191. [CrossRef] [PubMed]
39. Chen, T.L.-W.; Wong, D.W.-C.; Wang, Y.; Ren, S.; Yan, F.; Zhang, M. Biomechanics of fencing sport: A scoping review. *PLoS ONE* **2017**, *12*, e0171578. [CrossRef] [PubMed]

17

Changes in the Kinematic and Kinetic Characteristics of Lunge Footwork during the Fatiguing Process

Yanyan Du [1,2] and Yubo Fan [1,3,*]

1 Key Laboratory for Biomechanics and Mechanobiology of Ministry of Education, Beijing Advanced Innovation Centre for Biomedical Engineering, School of Biological Science and Medical Engineering, Beihang University, Beijing 100083, China; duyanyan@cupes.edu.cn
2 Beijing Key Laboratory of Sports Function Assessment and Technical Analysis, Capital University of Physical Education and Sports, Beijing 100191, China
3 School of Medical Science and Engineering, Beihang University, Beijing 100083, China
* Correspondence: yubofan@buaa.edu.cn

Featured Application: 1. The kinematic and kinetic characteristics of the lunge maneuver were gradually impaired in the fatiguing process. 2. Period IV (pre-drive-off) of the stance phase showed the most significant fatigue response. 3. Improving the strength of the knee extensor is important for the lunge maneuver, particularly in period IV. 4. It is important to improve the strength of hip extensors for the lunge maneuver. 5. The analysis of waveform data is more useful for the assessment of weak areas of the body and periods of motion.

Abstract: Fatigue is a major injury risk factor. The aim of this study was to investigate the effects of fatigue on lunging during the fatiguing process. The lower extremity joint kinematics and kinetics of fifteen male collegiate badminton players were simultaneously recorded by optical motion-capture and force plate systems during lunging. In addition to statistical analyses of discrete variables, one-dimensional statistical parametric mapping (SPM (1D)) was used to analyze the waveform data. The hypotheses were that the biomechanics of lunging maneuvers would change during the fatiguing process, and the fatigue effects would differ in different periods (I–V) of the stance phase and in different joints. Results showed that the initial contact angles, peak angles, moments, power, and time needed to reach the peak angles at the hip, knee, and ankle in the sagittal plane all decreased post-fatigue. A continuous decreasing tendency was reflected in the moments and power of hip and, in particular, knee joints (mostly $p < 0.001$). Period IV showed a significant fatigue response. In conclusion, both discrete and waveform data illustrated the effects of fatigue, however, the results of SPM (1D) analysis showed both the key period and body segments affected by the fatigue response.

Keywords: badminton; knee joint; injury; one-dimensional statistical parametric mapping

---

1. Introduction

Badminton, one of the most popular sports globally [1–4], is the fastest non-contact racket sport, and requires a combination of strength, speed, and stamina. While playing this sport, players must repetitively lunge, jump, and quickly change direction from a wide variety of positions. A previous epidemiology study conducted in Ireland reported that badminton was the sport with the most injuries [5]. Lower extremity injuries accounted for 43 to 86% of all injuries regardless of the nationality [6], and overuse is considered the major reason [7,8]. Ankles and knees are the most injured sites [1,7,9], particularly the knee joint [7,8]. Patellar tendinopathy [7] is the most common type of knee injury. As a specific and often-used example of footwork [10,11], the repetitive lunge is a likely cause of patellar tendinopathy, particularly for teenager players [3,12].

Moreover, epidemiology studies have also shown that a higher badminton injury rate was found at the end of a match or training [13], and higher rates have been found during training [7,14]. This could be explained by a higher intensity of training routine [7], which may induce fatigue. Because fatigue reduces the capacity of muscles to generate force, it may be an important factor causing injury. In badminton, increased ankle sprain injuries were found to occur at the end of a training or match session due to the accumulation of fatigue [6]. Due to fatigue caused by repeating the forward lunge, the activity of the vastus lateralis, vastus medialis, and biceps femoris showed a significant change [15], and knee injury risk was increased [16].

A number of studies [10,17–21] have investigated the biomechanical characteristics of the lunge, particularly its stance phase, which is defined as the period of time from initial contact to final lift-off from the ground by the dominant limb [10]. Ankle sprain [6] and patellar tendinopathy [14] may occur during the stance phase. However, the relationship between the repetitive lunge and injury is still not clear. A previous study examined the lunge under the condition of exhaustion to investigate the fatigue effect on the knee [16]. A limitation of this study is that the changes of lunge motion during the fatiguing process were ignored. Injury usually occurs at a certain time, instantaneously, and the factors inducing injury are prolonged. However, we are unaware of any studies that have investigated the biomechanical changes during the fatiguing process in badminton. Therefore, there is a lack of objective data on lower joint kinematics and kinetics of the lunge during the fatiguing process, which may provide essential insight into the understanding of the mechanism of injury.

Additionally, discrete data (related, for example, to the peak angle) has traditionally been used for statistical analysis to confirm the differences outlined above. However, it is worth noting that all kinematic and kinetic variables are continuous variables with time. Furthermore, as mentioned above, injury occurs partly due to the accumulation of changes. Thus, continuous data analysis may provide other useful information. In recent years, one-dimensional statistical parametric mapping (SPM (1D)) has been accepted as an effective method to analyze waveform data [22]. Kinematic waveform data of hip, knee, and ankle joints in three planes, measured in players with different levels, have been analyzed by SPM (1D) [18,19]. However, to the best of the authors' knowledge, no research has investigated the fatigue response by analyzing the biomechanics waveform data of the lunge.

Consequently, the purpose of this study was to investigate the changes of lunge biomechanical characteristics during the fatiguing process, from normal to fatigued states. To achieve this objective, a repetitive forehand forward lunge to exhaustion was proposed as the fatigue protocol. The fatiguing process was divided into sub-stages. In addition to the discrete data (ground reaction force (GRF), lower extremity joint angles, range of motion (RoM), moments, and power), waveform data (GRF and lower extremity joint angles, moments, and power) were also analyzed during different fatiguing stages. The hypotheses are (i) both discrete and waveform data of lunge biomechanical characteristics change significantly during the fatiguing process, especially post-fatigue; (ii) effects of fatigue vary with different periods of the stance phase; and (iii) the lower limb joints have different fatigue responses.

2. Materials and Methods

2.1. Participants

Fifteen male collegiate badminton players (age: 21.1 ± 2.2 years; height: 1.81 ± 0.04 m; weight: 72.5 ± 8.4 kg; years of badminton training: 8.9 ± 3.5 years) were recruited for the study. All participants were free from any injuries within the previous 3 months and did not take part in any high-intensity training or competitions during the two days prior to the experiment. All participants were informed of the procedures and requirements of the test, and written informed consent was obtained from each participant. In addition, a questionnaire about anthropometrics, health status, injury history, and physical activity level was completed. To minimize the potential effect of footwear, participants wore badminton shoes and socks of the same brand and series. The study was approved by the ethics committee of Beihang University (No. BM201900077).

2.2. Experimental Protocol

The test was conducted on a simulated badminton court of the biomechanics laboratory. Prior to the test, participants performed a familiarization of the forehand forward lunge and the study protocol, which included 10 min warm-up; tests of heart rate (HR), blood lactate (BL), and Borg 6–20 rating of perceived exertion (RPE); and a fatigue protocol. Considering the dependency of fatigue on the task being undertaken [23,24] and the aim of this study, repeating the forehand forward lunge until participants reached the state of exhaustion was proposed as the fatigue protocol [16]. More specifically, a forehand forward lunge cycle was defined as lunging from the starting position using the dominate limb with a sliding step, landing on the force plate positioned at the right front, hitting one shuttlecock, and then moving backward to the starting position. The degree of fatigue was estimated by values of HR [15], BL, and RPE [25], which were measured before (pre) and immediately after (post) the fatigue protocol.

A system of 9 optoelectronic cameras (Oqus 300+ Series, Qualisys AB®, Gothenburg, Sweden) and a Kistler mobile multi-component force plate (Type 9286A, Kistler, Kistler Instrument AG, Winterthur, Switzerland), integrated into the walkway, were used to record the marker position and ground reaction forces, and synchronized at 200 and 1000 Hz, respectively. According to the color atlas of skeletal (CAST) landmark definitions of the lower leg [26], twenty-eight reflective markers (diameter: 18 mm) were attached to the lower extremity for dynamic motion capture. The locations included anterior superior iliac spines, posterior superior iliac spines, thigh (markers cluster), shank (markers cluster), calcaneus, hallux, and 2nd and 5th metatarsal head of the left and right lower extremity. The markers on calcaneus, hallux, and 2nd and 5th metatarsal head were placed on the corresponding anatomical location of the badminton shoes.

2.3. Data Analysis

The kinematic and force data were obtained by the optical motion-capture system and then exported and saved as c3d files. Then, the hip, knee, and ankle joint angles, moments, power, and ground reaction force (GRF) were calculated using visual 3D software (V5, C-Motion, Bethesda, MD, USA). The raw kinematic data were filtered with a low-pass (Butterworth) filter with frequency of 20 Hz [10]. The threshold of the vertical ground reaction force (vGRF) data was set as 10 N.

The stance phase, from initial contact (heel strike) to final lift-off from the force-plate by the dominant limb, was determined by the vGRF value. During this phase, there were three vGRF peaks, namely, the initial impact peak (PF1) for heel strike transient, the secondary impact peak (PF2) for impact loading, and the third impact peak (PF3) for drive-off. Based on the classification of previous studies [10,20,21], five periods can be clearly identified in the stance phase: (I) initial contact (from heel strike to PF1); (II) impact loading (from PF1 to PF2); (III) weight acceptance (from PF2 to peak knee joint flexion angle (PAK)); (IV) pre drive-off (from PAK to PF3); and (V) drive-off (from PF3 to lift-off from ground). In addition, the fatiguing process was divided into four stages according to the slope of the HR–time curve. Six continuous lunging motions were assessed at the end of each stage, and the kinematic and kinetic data of three lunge motions were then averaged and normalized for further statistical analysis.

During the stance phase, the motion of lower extremity joints, particularly the knee, occurs primarily in the sagittal plane. This contributes to the major knee joint biomechanical characteristics in badminton research [10,21]. Based on the previous literature linked to the lunge in badminton [10,17–21,27], we analyzed the impact peak; duration of five sub-stance phases; hip, knee, and ankle joint initial contact angles; durations to peak angle; ranges of motion (RoM); peak angles; moments; and power in the sagittal plane.

2.4. Statistical Analysis

All variables of the fatiguing process were calculated during four sub-stages. The kinetic data were normalized by body weight. All discrete variables were reported as mean ± standard deviation (SD), and examined for normality using a Shapiro–Wilk test prior to statistical analysis. One-way repeated measures ANOVA was used for the analysis of the influence of fatigue on the related parameters and discrete biomechanical data. Paired *t*-tests were performed to identify the differences. All statistical procedures were performed with SPSS 25 (IBM SPSS Statistics for Window, IBM Corp., NY, USA). Additionally, the waveform data of joint angles, moments, and power in the sagittal plane were analyzed (paired *t*-test) and plotted using one-dimensional statistical parametric mapping (SPM (1D) (https://spm1d.org/)) in MATLAB (R2014b, Mathworks, Inc., Natick, MA, USA). In addition, prior to statistical analysis, normality tests were performed for the waveform data with SPM (1D). The statistical significance level was set at 0.05.

3. Results

3.1. Fatigue Protocol

After the fatigue protocol, the mean values of HR, BL, and RPE were greater than 185 beats/min, 14 mmol/L, and a score of 18, respectively. Results of repeated measurement indicated that HR, BL, and RPE were all affected by the fatigue protocol (partial η^2: 0.99, 0.876, and 0.994 respectively), and the p values were all less than 0.001 (Table 1).

Figure 1 illustrates the HR–time curve (mean) of four participants throughout the fatigue protocol. To divide the fatigue protocol into stages, time was normalized, the slope of the HR–time curve was calculated, and four stages were distinguished, namely, P1 (0–10% duration of fatiguing process (D)), P2 (10–30%D), P3 (30–60%D) and P4 (60–100%D).

Table 1. Values of heart rate (HR), blood lactate acid (BL), and rating of perceived exertion (RPE) pre- and post-fatigue protocol (mean ± SD).

	Mean ± SD			95% CI of the Difference			
	Pre	**Post**	η_p^2	**Lower**	**Upper**	t	p
HR (beats/min)	78.2 ± 9.4	185.8 ± 9.1	0.99	−115.013	−100.32	−32.256	<0.001
BL (mmol/L)	3 ± 2.4	14.3 ± 3.1	0.876	−14.241	−8.543	−8.801	<0.001
RPE	6 ± 0	18.4 ± 1	0.994	−13.05	−11.784	−43.176	<0.001

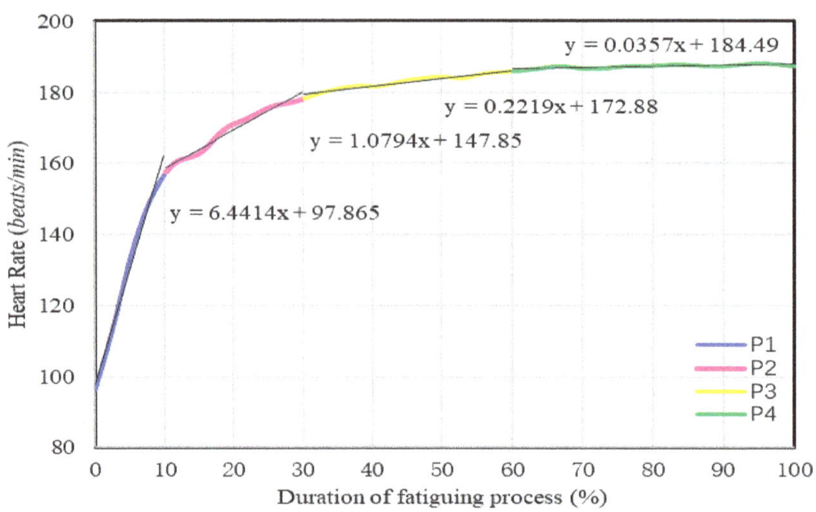

Figure 1. Heart rate (HR) of four participants during the fatiguing process (mean). According to the slope of the HR–time curve, the overall duration of the fatiguing process was divided into four stages, that is, P1, P2, P3, and P4. Duration of fatiguing process (%) vs. heart rate (beats/min).

3.2. *Kinematics of Lower Extremity Joints*

In the sagittal plane, Table 2 shows that the hip, knee, and ankle initial contact angle (CAH, CAK, CAA, respectively), peak angle (PAH, PAK, PAA, respectively), time to peak angle, and range of motion (RoM) all decreased during the process of the fatigue protocol (from P1 to P4).

Table 2. Kinematics variables in the four stages of fatiguing process (P1–P4) from pre- to post-fatigue protocol in the sagittal plane (mean ± SD).

	P1	P2	P3	P4	*p*
Joint angle at initial contact (°)					
CAH	46.08 ± 12.7	46.12 ± 10.32	42.2 ± 11.77	42.17 ± 11.77	*c*, *d**, *e**
CAK	13.11 ± 7.43	9.65 ± 7.55	7.82 ± 6.78	7.87 ± 6.09	*a*, *b*, *c**
CAA	10.35 ± 8.05	6.81 ± 8.25	8 ± 8.47	6.42 ± 9.11	
Peak joint angle (°)					
PAH	74.08 ± 11.94	73.3 ± 9.93	67.34 ± 11.74	67.84 ± 12.78	
PAK	69.46 ± 8.77	65.43 ± 9.44	64.17 ± 10.26	62.46 ± 8.84	*a**, *b*, *c**
PAA	−20.84 ± 5.7	−18.74 ± 5.2	−18.4 ± 4.9	−18.19 ± 6.55	
Time to peak joint angle (%)					
PAH	41.63 ± 6.59	42.13 ± 8.79	38.88 ± 7.55	36.75 ± 6.94	
PAK	45.88 ± 6.51	38.63 ± 9.12	37.25 ± 10.44	33.63 ± 9.43	*c**, *f*
PAA	14.13 ± 2.95	12.75 ± 2.82	12.38 ± 3.42	11.25 ± 2.71	*a*, *b*, *c*
Range of Motion (°)					
Hip joint	44.57 ± 10.44	39.16 ± 5.09	34.54 ± 6.85	38.67 ± 10.8	
Knee joint	59.32 ± 7.31	56.63 ± 6.84	56.74 ± 7.95	55.07 ± 6.28	*a*, *c*
Ankle joint	34.11 ± 8.09	29.82 ± 9.46	34.92 ± 9.68	31.98 ± 8.23	

Notes: CAH, CAK, and CAA: initial contact angle of hip, knee, and ankle joint, respectively; PAH, PAK, and PAA: peak joint angle of hip, knee, and ankle joint, respectively. P1–P4: the 1st, 2nd, 3rd, and 4th stages of the fatiguing process, respectively. *a*, *a**: significant differences between P1 and P2 at 0.05 and 0.01 levels, respectively; *b*: significant differences between P1 and P3 at 0.05 level; *c*: significant differences between P1 and P4 at 0.05 level; *d**: significant differences between P2 and P3 at 0.01 level; *e**: significant differences between P2 and P4 at 0.01 level; *f*: significant differences between P3 and P4 at 0.05 level.

At initial contact, a significant decrease was found for hip flexion (P1 vs. P4, $p = 0.044$; P2 vs. P3, $p = 0.009$; P2 vs. P4, $p = 0.003$) and knee flexion (P1 vs. P2, $p = 0.028$; P1 vs. P3, $p = 0.037$; P1 vs. P4, $p = 0.004$). Hip, knee, and ankle joints were all flexed (plantar-flexed) to the peak joint angle in less time. There were statistically significant differences in the time to peak value for the knee joint (P1 vs. P4, $p = 0.009$; P3 vs. P4, $p = 0.012$) and the ankle joint (P1 vs. P2, $p = 0.036$; P1 vs. P3, $p = 0.021$; P1 vs. P4, $p = 0.001$). The significance values (p) of the knee joint RoM were 0.013 (P1 vs. P2) and 0.048 (P1 vs. P4).

3.3. *Five Sub-Phases of the Stance Phase*

Table 3 shows that significant differences existed in the duration of the sub-stance phases II, III, IV, and V during the fatiguing process: durations were shorter for II (P1 vs. P3: $p = 0.012$), III (P1 vs. P4: $p = 0.041$; P3 vs. P4: $p = 0.005$), and V (P1 vs. P3: $p = 0.021$; P1 vs. P4: $p = 0.005$), and longer for IV (P1 vs. P2: $p = 0.022$; P1 vs. P3: $p = 0.024$; P1 vs. P4: $p = 0.002$; P2 vs. P4: $p = 0.002$; P3 vs. P4: $p = 0.036$).

3.4. *Kinetics of Lower Extremity Joints*

For the mean moments and power at the hip, knee, and ankle joints in the sagittal plane. Significant differences were found for moments at the hip (the 1st peak, P1 vs. P4: $p = 0.03$; the 2nd peak, P1 vs. P4: $p = 0.01$) and the knee (the 1st peak, P1 vs. P4: $p < 0.001$; the 2nd peak, P1 vs. P4: $p = 0.01$); power generation at the hip (P1 vs. P3: $p = 0.025$; P1 vs. P4: $p = 0.014$) and knee (P1 vs. P2, P1 vs. P3, P1 vs. P4: $p < 0.001$); and power consumption at the knee (P1 vs. P2: $p = 0.029$; P1 vs. P3: $p = 0.009$ and P1 vs. P4: $p < 0.001$) (details in Figure 4a).

3.5. *SPM (1D) of Kinematics of Lower Extremity Joints*

For the four stages of the fatiguing process (P1–P4), Figure 2a illustrates the joint angle–time curves in the sagittal plane (mean ± SD). SPM (1D) analysis results with significant differences are illustrated in Figure 2b. At the hip, significant differences exist in the initial contact (I), impact loading (II), weight acceptance (III), and pre-drive-off (IV) phases (P2 vs. P3 (I and II: $p = 0.01$; III and IV:

$p < 0.001$); P2 vs. P4 (I–IV: $p < 0.001$)). At the knee, significant differences were found mainly in the weight acceptance and pre-drive-off phases (P1 vs. P2 and P1 vs. P4: $p < 0.001$).

Table 3. Duration of five sub-phases (%) (mean ± SD).

	P1	P2	P3	P4	*p*
Duration of Five Sub-Phases (%)					
I (0-PF1)	3.88 ± 0.64	4 ± 0.93	4 ± 0.76	3.75 ± 0.71	
II (PF1-PF2)	11.13 ± 2.75	8.63 ± 4.44	8 ± 3.55	8.88 ± 3.31	*b*
III (PF2-PAK)	30.88 ± 6.03	26 ± 7.11	25.25 ± 9.25	21 ± 9.3	*c*, *f**
IV (PAK-PF3)	27.25 ± 10.69	36.5 ± 14.32	39.25 ± 17.17	43.38 ± 15.24	*a*, *b*, *c**, *e**, *f*
V (PF3-FO)	26.88 ± 5.57	24.88 ± 7.24	23.5 ± 7.23	23 ± 6.68	*b*, *c**

Notes: PF1: initial impact peak (the 1st peak vertical ground reaction force, vGRF); PF2: secondary impact peak (the 2nd peak vGRF); PF3: third impact peak (the 3rd peak vGRF); PAK: peak knee joint flexion angle. FO: foot off. The stance phase was divided into five sub-phases (I–V) according to impact peak and PAK. P1–P4: the 1st, 2nd, 3rd, and 4th stages of the fatiguing process, respectively. *a*, *a**: significant differences between P1 and P2 at 0.05 and 0.01 levels, respectively; *b*: significant differences between P1 and P3 at 0.05 level; *c*, *c**: significant differences between P1 and P4 at 0.05 and 0.01 levels, respectively; *e**: significant differences between P2 and P4 at 0.01 level; *f*, *f**: significant differences between P3 and P4 at 0.05 and 0.01 levels, respectively.

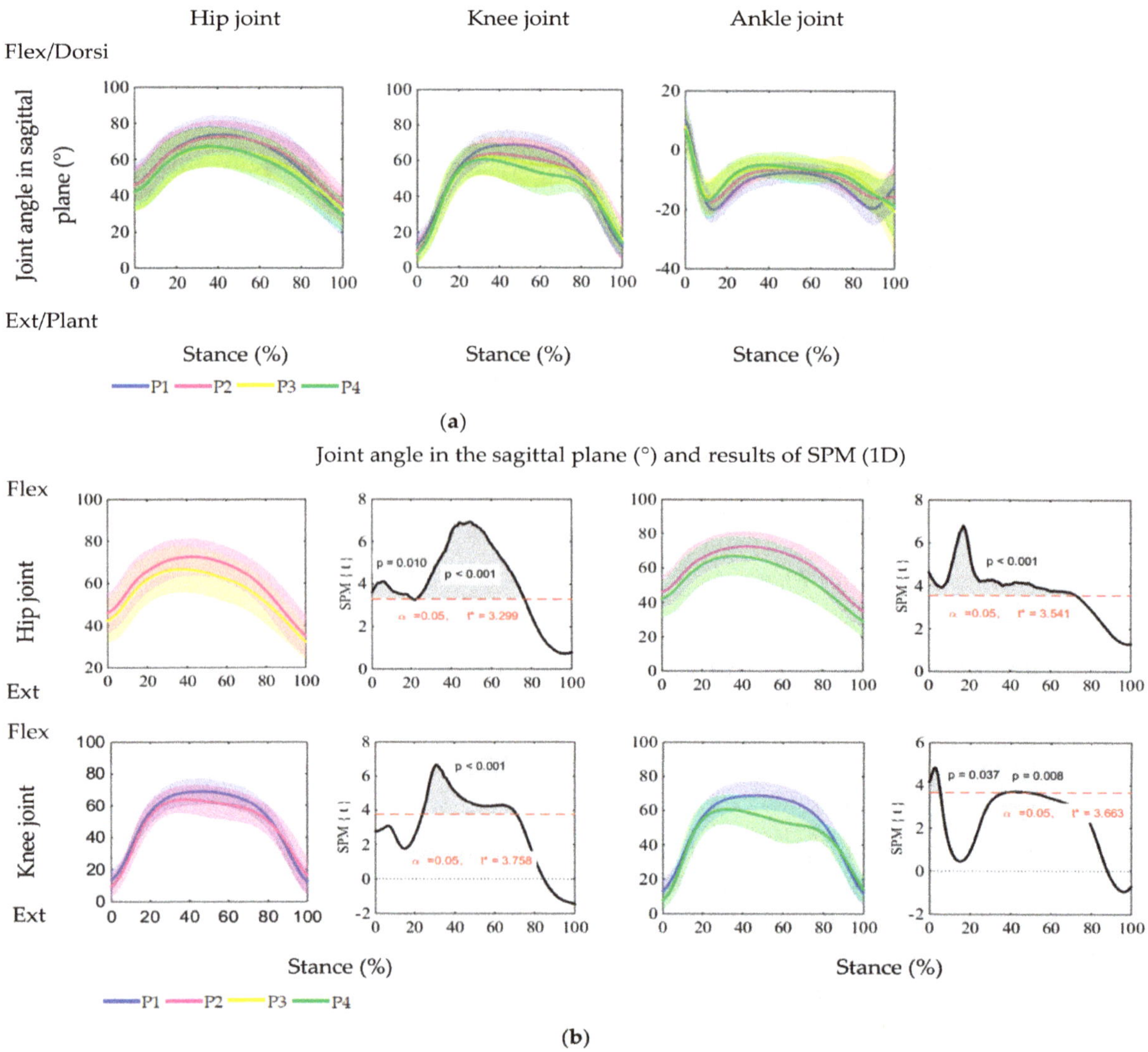

Figure 2. (**a**) Summary of the joint angles (mean ± SD) of lower limbs in the sagittal plane. (**b**) Results with significant differences of one-dimensional statistical parametric mapping (SPM (1D)) for hip and knee joint angles. Positive angles represent hip and knee flexion and ankle dorsi-flexion. P1–P4: the 1st, 2nd, 3rd, and 4th stages of the fatiguing process, respectively.

3.6. SPM (1D) of Kinetics of Lower Extremity Joints

Figure 3 illustrates the vGRF waveform data of P1, P2, P3, and P4, and the results of SPM (1D) analysis with significant differences, which are shown mainly in the pre-drive-off phases between P1 and P4 ($p < 0.001$).

Figure 4a illustrates the waveform data of the hip, knee, and ankle joint moments and power in the sagittal plane (mean ± SD) in P1, P2, P3, and P4. SPM (1D) analysis results of moments and power with significant differences are illustrated in Figure 4b,c, respectively. For hip and knee moments, significant differences exist in the partial period of the pre-drive-off phase (IV) between P1 and P3 ($p < 0.001$), and in the IV phase between P1 and P4 ($p < 0.001$). Moreover, Figure 4c illustrates that significant differences exist in the partial IV and drive-off (V) phases for hip power (P1 vs. P4: $p < 0.05$) and knee power (P1 vs. P3: $p < 0.001$; P1 vs. P4: $p < 0.001$).

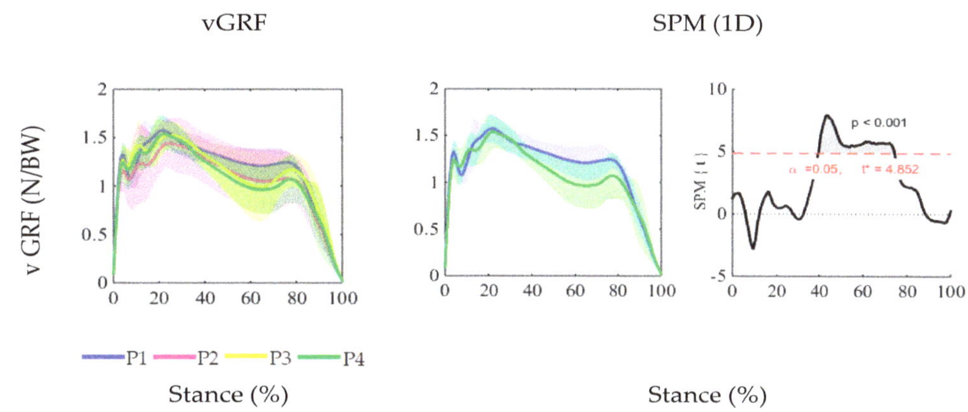

Figure 3. Vertical ground reaction force (vGRF) and results with significant differences of one-dimensional statistical parametric mapping (SPM (1D)). P1–P4: the 1st, 2nd, 3rd, and 4th stages of the fatiguing process, respectively.

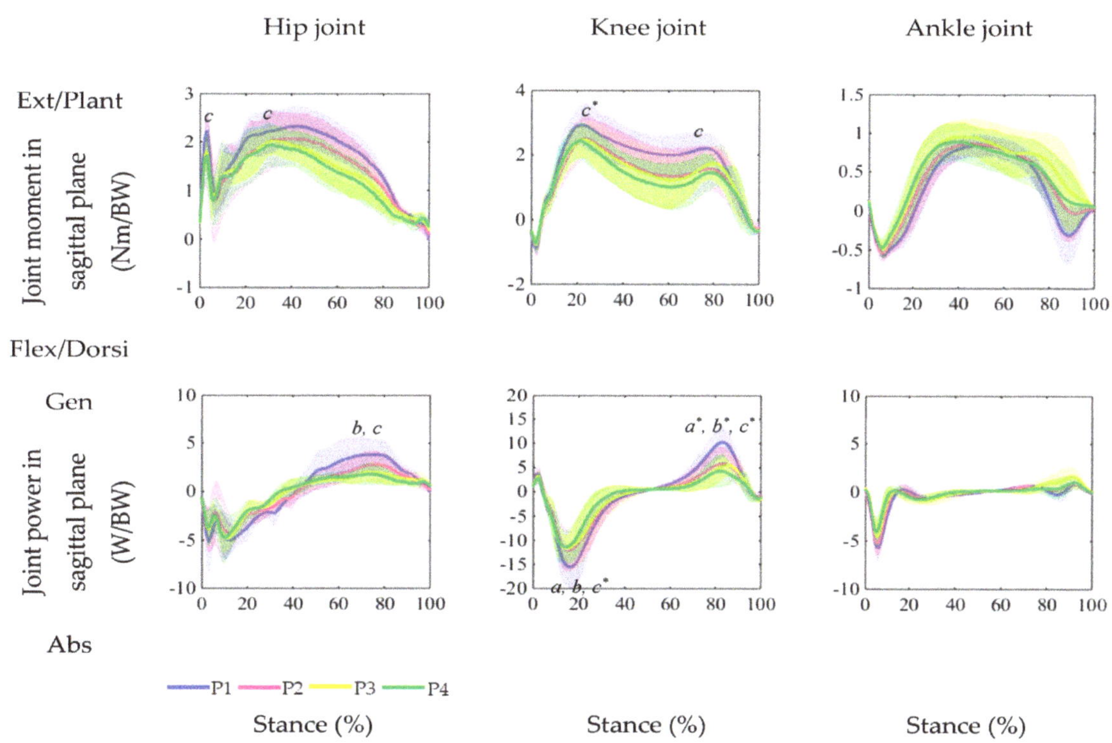

(a)

Figure 4. *Cont.*

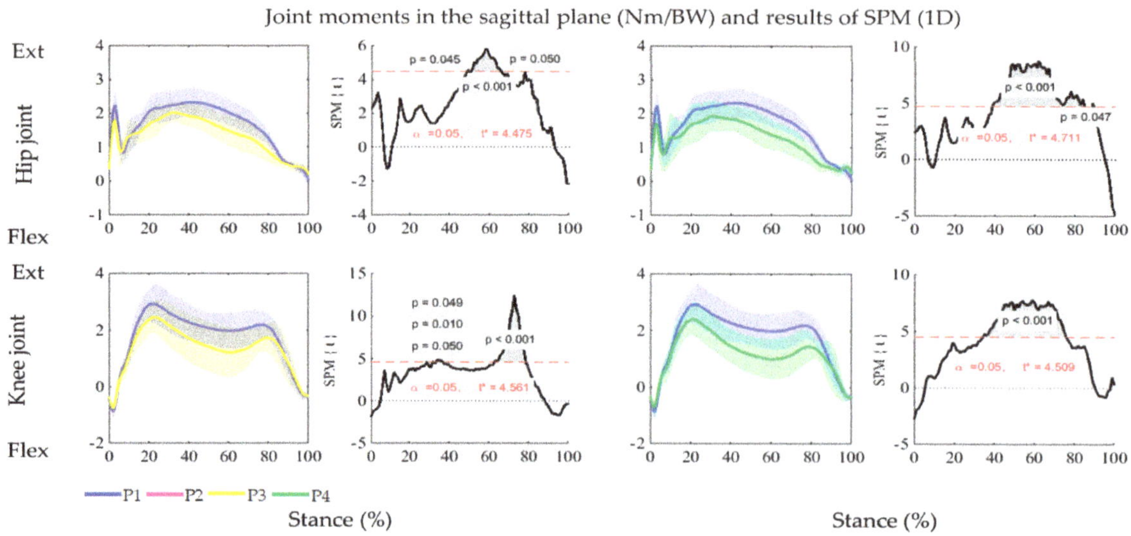

(b)

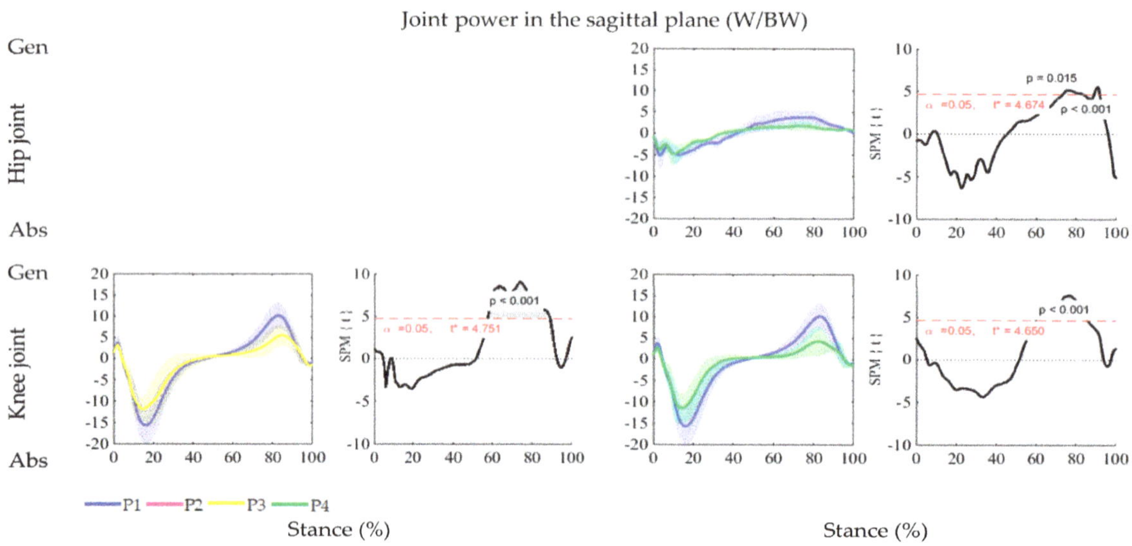

(c)

Figure 4. (**a**) Summary of joint moments and power (mean ± SD) of lower extremities in the sagittal plane during the lunge. (**b**) Results with significant differences of one-dimensional statistical parametric mapping (SPM (1D)) for hip and knee joint moments. (**c**) Results with significant differences of SPM (1D) for hip and knee joint power. Positive moments represent hip and knee extensor and ankle plantar flexor moments, and positive joint power indicates periods of power generation. P1–P4: the 1st, 2nd, 3rd, and 4th stages of the fatiguing process, respectively. *a*, *a**: significant differences between P1 and P2 at 0.05 and 0.01 levels, respectively; *b*: significant differences between P1 and P3 at 0.05 level; *c*, *c**: significant differences between P1 and P4 at 0.05 and 0.01 levels, respectively.

4. Discussion

An increasing number of people now play badminton. Both athletes and recreational players attempt to optimize their performance, thus increasing the risk of injury. Prevention of sports-related injuries is an important challenge. Fatigue is a major factor causing injury. Consequently, this study investigated the fatigue effects on a specific movement in badminton, i.e., the footwork associated with the lunge, which is one of the most used and integral movements [10,11].

Considering the task dependency of fatigue, a repeated forehand forward lunge, until reaching exhaustion, was proposed as the fatigue protocol, which was subdivided into four stages (P1, P2, P3, and P4) according to the slope of the heart rate (HR)–time curve. After the protocol, the mean values of HR, blood lactate (BL), and rating of perceived exertion (RPE) increased significantly at the significance level of 0.001; in particular, the mean HR was greater than 185 beats/min, the mean BL value was greater than 14 mmol/L, and the mean RPE score was greater than 18, indicating that all participants were fatigued. At P1, the first stage of the fatigue protocol, all participants were in a pre-fatigue state and, at P4, the final stage of the fatigue protocol, they were fatigued. In addition, according to previous studies [10,20,21], the first, second, and third impact peak (PF1, PF2, and PF3) and knee flexion peak angle (PAK) were used to subdivide the lunge stance phase into initial contact (I: 0-PF1)), impact loading (II: PF1-PF2), weight acceptance (III: PF2-PAK), pre drive-off (IV: PAK-PF3), and drive-off (V: PF3-end) periods. Then, statistical analyses were undertaken for both discrete and waveform kinematic and kinetic data in the sagittal plane, in which the largest movements occurred, comparing not only the pre- and post-fatigue states, but also the four stages of the fatiguing process.

The results supported the hypothesis that the biomechanical characteristics of the lunge change significantly during the fatiguing process. At the initial contact time, participants exhibited a more "erect" posture for the lunge, which is usually observed by coaches, and was shown as less hip and knee flexion, and ankle dorsi-flexion. Less dorsi-flexion at the foot strike has been found for recreational players with a relative lack of muscle power compared to national-level badminton athletes [19]. In the lateral jump performed in badminton, Herbaut et al. [27] found a decreased plantar-flexion angle at the foot strike post-fatigue. These changes may be induced by muscle fatigue caused by repeated stretch-shortening. Furthermore, the range of motion (RoM) of hip, knee, and ankle joints was decreased due to the fatiguing process.

Smaller peak joint angles were found at hip, knee, and ankle joints in the sagittal plane, particularly at the knee joint (with significant differences between P1 and the other three stages of the fatiguing process). After fatigue, a decrease in the knee peak angle was also found by Valldecabres et al. [16], however, no significant difference was found. The discrepancy may be due to the participant's sports level [24]. The decrease in the peak angle could be explained by the decrease in joint moments (details in Figure 4). There were significant differences in peak joint moments at the hip and knee extensor (P1 vs. P4: hip ($p = 0.03$), knee ($p < 0.001$)). A similar relationship was illustrated by Fu et al. [19] between professional and amateur badminton players; that is, professional players with greater muscle strength and better performance showed higher knee and ankle joint moments. Additionally, a shorter time was taken to flex to the peak angle, with significant decreases in time shown at the knee and ankle. This may be caused by impaired control due to fatigue. This can also be explained in this study by the decrease in joint moments and power.

In addition to the angles, the durations of the four sub-stance phases (II–V) changed during the process of the fatigue protocol. The shorter durations of II and III indicate that less time was taken to reach PF2 and PAK, respectively; that is, due to the fatiguing process, the participant placed his foot flat and flexed his knee more quickly. This is consistent with the increased ankle plantar flexor and knee flexor moments in the present study (Figure 4a), and with the opinion that fatigue reduces the capacity of muscles to generate force. The most significant increase was found in the IV phase (pre-drive-off), increasing from 27.25 ± 10.69% stance to 43.38 ± 15.24% stance. Significantly decreased hip and knee peak power in this phase provided sufficient support for this change. Less power was generated for players for the drive-off. Kuntz et al. [10] indicated that a hop style lunge generates higher peak vertical force during loading. In this study, three participants used the hop style at the final stage of the fatigue protocol. The change of lunge style may be a strategy to generate more power for driving-off and returning to the starting position [14].

Furthermore, considering the time continuity of biomechanical variables of the lunge motion, one-dimensional statistical parametric mapping SPM (1D) was used to analyze the biomechanical waveform data in the sagittal plane. Most of the joint angle, moment, and power waveforms decreased consistently during the process of the fatigue protocol (among P1, P2, P3, and P4). Significant differences were found in the hip and knee joint angles, mainly in the pre-drive-off phase (IV) (most p values were less than 0.001). The results support the hypothesis that the fatigue effects were different in the five periods of the lunge. Moreover, these results support the view that lunge characteristics change due to fatigue.

Taking into account the joint moments, both the hip and knee joints showed a significant response to the fatigue protocol. Significant differences were found between P1 and P3 in part of the period of IV, and between P1 and P4 in IV. The hip moments had a larger effective scope. However, there were only significant differences in the hip power between P1 and P4. For knee power, the significant differences were seen between P1 and P3, and also between P1 and P4, with a larger effective scope of the period. This indicates that the significant decrease in joint power occurred earlier and was mostly evident at the knee; that is, the fatigue responses manifested mostly at the knee joint. This result is consistent with a previous epidemiology study that reviewed musculoskeletal injuries among Malaysian badminton players, which reported that the majority of injuries sustained by players were due to overuse, primarily of the knee [7]. Another study [28] suggested that the rapidly changing eccentric/concentric work of the quadriceps in the varying degree of knee flexion was probably associated with patellar tendon injury. This may be why patellar tendinopathy is the most common injury of lower limbs among badminton players, and this result also supports our third hypothesis. Coaches and players should pay more attention to the training of the knee, and particularly the knee extensors.

Additionally, a comparison indicates that the discrete and waveform results are consistent. There are significant differences in CAH (P2 vs. P3), CAK (P2 vs. P4), PAK (P1 vs. P2; P1 vs. P4), knee peak moment (P1 vs. P4), hip peak power (P1 vs. P4), and knee peak power (P1 vs. P3; P1 vs. P4). In addition, significant differences were shown in these periods of stance phase in the discrete data. The results of SPM (1D) analysis clearly provided more information, indicating the period rather than a point of time in the fatigue response. This is also helpful in identifying the key body segments affected by fatigue. Thus, it is important for coaches and players to design a corresponding training program to improve the technique and muscle strength. Moreover, the results of SPM (1D) can provide support for monitoring of training.

Considering the key findings of this study, a few limitations should be noted when interpreting the results. First, the participants were male badminton players with at least 8 years of special badminton training. Results may differ for players of different levels, ages, and gender, thus studies of players with a range of abilities and ages, including female players, should be considered. Second, all tests were conducted on a simulated badminton court. Third, the sample size was limited. Fourth, the changing slope of the HR–time curve was used to subdivide the fatiguing process. However, it is not sufficient to explain the status of fatigue. Electromyography (EMG) data might be more suitable and could be used in future work. Finally, although joint moments and power allow further assessment of the functional contribution of the joints, EMG and musculoskeletal system simulations would help understand movement changes during the fatiguing process.

5. Conclusions

This study investigated the changes in the kinematic and kinetic characteristics of lunge footwork during the fatiguing process. To the best of our knowledge, this study was the first to subdivide the fatiguing process and analyze the changes among different sub-stages. It was also the first study to use one-dimensional statistical parametric mapping (SPM (1D)) to analyze the effect of fatigue on the lunge footwork in badminton. Statistically significant differences were found in both the discrete and waveform data. Moreover, these differences were shown not only between pre- and post-fatigue, but also among other sub-stages.

Overall, the results presented in this study confirm that period IV of the stance phase is more sensitive to fatigue than the other periods. In addition, the training program should focus on muscular strengthening of the knee extensor, particularly in period IV. It is also important to improve the strength of hip extensors. Furthermore, although the results show consistent changes between the discrete and waveform data, findings from this study highlight that results of SPM (1D) are more useful for the assessment of weak areas of the body and periods of motion. This information may contribute to the future design and development of training plans and to the monitoring of training.

Author Contributions: Y.D. designed, carried out the experiments, analyzed the data and wrote the paper, Y.F. designed the experiments, reviewed and revised the paper. All authors have read and agreed to the published version of the manuscript.

Acknowledgments: We thank Changhao Jiang from Capital University of Physical Education and Sports and Huijuan Tian from Tianjin Polytechnic University for giving suggestions for the analysis. We thank all the participants in this study.

References

1. Krøner, K.; Schmidt, S.A.; Nielsen, A.; Yde, J.; Jakobsen, B.W.; Møller-Madsen, B.; Jensen, J. Badminton injuries. *Br. J. Sports Med.* **1990**, *24*, 169–172. [CrossRef] [PubMed]
2. Fahlstrom, M.; Bjornstig, U.; Lorentzon, R. Acute badminton injuries. *Scand. J. Med. Sci. Sports* **1998**, *8*, 145–148. [CrossRef] [PubMed]
3. Yung, P.S.; Chan, R.H.; Wong, F.C.; Cheuk, P.W.; Fong, D.T. Epidemiology of injuries in Hongkong elite badminton athletes. *Res. Sports Med.* **2007**, *15*, 133–146. [CrossRef] [PubMed]
4. Badminton World Federation. Players Worldwide. In Badminton World Federation [Online]. Available online: http://smj.sma.org.sg/5011/5011a10.pdf (accessed on 25 June 2009).
5. Weir, M.A.; Watson, A.W. A twelve month study of sports injuries in one Irish school. *Irish J. Med. Sci.* **1996**, *165*, 165–169. [CrossRef] [PubMed]
6. Herbaut, A.; Delannoy, J.; Foissac, M. Injuries in French and Chinese regular badminton players. *Sci. Sport* **2018**, *33*, 145–151. [CrossRef]
7. Shariff, A.H.; George, J.; Ramlan, A.A. Musculoskeletal injuries among Malaysian badminton players. *Singap. Med. J.* **2009**, *50*, 1095–1097.
8. Goh, S.L.; Mokhtar, A.H.; Mohamad Ali, M.R. Badminton injuries in youth competitive players. *J. Sports Med. Phys. Fit.* **2013**, *53*, 65–70.
9. Hensley, L.D.; Paup, D.C. A survey of badminton injuries. *Brit. J. Sports Med.* **1979**, *13*, 156–160. [CrossRef]
10. Kuntze, G.; Mansfield, N.; Sellers, W. A biomechanical analysis of common lunge tasks in badminton. *J. Sports Sci.* **2010**, *28*, 183–191. [CrossRef]
11. Phomsoupha, M.; Laffaye, G. The science of badminton: Game characteristics, anthropometry, physiology, visual fitness and biomechanics. *Sports Med.* **2015**, *45*, 473–495. [CrossRef]
12. Muttalib, A.; Zaidi, M.; Khoo, C. A survey on common injuries in recreational badminton players. *Malays. Orthop. J.* **2009**, *3*, 8–11. [CrossRef]
13. Kondric, M.; Matković, B.R.; Furjan-Mandić, G.; Hadzić, V.; Dervisević, E. Injuries in racket sports among Slovenian players. *Coll Antropol.* **2011**, *35*, 413–417. [PubMed]
14. Jørgensen, U.J.; Winge, S.J. Injuries in Badminton. *Sports Med.* **1990**, *10*, 59–64. [CrossRef] [PubMed]
15. Pincivero, D.M.; Aldworth, C.; Dickerson, T.; Petry, C.; Shultz, T. Quadriceps-hamstring EMG activity during functional, closed kinetic chain exercise to fatigue. *Eur. J. Appl. Physiol.* **2000**, *81*, 504–509. [CrossRef] [PubMed]
16. Valldecabres, R.; De Benito, A.M.; Littler, G.; Richards, J. An exploration of the effect of proprioceptive knee bracing on biomechanics during a badminton lunge to the net, and the implications to injury mechanisms. *Peer J.* **2018**, *6*, e6033. [CrossRef]
17. Hong, Y.; Wang, S.J.; Lam, W.K.; Cheung, J.T.M. Kinetics of badminton lunges in four directions. *J. Appl. Biomech.* **2014**, *30*, 113–118. [CrossRef]
18. Mei, Q.; Gu, Y.; Fu, F.; Fernandez, J. A biomechanical investigation of right-forward lunging step among badminton players. *J. Sports Sci.* **2017**, *35*, 457–462. [CrossRef]
19. Fu, L.; Ren, F.; Baker, J.S. Comparison of joint loading in badminton lunging between professional and amateur badminton players. *Appl. Bionics Biomech.* **2017**, *2017*, 5397656. [CrossRef]

20. Lees, A.; Hurley, C. Forces in a badminton lunge movement. In *Science and Racket Sports*; Reilly, T., Hughes, M., Lees, A., Eds.; E & FN Spon: London, UK, 1994; pp. 249–256.
21. Lam, W.K.; Ding, R.; Qu, Y. Ground reaction forces and knee kinetics during single and repeated badminton lunges. *J. Sports Sci.* **2017**, *35*, 587–592. [CrossRef]
22. Pataky, T.C. Generalized n-dimensional biomechanical field analysis using statistical parametric mappin. *J. Biomech.* **2010**, *43*, 1976–1982. [CrossRef]
23. Barber-Westin, S.D.; Noyes, F.R. Effect of fatigue protocols on lower limb neuromuscular function and implications for anterior cruciate ligament injury prevention training: A systematic review. *Am. J. Sports Med.* **2017**, *45*, 3388–3396. [CrossRef] [PubMed]
24. Roth, R.; Donath, L.; Zahner, L.; Faude, O. Acute leg and trunk muscle fatigue differentially affect strength, sprint, agility, and balance in young adults. *J. Strength Cond. Res.* **2019**. [CrossRef] [PubMed]
25. Borg, G.A.V. Psychophysical bases of perceived exertion. *Med. Sci. Sports Exerc.* **1982**, *14*, 377–381. [CrossRef] [PubMed]
26. Cappozzo, A.; Catani, F.; Della Croce, U.; Leardini, A. Position and orientation in space of bones during movement: Anatomical frame definition and determination. *Clin. Biomech.* **1995**, *10*, 171–178. [CrossRef]
27. Herbaut, A.; Delannoy, J. Fatigue increases ankle sprain risk in badminton players: A biomechanical study. *J. Sports Sci.* **2020**, *38*, 1560–1565. [CrossRef]
28. Peers, K.H.; Lysens, R.J. Patellar tendinopathy in athletes: Current diagnostic and therapeutic recommendations. *Sports Med.* **2005**, *35*, 71–87. [CrossRef]

Permissions

All chapters in this book were first published by MDPI; hereby published with permission under the Creative Commons Attribution License or equivalent. Every chapter published in this book has been scrutinized by our experts. Their significance has been extensively debated. The topics covered herein carry significant findings which will fuel the growth of the discipline. They may even be implemented as practical applications or may be referred to as a beginning point for another development.

The contributors of this book come from diverse backgrounds, making this book a truly international effort. This book will bring forth new frontiers with its revolutionizing research information and detailed analysis of the nascent developments around the world.

We would like to thank all the contributing authors for lending their expertise to make the book truly unique. They have played a crucial role in the development of this book. Without their invaluable contributions this book wouldn't have been possible. They have made vital efforts to compile up to date information on the varied aspects of this subject to make this book a valuable addition to the collection of many professionals and students.

This book was conceptualized with the vision of imparting up-to-date information and advanced data in this field. To ensure the same, a matchless editorial board was set up. Every individual on the board went through rigorous rounds of assessment to prove their worth. After which they invested a large part of their time researching and compiling the most relevant data for our readers.

The editorial board has been involved in producing this book since its inception. They have spent rigorous hours researching and exploring the diverse topics which have resulted in the successful publishing of this book. They have passed on their knowledge of decades through this book. To expedite this challenging task, the publisher supported the team at every step. A small team of assistant editors was also appointed to further simplify the editing procedure and attain best results for the readers.

Apart from the editorial board, the designing team has also invested a significant amount of their time in understanding the subject and creating the most relevant covers. They scrutinized every image to scout for the most suitable representation of the subject and create an appropriate cover for the book.

The publishing team has been an ardent support to the editorial, designing and production team. Their endless efforts to recruit the best for this project, has resulted in the accomplishment of this book. They are a veteran in the field of academics and their pool of knowledge is as vast as their experience in printing. Their expertise and guidance has proved useful at every step. Their uncompromising quality standards have made this book an exceptional effort. Their encouragement from time to time has been an inspiration for everyone.

The publisher and the editorial board hope that this book will prove to be a valuable piece of knowledge for researchers, students, practitioners and scholars across the globe.

List of Contributors

Brooke L. Devlin and Adrienne K. Forsyth
Department of Rehabilitation, Nutrition and Sport, La Trobe University, Bundoora, VIC 3068, Australia

Sarah L. Jenner
Department of Rehabilitation, Nutrition and Sport, La Trobe University, Bundoora, VIC 3068, Australia
Carlton Football Club, Ikon Park, Carlton, VIC 3053, Australia

Georgina L. Buckley and Regina Belski
School of Health Sciences, Swinburne University of Technology, Hawthorn, VIC 3122, Australia

Filip Ujaković
Faculty of Kinesiology, University of Zagreb, 10110 Zagreb, Croatia
Basketball Club Cedevita Olimpija Ljubljana, 1000 Ljubljana, Slovenia

Nejc Šarabon
Faculty of Health Sciences, University of Primorska, Polje 42, 6310 Izola, Slovenia
S2P, Science to Practice, Ltd., Laboratory for Motor Control and Motor Behavior, 1000 Ljubljana, Slovenia

Joelle Leonie Flueck and Claudio Perret
Institute of Sports Medicine, Swiss Paraplegic Centre Nottwil, CH-6207 Nottwil, Switzerland

Alessandro Gallo
Department of Health and Technology, ETH Zurich (Swiss Federal Institute of Technology Zurich), CH-8003 Zurich, Switzerland

Nynke Moelijker, Nikolay Bogdanov and Anna Bogdanova
Institute of Veterinary Physiology, Vetsuisse Faculty and the Zurich Center for Integrative Human Physiology (ZIHP), University of Zurich, CH-8057 Zurich, Switzerland

Matej Supej and Jan Ogrin
Faculty of Sport, University of Ljubljana, 1000 Ljubljana, Slovenia

Hans-Christer Holmberg
Department of Physiology and Pharmacology, Biomedicum C5, Karolinska Institute, 171 77 Stockholm, Sweden
China Institute of Sport and Health Science, Beijing Sport University, Beijing 100084, China

Pedro L. Valenzuela
Department of Systems Biology, University of Alcalá, 28805 Madrid, Spain

Fernando Mata
NutriScience, Nutrition & Health Sciences, 14002 Córdoba, Spain

Javier S. Morales and Alejandro Lucia
Faculty of Sport Sciences, Universidad Europea de Madrid and Research Institute 'i+12' (Hospital 12 de Octubre), 28670 Madrid, Spain

Adrián Castillo-García
Fissac-Physiology, health and physical activity, 28015 Madrid, Spain

Abedin Bahtiri
Department of Physical Culture, Sport and Recreation, Kolegji Universi (Universi College) Prishtina, 10000 Prishtina, Kosovo

Jeton Havolli
Department of Physical Culture, Sport and Recreation, Kolegji Universi (Universi College) Prishtina, 10000 Prishtina, Kosovo
Faculty of Sport and Physical Education, 81400 Nikšić, Montenegro

Kemal Idrizović and Duško Bjelica
Faculty of Sport and Physical Education, 81400 Nikšić, Montenegro

Tim Kambič
Department of Research and Education, General Hospital Murska Sobota, 9000 Murska Sobota, Slovenia
Department of Sports Medicine, Faculty of Sport, University of Ljubljana, 1000 Ljubljana, Slovenia

Primož Pori
Department of Sports Medicine, Faculty of Sport, University of Ljubljana, 1000 Ljubljana, Slovenia

Justin Roberts, James Johnstone, Lee Smith and Viviane Merzbach
School of Psychology and Sport Science, Cambridge Centre for Sport and Exercise Sciences, Anglia Ruskin University, East Road, Cambridge CB1 1PT, UK

Anastasia Zinchenko
Department of Biochemistry, Kings College, University of Cambridge, Kings Parade, Cambridge CB2 1ST, UK
International Scientific Research Foundation for Fitness and Nutrition, 1073 LC Amsterdam, The Netherlands

Miguel Blacutt, Oscar Banderas, Luis Villasenor, Fredrik T. Vårvik and Menno Henselmans
International Scientific Research Foundation for Fitness and Nutrition, 1073 LC Amsterdam, The Netherlands

Krishnaa T. Mahbubani
Department of Surgery, Addenbrookes Hospital, Cambridge CB2 0QQ, UK

Goichi Hagiwara and Hirotoshi Mankyu
National Institute of Fitness and Sports in Kanoya, 1 Shiromizucho, Kanoya-shi, Kagoshima 891-2393, Japan

Takaaki Tsunokawa
Faculty of Health and Sport Science, University of Tsukuba, 1-1-1 Tennodai, Tsukuba-shi, Ibaraki 305-8574, Japan

Masaru Matsumoto and Hirokazu Funamori
Sharp Corporation, 3-1-72 Kitakamei-cho, Yao-shi, Osaka 581-8585, Japan

Rachel Lohman and Amelia Carr
Centre for Sport Research, School of Exercise and Nutrition Sciences, Faculty of Health, Deakin University, 221 Burwood Highway, Burwood, Melbourne, VIC 3125, Australia

Dominique Condo
Centre for Sport Research, School of Exercise and Nutrition Sciences, Faculty of Health, Deakin University, 221 Burwood Highway, Burwood, Melbourne, VIC 3125, Australia
Institute for Physical Activity and Nutrition, School of Exercise and Nutrition Sciences, Faculty of Health, Deakin University, 221 Burwood Highway, Burwood, Melbourne, VIC 3125, Australia
Geelong Football Club, GMHBA Stadium, Geelong, VIC 3125, Australia

Monica Kelly
Geelong Football Club, GMHBA Stadium, Geelong, VIC 3125, Australia

Bernardino J. Sánchez-Alcaraz and Alejandro Sánchez-Pay
Department of Physical Activity and Sport, Faculty of Sport Sciences, University of Murcia, C/Argentina, s/n, 30720 San Javier, Murcia, Spain

Diego Muñoz
Department of Didactic of Musical, Plastic and Corporal Expression, Faculty of Sports Science, University of Extremadura, Avda de la Universidad, s/n, 10003 Cáceres, Spain

Francisco Pradas
Department of Musical, Plastic and Corporal Expression, Faculty of Human Sciences and Education, University of Zaragoza, C/Pedro Cerbuna, 12, 50009 Zaragoza, Spain

Jesús Ramón-Llin
Department of Musical, Plastic and Corporal Expression, Faculty of Education, University of Valencia, Av. Dels Tarongers, 4, 46022 Valencia, Spain

Jerónimo Cañas
Department of Physical Education and Sport, Faculty of Sport Sciences, University of Granada, Carretera de Alfacar, 21, 18071 Granada, Spain

Samuel P. Hills, Peter Mitchell, Christine Wells and Mark Russell
School of Social and Health Sciences, Leeds Trinity University, Horsforth, Leeds LS18 5HD, UK

Milan Čoh, Nejc Bončina and Stanko Štuhec
Faculty of Sport, University of Ljubljana, Gortanova ul. 22, 1000 Ljubljana, Slovenia

Krzysztof Mackala
Department of Track and Field, University School of Physical Education, Al. Ignacego Paderewskiego 35, 51-612 Wrocław, Poland

Nida Murtaza, Lutz Krause and Mark Morrison
Faculty of Medicine, Translational Research Institute, University of Queensland Diamantina Institute, Brisbane, QLD 4102, Australia

Louise M. Burke and Megan L. Ross
Australian Institute of Sport, Canberra, ACT 2617, Australia
Centre for Exercise & Nutrition, Mary MacKillop Institute for Health Research, Australian Catholic University, Melbourne, VIC 3000, Australia

Nicole Vlahovich
Australian Institute of Sport, Canberra, ACT 2617, Australia
Faculty of Health Sciences & Medicine, Bond University, Robina, QLD 4226, Australia

Bronwen Charlesson
Australian Institute of Sport, Canberra, ACT 2617, Australia

Hayley M. O'Neill and Katrina L. Campbell
Faculty of Health Sciences & Medicine, Bond University, Robina, QLD 4226, Australia

Attilio Carraro
Faculty of Education, Free University of Bolzano, 39042 Bressanone (Bolzano), Italy

Martina Gnech and Diego Sarto
School of Human Movement Sciences, University of Padova, 35122 Padova, Italy

Fabio Sarto
Department of Biomedical Sciences, University of Padova, 35131 Padova, Italy

Jörg Spörri
Sports Medical Research Group, Department of Orthopaedics, Balgrist University Hospital, University of Zurich, 8006 Zurich, Switzerland
University Centre for Prevention and Sports Medicine, Department of Orthopaedics, Balgrist University Hospital, University of Zurich, 8006 Zurich, Switzerland

Stefano Masiero
Department of Neurosciences, Section of Rehabilitation, University of Padova, 35128 Padova, Italy

Chun-Fang Hsueh
Graduate Institute of Sport Coaching Science, Chinese Culture University, Taipei 114, Taiwan

Huey-June Wu
Department of Combat Sports and Martial Arts, Chinese Culture University, Taipei 114, Taiwan

Tzu-Shiou Tsai
Taipei Municipal Nan Gang High School, Taipei 115, Taiwan

Ching-Lin Wu
Graduate Institute of Sports and Health Management, National Chung Hsing University, Taichung 402, Taiwan

Chen-Kang Chang
Department of Sport Performance, National Taiwan University of Sport, 16, Section 1, Shaun-Shih Road, Taichung 404, Taiwan

Tony Lin-Wei Chen and Qitao Tan
Department of Biomedical Engineering, Faculty of Engineering, The Hong Kong Polytechnic University, Hong Kong 999077, China

Duo Wai-Chi Wong, Yan Wang and Ming Zhang
Department of Biomedical Engineering, Faculty of Engineering, The Hong Kong Polytechnic University, Hong Kong 999077, China
The Hong Kong Polytechnic University Shenzhen Research Institute, Shenzhen 518057, China

Wing-Kai Lam
Guangdong Provincial Engineering Technology Research Center for Sports Assistive Devices, Guangzhou Sport University, Guangzhou 510000, China
Department of Kinesiology, Shenyang Sport University, Shenyang 110102, China
Li Ning Sports Science Research Center, Li Ning (China) Sports Goods Company, Beijing 101111, China

Yanyan Du
Key Laboratory for Biomechanics and Mechanobiology of Ministry of Education, Beijing Advanced Innovation Centre for Biomedical Engineering, School of Biological Science and Medical Engineering, Beihang University, Beijing 100083, China
Beijing Key Laboratory of Sports Function Assessment and Technical Analysis, Capital University of Physical Education and Sports, Beijing 100191, China

Yubo Fan
Key Laboratory for Biomechanics and Mechanobiology of Ministry of Education, Beijing Advanced Innovation Centre for Biomedical Engineering, School of Biological Science and Medical Engineering, Beihang University, Beijing 100083, China
School of Medical Science and Engineering, Beihang University, Beijing 100083, China

Index

Printed in the USA
CPSIA information can be obtained
at www.ICGtesting.com
LVHW010847011123
762637LV00010B/405

9 798887 404684